# Family
# Health

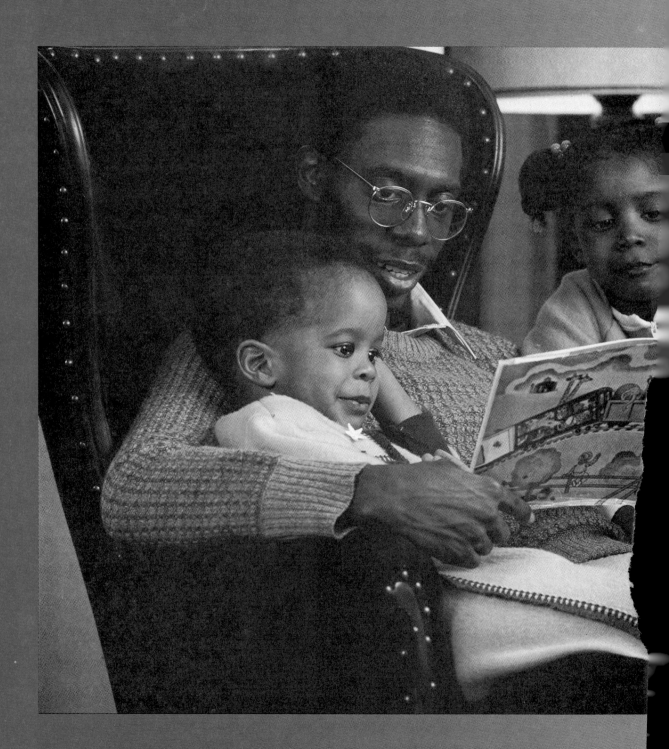

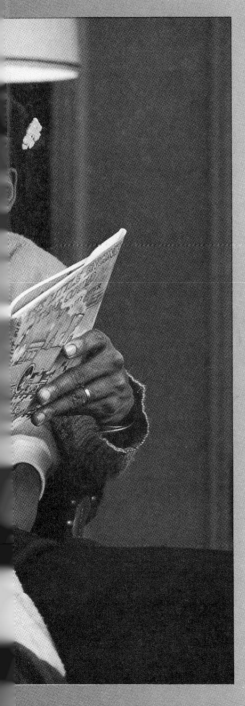

# Family Health

Written by:

**Roberta Larson Duyff, M.S., R.D., C.H.E.**
Nutrition Education Consultant
St. Louis, Missouri

**Margaret Wichard, R.N., M.S.N.**
Director of Emergency Training
St. Louis Bi-State Chapter, American Red Cross
St. Louis, Missouri

**Patsy Johnson Hallman, Ph.D., C.H.E.**
Professor of Home Economics
Stephen F. Austin State University
Nacogdoches, Texas

**Joanne C. Reid, M.Ed., C.H.E.**
Home Economics Supervisor
Evansville-Vanderburgh School Corporation
Evansville, Indiana

Edited by:

Roberta Larson Duyff

**GLENCOE PUBLISHING COMPANY**
BENNETT & McKNIGHT DIVISION

# Reviewers

Annetta Bailey
Aqua Dulce High School
Aqua Dulce, TX

Maurie Carpenter
Waltrip High School
Houston, TX

Nadene Davidson
Malcolm Price
Laboratory School
Cedar Falls, IA

Susan Davis
Pleasant Grove High School
Texarkana, TX

Ann A. Hagan
Assistant Professor
American University
Washington, D.C.

Janet Hogan
Clinton High School
Clinton, IL

Janie King
Glen Cliff High School
Nashville, TN

Marilyn Lanier
Whites Creek High School
Nashville, TN

Linda Valiga
Streamwood High School
Streamwood, IL

# Chart Credits

**Page 16** Reprinted by permission of the American Alliance for Health, Physical Education, Recreation and Dance, 1900 Association Drive, Reston, Virginia 22091.

**Page 72** The Metropolitan Life Insurance Company's Desirable Weight table, 1983.

**Page 73** Copyright © 1981 by Jack H. Wilmore, Department of Physical and Health Education, The University of Texas at Austin.

**Pages 121 and 123** *Jane Brody's The New York Times Guide to Personal Health* © 1982 by *The New York Times*.

Send inquiries to:
Glencoe Publishing Company
15319 Chatsworth Street
Mission Hills, California 91345

Printed in the United States of America

ISBN 0-02-675920-9 (Text)
ISBN 0-02-675940-3 (Teacher's Resource Guide)

1  2  3  4  5  6  7  8  9  10  91  90  89  88  87

# Contents

# Physical Wellness

After reading this chapter, you should be able to:

- explain the meaning of wellness.

- state factors which promote physical wellness.

- explain the relationships of exercise, diet, and health.

- use the decision-making process to make choices that promote wellness.

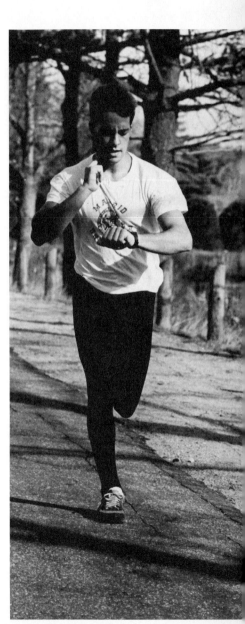

## Terms to Understand

| | |
|---|---|
| acne | flossing |
| aerobic exercise | hygiene |
| calories | nutrient density |
| cholesterol | nutrients |
| Daily Food Guide | plaque |
| empty-calorie foods | wellness |

Suppose someone offered you a "deal" which could save you money, give you more energy to study and play hard, and improve your chances of living a longer, more productive life. That "deal" would help you look and feel great. Would you be interested?

This "deal" can be yours right now! By learning about healthful lifestyles and making smart choices, you can feel and look your best and also have energy for top personal performance!

## Wellness

*Wellness* is the process of becoming and staying healthy. It's much more than not being sick. To be well, you need to take personal responsibility for your own health and practice healthful lifestyles. In this way you can reach and help maintain your highest level of physical, emotional, and social health.

Being healthy doesn't mean having a perfect body. Almost no one has that. In fact, most people have some limitations, perhaps even a physical impairment. The key to wellness is controlling your limitations and making the most of what you have.

### Signs of Wellness

How do you know if you're well? The signs of good health usually relate to your appearance, your vitality or energy, and the absence of illness. Being at your desirable body weight, for example, is one sign of good health and fitness. Good health also includes greater resistance to disease, and when illness does strike, quicker recovery.

Emotional and social health are evident when you can handle life with ease, have a zest for living, and express a direction in your life. This chapter will deal mostly with physical health. Chapter 2 will deal more fully with social and emotional health.

For a detailed list of the signs of wellness, see the chart, "Good Health Shows All Over", on page **19**.

## Nutrition

Your food choices are some of the most important decisions you make each day. The food you eat affects your energy level, your appearance, and your overall well-being. That's because food contains substances called nutrients. *Nutrients* are chemicals the body must have to function, grow, repair itself, and make energy. The food you eat is broken down during the digestive process so that the nutrients from food can be released into the bloodstream and carried through the body to cells where they are used. Nutrition is the study of how your body uses the nutrients in the food.

## Nutrients

There are over 40 different nutrients in food. All these nutrients are grouped into six categories—protein, carbohydrate, fat, vitamins, minerals, and water. Each has a specific role in keeping you healthy. The chart on page **3** lists many important nutrients, their sources, and their functions.

### PROTEIN

Protein is the nutrient used to build and repair body cells. Protein is broken down by the digestive process into amino acids. Amino acids are one type of building block of all body cells. There are many different amino acids, and each has a specialized function. Foods that supply all the amino acids essential to your body are called complete proteins. Complete proteins are essential for growth and body repair. Food sources of complete proteins include meat, fish, poultry, eggs, and dairy products.

Other good protein sources don't have all the essential amino acids. These incomplete

## These Nutrients Keep You Healthy!

| Nutrient | Key Functions | Food Sources |
|---|---|---|
| Protein | Promotes growth; builds and repairs body tissues | Meat, poultry, fish, nuts, eggs, legumes, cheese. (Legumes are seeds which grow in pods, such as kidney beans and black-eyed peas.) |
| Carbohydrate | Provides energy; aids digestion by providing fiber | Sugar: fruit, honey, jelly, desserts, soft drinks<br><br>Starch: breads, potatoes, cereal, pasta, rice, legumes<br><br>Fiber: bran, whole-grain products, raw fruits and vegetables, popcorn, nuts |
| Fat | Provides energy; carries fat-soluble vitamins | Butter, margarine, oils, nuts, egg yolks, chocolate, fried foods, cream, whole milk |
| Vitamin A | Promotes good vision; promotes healthy skin; aids healing; promotes growth | Green, leafy vegetables, deep-yellow vegetables, egg yolk, milk, liver |
| Vitamin B Complex (thiamin, riboflavin, niacin) | Help maintain healthy nervous system; promote energy production; help resist infection; provide healthy skin | Breads and cereals, pork, liver, dried legumes. (Many dairy products are a good source of riboflavin.) |
| Vitamin C | Increases resistance to infection; maintains healthy teeth and gums; helps keep blood vessels firm | Citrus fruits, cantaloupe, tomatoes, strawberries, raw cabbage, broccoli |
| Vitamin D | Helps build strong bones and teeth | Milk |
| Vitamin E | Preserves cell tissues | Egg yolks, milk, whole-grain cereals, greens, vegetable oils |
| Vitamin K | Helps blood clot | Leafy green vegetables, cabbage, cauliflower |
| Calcium | Builds strong bones and teeth; helps muscles contract | Milk, cheese, ice cream, yogurt |
| Iron | Carries oxygen in the blood | Meat (especially liver), eggs, greens |
| Phosphorus | Helps calcium work | Milk, meat, grain products |
| Water | Carries nutrients to body cells | Water, other beverages |

proteins are found in some plant sources of food, such as dry peas and beans, nuts, and seeds. When foods with incomplete protein are combined with complete protein from animal sources or with grain products, the body gets all the essential amino acids. Grain products include cereals, rice, and products made with flour, such as bread and pasta. Grains have a small amount of protein, including the amino acids missing from dry beans and peas, nuts, and seeds.

Although not the best source, protein can provide energy for your body cells, but carbohydrate and fat are the preferred fuels.

## CARBOHYDRATE

Carbohydrate is the body's main energy source. There are simple carbohydrates—sugars—and complex carbohydrates—starches. Good sources of carbohydrate include fruit, vegetables, dry peas and beans, pasta, rice, and other grain products.

Many carbohydrate-rich foods are also rich in fiber. Fiber, which isn't digestible, supplies bulk that helps move food through the digestive tract. Edible peels and whole-grain foods are especially good sources of fiber.

## FAT

Fat is another nutrient which supplies energy. It also carries fat-soluble vitamins and acts as a source of essential fatty acids necessary for growth and body maintenance. Fat in the diet comes from meat, poultry, fried foods, whole milk, nuts, gravy, butter or margarine, and salad oils. Fats are classified as saturated and unsaturated. The difference is in the chemical makeup of the fats. Saturated fats are solid at room temperature, and unsaturated fats are soft or liquid.

*Cholesterol* is a fat-like substance that the body uses to help make some body chemicals. Cholesterol comes from foods of animal origin, such as egg yolk, liver, red meat, and cheese. The body also makes cholesterol. There is some evidence that a high level of cholesterol in the blood leads to a greater risk of heart disease. For this reason, experts recommend that many people limit their cholesterol intake.

## VITAMINS

Vitamins help regulate body processes. They have many different body functions. For example, B vitamins help produce energy, and vitamin C helps the body resist infection. Without vitamins, your body couldn't function properly or use other nutrients in food. Vitamins work together. The lack of one vitamin may affect the work of another. Almost all foods have vitamins, but the specific kind and amount differs from food to food.

## MINERALS

Like vitamins, minerals also regulate body processes. However, unlike vitamins, they become part of the body's bones, tissues, and fluids. Calcium and phosphorus, for example, help build and become part of bones and teeth. Iron becomes part of the blood.

Minerals often work with other nutrients to help the body function normally. For example, sodium works with two other minerals, chloride and potassium, to help regulate body fluids. Calcium teams with vitamin C to maintain and repair bones.

## WATER

Water is part of many body fluids, such as your blood, saliva, and perspiration. As part of blood, water carries nutrients and other body chemicals to cells and removes waste. Beverages and soups are excellent water sources. But many foods, such as lettuce and celery, are good sources, too. You need about six to eight glasses of water a day.

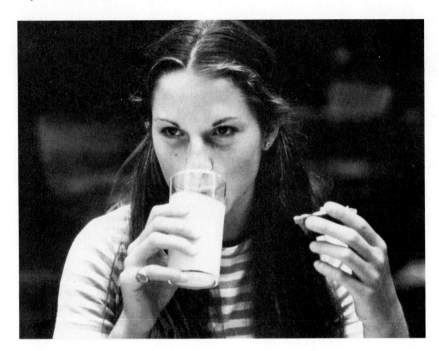

*By consuming enough calcium as a teenager, you help your bones grow stronger and more dense. This will help protect you from bone disease later in life.*

## Calories

You've heard the term calories many times. *Calories* refer to the measurement of energy in food and the energy your body uses.

Calories for your body come from the various foods you eat. Carbohydrate and protein yield four calories per gram. Fat yields nine calories per gram.

You can estimate the number of calories in your food choices by recording all the foods you eat, including snacks, for one typical day. Write down how much of each food you eat. Then look up the amount of calories in each food using a calorie guide. Total these amounts.

People need calories for metabolism, physical exercise, and the digestion of food. The term metabolism refers to all your body processes, such as breathing, circulating blood, and building and repairing cells and tissues.

The number of calories you burn for ex-ercise depends on the type of activities you that are doing, their duration, and their intensity. The harder you exercise, the more calories you burn. The chart on page **6** shows how many calories the body uses for various activities.

Every day the average 15 to 18 year-old male uses about 19 calories per pound of body weight. The average female of the same age uses about 18 calories per pound. Moderate to heavy exercise adds about two more calories per pound. An inactive person should subtract two calories per pound. Calculate the calories you use: your weight in pounds times the calories per pound equals your approximate daily calorie use.

These calculations are just averages. You may need more or less. People with a faster metabolic rate may burn more. Metabolic rate is the rate at which your body burns calories. And people with more muscle mass burn calories more efficiently.

## Calories Used for Activities

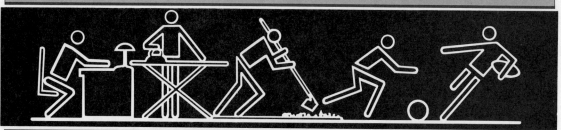

| Type of Activity | Calories per hour |
|---|---|
| **Sedentary**<br>Activities done while sitting, with little or no arm movement. Reading; writing; eating; watching television or movies; sewing; playing cards. | 80 to 100 |
| **Light**<br>Activities done while standing that require some arm movement, and strenuous activities done while sitting. Preparing food; doing dishes; dusting; handwashing small articles of clothing; ironing; walking slowly; personal care; rapid typing; filing in an office. | 110 to 160 |
| **Moderate**<br>Activities done while standing that require moderate arm movement and activities done while sitting that require vigorous arm movement. Making beds, mopping, and scrubbing; sweeping; light polishing and waxing; laundering by machine; light gardening and carpentry work; walking moderately fast. | 170 to 240 |
| **Vigorous**<br>Heavy scrubbing and waxing; handwashing large articles of clothing; hanging out clothes; walking fast; bowling; golfing; gardening. | 250 to 350 |
| **Strenuous**<br>Swimming; tennis; running; bicycling; dancing; skiing; football. | 360 or more |

*Source: U.S. Department of Agriculture*

## Guidelines to Healthful Eating

Calories supply the energy your body needs. However, it is possible to get all the calories you need and still not get all the nutrients you need. When people don't get adequate amounts of nutrients, their bodies don't work properly. Deficiency diseases develop when nutrient intake is significantly lower than needed. People can also develop poor health by consuming too much of some nutrients. A varied diet can provide you with adequate amounts of essential nutrients. Several guidelines can help you make nutritious food selections without consuming too much.

### DAILY FOOD GUIDE

The *Daily Food Guide,* shown on pages **7–9,** is a guideline for making wise and varied

## Daily Food Guide

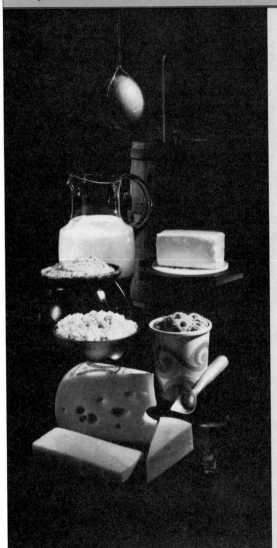

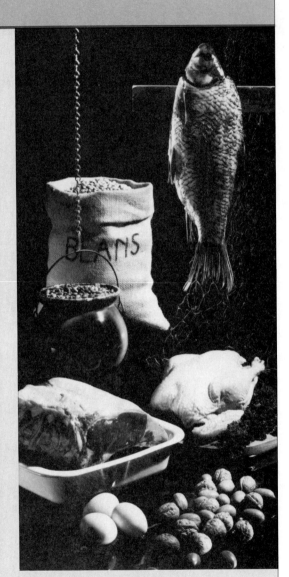

Number of servings daily: Teens—4; Adults—2

This group includes milk in any form: whole, skim, lowfat, evaporated, buttermilk, and nonfat dry milk in addition to yogurt, ice cream and cheese.

Two servings daily.

Included in this group are beef, veal, lamb, pork, poultry, fish, shellfish (shrimp, oysters, crab, etc.), organ meats (liver, kidneys, etc.), dry beans or peas, soybeans, lentils, eggs, seeds, nuts, peanuts, and peanut butter.

## Daily Food Guide (continued)

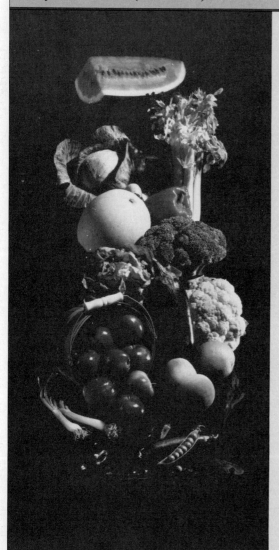

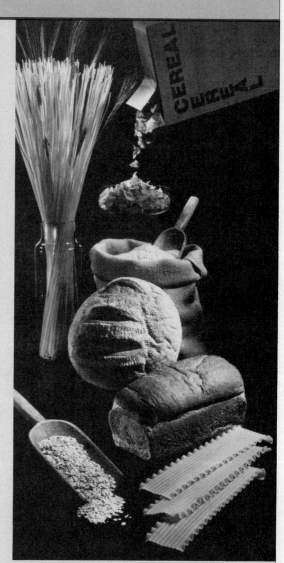

Four servings daily.

All vegetables and fruits belong in this group. Include one good vitamin C source each day. Deep-yellow or dark-green vegetables provide vitamin A and unpeeled fruits and vegetables and those with edible seeds (such as berries) provide fiber.

Four servings daily.

Included in this group are all products made with whole grains or enriched flour. Some of these products are bread, biscuits, muffins, waffles, pancakes, cooked and ready-to-eat cereals, grits, macaroni, spaghetti, noodles, and rice.

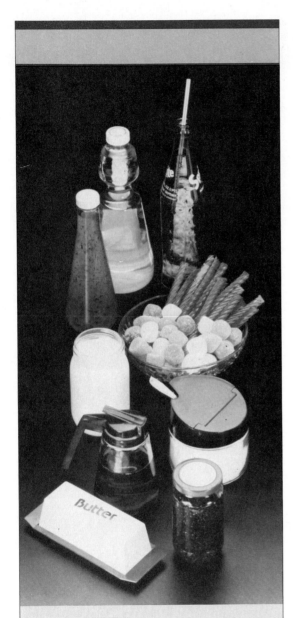

This group includes butter, margarine, mayonnaise, salad dressings, oils, candy, sugar, jams, syrups, and soft drinks.

food choices. It divides food into five food groups according to the nutrients that they contain:

- **Milk and Cheese Group** provides protein, calcium, phosphorus, vitamins A and D, and riboflavin.
- **Meat, Poultry, Fish, and Beans Group** provides protein, thiamin, niacin, and iron.
- **Vegetable and Fruit Group** provides vitamins A and C, carbohydrate, and fiber.
- **Bread and Cereal Group** provides carbohydrate, B vitamins, and iron.
- **Fats and Sweets Group** provides fat and carbohydrate.

Foods from the first four food groups are nutrient dense. *Nutrient density* means that foods are rich sources of nutrients, yet they have relatively few calories. The more nutrients a food has in relation to calories, the higher its nutrient density. Orange juice has a high nutrient density. On the other hand, a danish pastry has a low nutrient density because it is high in calories but has few nutrients.

The Fats and Sweets Group contains foods with low nutrient density. Most of these foods are high in fat, sugar, or both. They're called *empty-calorie* foods because they have few nutrients besides fat or carbohydrate. Some, such as a diet soft drink, don't have any calories. In limited amounts, empty-calorie foods offer flavor, interest, and calories to food choices.

A diet that promotes wellness is balanced. That means it provides adequate amounts of nutrients needed each day and it meets the recommendations of the Daily Food Guide. The chart on pages **7–9** shows how many servings you need daily from each food group.

To evaluate your food choices, keep a record of the foods you eat for a day. Record the serving size. Then you can compare your meals and snacks with the recommendations from the Daily Food Guide.

## RECOMMENDED DIETARY ALLOWANCES

The Recommended Dietary Allowances (RDA) are another guide for planning and evaluating food choices. These guidelines are recommendations for the amount of key nutrients, as well as calories, you need each day for good health. The chart on this page shows the RDA for teenagers. Recommendations have also been established for other age groups and for pregnant and breast-feeding women. The RDA are revised periodically as scientists learn more about nutrition and health.

The nutrient guidelines given in the RDA are somewhat higher than what most people actually need. This provides a margin of safety for those who need more. Even your own needs may go up when you are sick, injured, or under stress.

You can use the RDA to evaluate your food choices by first keeping a record of everything you eat and the amount. Using a nutrient composition guide, you then write the nutrient value of each food and total each nutrient amount. The last step is to compare the totals to your RDA.

The RDA is the basis for the U.S. Recommended Daily Allowances (U.S. RDA) These standards are used for nutrient labeling on food packages. You can use nutrient labels to compare the amounts of selected nutrients and calories in different food products and to choose the foods that best fit your nutritional needs.

## DIETARY GUIDELINES

Health professionals recognize that many Americans consume more fat, sugar, and sodium than they need and not enough of some

## Recommended Dietary Allowances (1980) for Selected Nutrients

| | Males | | Females | |
|---|---|---|---|---|
| | 11–14 Years | 15–18 Years | 11–14 Years | 15–18 Years |
| Calories* | 2700 | 2800 | 2200 | 2100 |
| Protein (grams) | 45 | 56 | 46 | 46 |
| Vitamin A (micrograms of retinol equivalents) | 1000 | 1000 | 800 | 800 |
| Thiamin (milligrams) | 1.4 | 1.4 | 1.1 | 1.1 |
| Riboflavin (milligrams) | 1.6 | 1.7 | 1.3 | 1.3 |
| Niacin (milligrams of niacin equivalents) | 18 | 18 | 15 | 14 |
| Vitamin C (milligrams) | 50 | 60 | 50 | 60 |
| Vitamin D (micrograms) | 10 | 10 | 10 | 10 |
| Vitamin E (milligrams of alpha-tocepherol equivalents) | 8 | 10 | 8 | 8 |
| Calcium (milligrams) | 1200 | 1200 | 1200 | 1200 |
| Phosphorus (milligrams) | 1200 | 1200 | 1200 | 1200 |
| Iron (milligrams) | 18 | 18 | 18 | 18 |

*Calories are given as an average for people who don't get much exercise. People who get moderate or strenuous daily exercise need more calories.

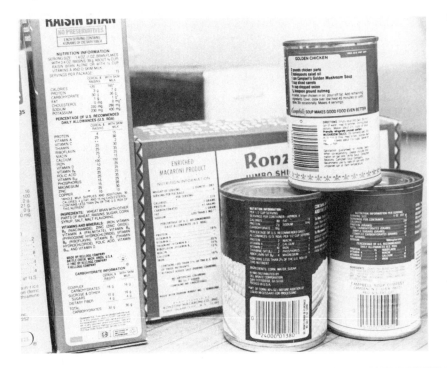

*By using nutritient labels, you can make wise decisions in the supermarket. What does this label tell you?*

other nutrients. On the average, people get about 37 percent of their calories from fat, about 46 percent from carbohydrate, and about 16 percent from protein. A much healthier guideline is to eat less fat and more complex carbohydrate: about 30–33 percent calories from fat, 55–60 percent from complex carbohydrates, and 12–15 percent from protein.

The Dietary Guidelines for Americans on page **12** are recommendations developed to help average Americans make healthful food choices. These guidelines should be considered along with the Daily Food Guide and the RDA.

## Meals and Snacks

Healthful meals have a variety of foods from the four main food groups. Variety at each meal is important since nutrients from

### PERCENTAGE OF U.S. RECOMMENDED DAILY ALLOWANCES (U.S. RDA)

| | CEREAL & RAISINS | WITH SKIM MILK |
|---|---|---|
| PROTEIN | 4 | 15 |
| VITAMIN A | 25 | 30 |
| VITAMIN C | ** | 2 |
| THIAMIN | 25 | 30 |
| RIBOFLAVIN | 25 | 35 |
| NIACIN | 25 | 25 |
| CALCIUM | 2 | 15 |
| IRON | 100 | 100 |
| VITAMIN D | 10 | 25 |
| VITAMIN $B_6$ | 25 | 25 |
| FOLIC ACID | 25 | 25 |
| VITAMIN $B_{12}$ | 25 | 35 |
| PHOSPHORUS | 15 | 25 |
| MAGNESIUM | 15 | 20 |
| ZINC | 25 | 30 |
| COPPER | 10 | 10 |

*WHOLE MILK SUPPLIES AND ADDITIONAL 30 CALORIES, 4 g FAT, AND 15 mg CHOLESTEROL.
**CONTAINS LESS THAN 2% OF THE U.S. RDA OF THIS NUTRIENT

# Dietary Guidelines for Americans

The average American eats too much fat, sugar, and sodium and too little fiber. Forty percent of Americans are overweight. These factors have been linked to various health problems, such as high blood pressure, heart disease, and cancer. To encourage people to improve their eating habits, the United States Government developed the Dietary Guidelines for Americans.

The Guidelines are listed below, along with explanations of why they are important and how to put them into practice. Keep in mind that these are general guidelines based on the average American diet. You must assess your individual diet to determine how the Dietary Guidelines apply to you.

No diet can guarantee health or well-being. These depend on heredity, lifestyle, and mental attitudes as well as diet. But good eating habits are based on moderation. Variety can do a lot to help you stay healthy. Make the Dietary Guidelines a part of your overall wellness program!

| Guideline | Why | How |
|---|---|---|
| 1. Eat a variety of foods. | • Most foods contain several nutrients, but no single food can give you all the nutrients you need. The greater the variety, the less likely you are to develop either a deficiency or an excess of any single nutrient.<br>• Eating a variety of foods reduces the likelihood of being exposed to excessive amounts of contaminants. | • Select foods each day from each of the four major food groups: Milk—Cheese, Fruit—Vegetable, Meat—Poultry—Fish—Beans, Bread—Cereal. |
| 2. Maintain desirable weight. | • If you are overweight, your chances of developing certain disorders are increased. These include high blood pressure, increased level of blood fats and cholesterol, and diabetes. These disorders, in turn, increase your risk of heart attacks and strokes.<br>• If you are much underweight, you will have little strength and tire easily. Your resistance to infection may be lowered. | • Eat in moderation, neither too much nor too little, according to the Daily Food Guide.<br>• Choose foods that provide a high amount of nutrition in relation to calories.<br>• Exercise. |
| 3. Avoid too much fat, saturated fat, and cholesterol. | • High blood cholesterol levels increase the risk of heart attacks. In some people, high blood cholesterol levels are related to a high intake of fats, particularly saturated fats, and cholesterol in the diet. | • Choose lean meats, fish, poultry, and dried beans and peas as your protein sources.<br>• Eat eggs and organ meats occasionally.<br>• Limit your intake of butter, cream, shortening, and hydrogenated margarine.<br>• Trim excess fat off meats.<br>• Broil, bake, or boil rather than fry.<br>• Read labels to determine amounts and types of fat in foods. |
| 4. Eat foods with adequate starch and fiber. | • Complex carbohydrates—starches—provide more nutrients per calorie than simple carbohydrates—sugars.<br>• Certain complex carbohydrates provide fiber. High-fiber foods help reduce the symptoms of chronic constipation, diverticulosis, and some types of "irritable bowel."<br>• Some researchers believe a diet *low* in fiber increases the risk of colon cancer. | • Select foods which are good sources of fiber and starch. These include whole-grain breads and cereals, fruits, vegetables, beans, peas, and nuts. |
| 5. Avoid too much sugar. | • Eating too much sugar, especially sticky sweets and sugared soft drinks, increases the likelihood you will get cavities in your teeth.<br>• Too much sugar may cause hyperactivity. | • Use less of all sugars—white sugar, brown sugar, honey, and syrups.<br>• Eat less of the foods that contain these sugars, such as candy, cakes, sugared soft drinks, and fruits canned in heavy syrup.<br>• Read food labels. If sucrose, glucose, maltose, dextrose, lactose, fructose, or syrups are first, then the food has a lot of sugar. |
| 6. Avoid too much sodium. | • A little sodium is essential for health, but most Americans consume far more than they need. Excess sodium intake may increase the likelihood of developing high blood pressure. | • Reduce the amount of salt used.<br>• Limit your intake of salty foods, such as potato chips, and pickled foods.<br>• Read food labels to find out the amount of sodium in processed foods and snacks. |

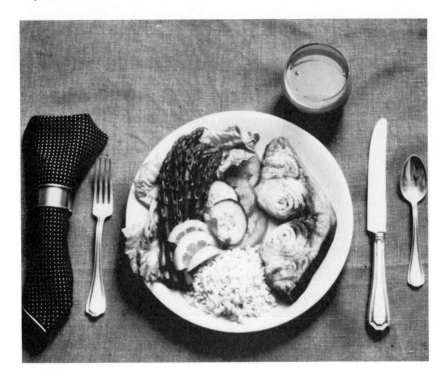

*A well-balanced meal that includes a variety of foods provides the wide assortment of nutrients your body needs.*

different types of food must be available to work together to help the body to function normally.

A good breakfast provides about one-fourth of the day's nutrient and calorie needs. Breakfast replenishes the body's nutrient supply after 10 to 14 hours without eating. People who skip breakfast, or other meals, don't get all the nutrients their bodies need. Without breakfast, they may run out of energy for mental and physical work by midmorning. Both noon and evening meals should provide about one-third of the day's nutrient and calorie needs.

Snacking in moderation can provide nutrients missed at mealtime when nutrient-dense foods are chosen. Too much snacking, however, can add up to excess calories and cause weight problems.

With a balanced day's food intake, vitamin pills and other nutrient supplements usually aren't necessary. In fact, taking them may give you more vitamins or minerals than you need. Too many vitamins and minerals can be unhealthy. For example, very large amounts of vitamin A can cause headaches, nausea, yellowish skin, and can stunt growth in children. Supplements cannot be a substitute for a balanced diet because they don't provide all the nutrients that food does, and they have no calories.

## Nutrition for Sports

Athletes need a balanced diet to get the nutrients they need for top performance. Their nutrient needs are about the same as those of nonathletes. However, they need more calories for physical energy. Some athletes believe that extra protein will build muscle. Exercise, not protein, builds muscle. The best diet for training and competition is a balanced one.

Eating a high-carbohydrate meal three or four hours before competition or a strenuous physical workout is best. It takes that long before nutrients pass through the stomach and begin to be absorbed. Food eaten an hour prior to competition, including candy bars, will not have time to be digested, absorbed, then used as an energy source for that sporting event.

Contrary to popular myths, high-protein liquid diets are no substitute for a balanced diet. Crash diets to make weight for sports, such as wrestling, are unhealthy because they may cause too much water loss. Both practices may lower athletic performances. Taking vitamin pills won't give extra energy—vitamins are not an energy source.

Athletes often lose a lot of water as they perspire, so drinking beverages to replace fluids is essential during and after strenuous activity. Plain, cold water is better than juices or sports drinks since it cools the body more efficiently. Serious health problems such as dehydration, organ damage, and heat stroke can develop if the body loses too much water. These conditions will be discussed in later chapters.

Sodium and potassium are lost through perspiration. Since most athletes get more than enough sodium in their meals and snacks, they don't need salt tablets. Salt is made of sodium and chloride. Eating foods high in potassium every day is the best way to replace potassium. Foods high in potassium include oranges, bananas, fish, and milk.

## Exercise

More than ever, people today realize the value of exercise to health. In record numbers, they're jogging, working out in health clubs, and finding other ways to be physi-

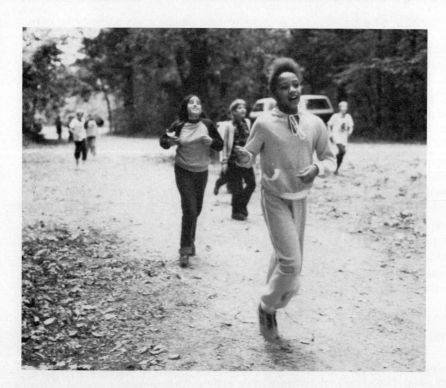

*When you exercise, your body perspires to keep itself cool. The perspiration causes a loss of water in the body, which then must be replaced.*

cally active. Through exercise, people are trying to make up for inactive patterns of work, study, and recreation. Some experts, however, feel that teenagers, on the average, are not exercising enough.

## Benefits of Exercise

Why is exercise so important to wellness? Exercise has many benefits. It:

- helps develop and maintain muscle mass and tone. Muscle helps give the body its shape. A lean body with a high proportion of muscle mass to body fat is healthier and looks better.
- improves muscular strength, making it easier to move and lift objects.
- increases physical endurance. This allows you to work and play longer and harder.
- improves coordination and flexibility. You move more gracefully and easily.
- helps control body weight. Exercise burns calories which might otherwise be stored as body fat. Strenuous exercise also increases metabolic rate for a short time so calories are burned at a faster rate.
- helps regulate appetite.
- improves posture. Well-developed muscles help a person stand, sit, and walk erect!
- strengthens the heart muscle. A healthy heart is efficient. It doesn't have to pump as fast to circulate blood.
- improves the lungs' capacity to inhale oxygen and exhale carbon dioxide.
- helps maintain bone mass. Weightbearing exercises help strengthen the bones.
- helps you relax. Exercise helps relieve stress and tension, which, in turn, helps you sleep.
- contributes to positive attitudes. That's because people who exercise tend to be more relaxed, tire less easily, and feel good all over!

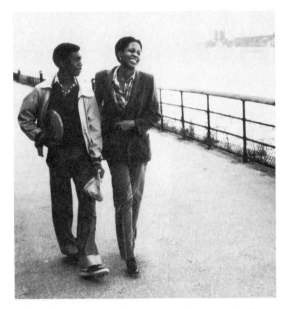

*Exercise is an important part of losing weight. Try walking rather than taking a car—and including a friend can make it all the more enjoyable.*

## Kinds of Exercise

Many types of exercise promote good health. Each type has a different function—endurance, strength, flexibility, and coordination. The best exercise progam includes a balanced selection of exercises.

### EXERCISES FOR MUSCULAR STRENGTH

Strength is your muscles' ability to apply force. Push-ups, bent-knee sit-ups, pull-ups, and running up stairs develop muscular strength. Handball, racquetball, soccer, and tennis are sports that develop muscular strength.

### ENDURANCE EXERCISES

Endurance is the length of time you can continue exercise or hard work. There are two kinds of endurance—cardiorespiratory and muscular endurance.

## How Fit Are You?

These three tests can help you determine if you're really in shape or if you need to improve your physical fitness.

| Test for These Qualities | Take the Test | Score the Test | |
|---|---|---|---|
| | | Females | Males |
| Flexibility | This **sit-and-reach test** measures the flexibility of your lower back and the back of your thighs.<br><br>Place the end of a ruler on top of a 12"-high box. Sit on the floor. Place your feet (no shoes) against the box, shoulder-width apart. Place your arms in front of you with one hand on top of the other. Reach forward as far as possible three times without bending your knees or bouncing. On the fourth reach, hold the forward reach for at least 1 second. Check the ruler to see how far you reached. | How far did your fingertips reach?<br><br>Excellent shape: $6\frac{1}{4}''$ or more<br><br>Good shape: $4\frac{1}{4}''$–$6''$<br><br>Fair shape: $2\frac{3}{4}''$–$4''$<br><br>Out-of-shape: less than $2\frac{3}{4}''$ | How far did your fingertips reach?<br><br>Excellent shape: $5''$ or more<br><br>Good shape: $2\frac{3}{4}''$–$4\frac{3}{4}''$<br><br>Fair shape: $\frac{3}{4}''$–$2\frac{1}{2}''$<br><br>Out-of-shape: less than $\frac{3}{4}''$ |
| Muscular Strength and Endurance | **Bent-knee sit-ups** test the strength and endurance of your abdominal muscles.<br><br>Lie on the floor, with your knees bent. Cross your arms and place your hands on opposite shoulders. Have someone hold your feet. Sit up and touch your elbows to your thighs. Return to the starting position. Count the number of sit-ups you do in 1 minute. | How many did you do in 60 seconds?<br><br>Excellent shape: 42 or more<br><br>Good shape: 33–41<br><br>Fair shape: 29–32<br><br>Out-of-shape: 28 or less | How many did you do in 60 seconds?<br><br>Excellent shape: 51 or more<br><br>Good shape: 45–50<br><br>Fair shape: 38–44<br><br>Out-of-shape: 37 or less |
| Cardiorespiratory Endurance | The **12-minute run/walk** tests the capacity and endurance of your heart and lungs.<br><br>Use the yard lines on a football field or have someone follow you in a car, watching the mileage. After warming up with some stretches, see how far you can run (or walk if you have to) in 12 minutes. | How many yards (or miles) did you cover?<br><br>Excellent shape: 2100 yards (1.2 miles) or more<br><br>Good shape: 1861–2099 yards (1.1–1.2 miles)<br><br>Fair shape: 1622–1860 yards (.9–1.1 miles)<br><br>Out-of-shape: less than 1622 yards (.9 miles) | How many yards (or miles) did you cover?<br><br>Excellent shape: 2879 yards (1.6 miles) or more<br><br>Good shape: 2592–2878 yards (1.5–1.6 miles)<br><br>Fair shape: 2305–2591 yards (1.3–1.5 miles)<br><br>Out-of-shape: less than 2305 yards (1.3 miles) |

The strength of your heart and lungs and their ability to deliver nutrients and oxygen to your body tissues and remove wastes is cardiorespiratory endurance. "Cardio" refers to the heart and the blood vessels, and "respiratory" refers to the lungs. Aerobic exercises help develop cardiorespiratory endurance. *Aerobic exercise* is vigorous, sustained exercise. Some examples of aerobic exercises can be running, jogging, bicycling, walking, swimming, jumping rope, and aerobic dancing. Some aerobic sports are basketball, handball, racquetball, and cross-country skiing.

Other exercises promote muscular endurance. This is the ability to apply force for a period of time. To develop this type of endurance, do exercises for muscular strength. Then gradually increase the number of times, the difficulty, or the length of time you do these exercises.

### FLEXIBILITY EXERCISES

Flexibility is the ability to move your muscles to their fullest extent. It enables you to move, bend, stretch, and twist easily. Being flexible helps you move more gracefully and prevents sore muscles. Yoga and stretching exercise, such as trunk twists, arm circles, and hamstring stretches, all develop flexibility.

### EXERCISES FOR COORDINATION

Coordination is the ability to move muscles in a harmonious way. Many exercises promote physical coordination: tennis, swimming, softball, dancing, soccer, skating, and basketball.

*During aerobic activity, take your exercise heart rate, but don't stop moving. Your training heart rate should increase slowly.*

## An Exercise Program

People who are physically fit participate in a variety of exercises. They also exercise regularly and strenuously at least three times a week, 20 to 30 minutes at a time.

A good exercise pattern starts with 10 minutes of warm-up exercises. These are moderate exercises which include stretching to "warm up" the muscles and to slowly increase the heart rate. Warm-ups help reduce injury. Then 10 to 30 minutes of strenuous, continuous aerobic activity exercises the heart. This is followed by 10 minutes of cooldown exercise which gradually brings down the heart rate.

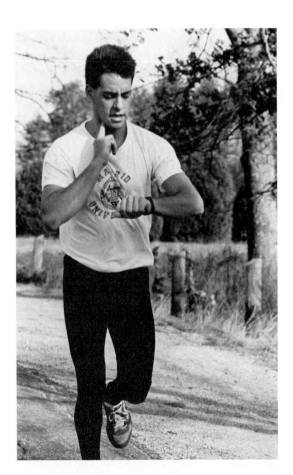

Aerobic exercises raise the heartbeat from a resting heart rate to a training heart rate. For people age 14 to 29, resting heart rate is about 70 to 80 heartbeats per minute. The low training heart rate is 140 heartbeats per minute, the moderate rate is 155, and the high rate is 170. When you start an aerobic exercise program, aim for the low rate and only continue for 10 minutes at first. Then increase the time slowly as you feel your body develop more endurance.

Before you start your warm-up exercises, take your resting heart rate. Place the flat side of the first two fingers of one hand in the hollow of the neck below the jaw. Count your heartbeats for 15 seconds, then multiply by four to find out how many times your heart beats in one minute. After you work into the strenuous part of exercise, use the same technique to measure your training heart rate. But don't stop moving while you check your training heart rate. If your heartbeat was too slow, speed up. If it was too fast, slow down. You shouldn't feel too uncomfortable or out of breath. After a few days, you often can estimate your heart rate without counting. As you cool down, your heart rate should gradually return to a resting heart rate.

## Exercise and Lifestyle

Many people live sedentary, or inactive, lifestyles. At school or at the office, much of the day is spent sitting. They sit in a car or bus. They sit to watch television. They sit while they socialize. Too much sitting means too little exercise.

Most people can add exercise to their lifestyle without much extra planning. You might walk to school, climb stairs, dance, or participate in sports instead of just watching. Consult with your doctor if you have any special medical problems to find activities that are right for you. Then make exercise a lifelong habit!

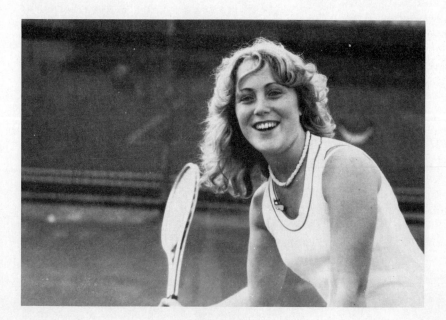

*People need to be physically active throughout life to maintain their health. Learn a sport which you can enjoy for a lifetime.*

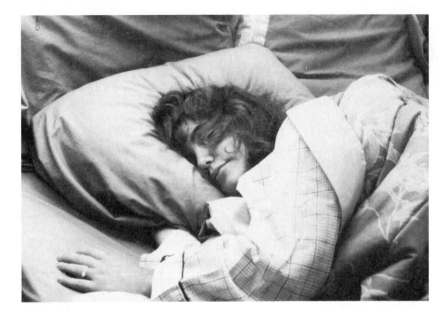

*While you are sleeping or resting, your body is storing energy for the next day's activities.*

## Rest

Rest and relaxation are important for maintaining wellness. Rest is needed after working, studying, and playing hard. During sleep, the body slows down its activities, but it does not stop working. It continues to build and repair tissue while you rest. The body also builds up energy stores to use when a person awakens.

People differ in the amount of sleep they need. Seven hours is average for adults, but children need more. Everyone needs a regular sleep schedule. Irregular sleep hours interrupt the body's rhythms. As a result, a person may feel tired and irritable even with enough total sleep hours. Insomnia is the inability to fall asleep. It may be caused by being overtired, tense, overeating before bedtime, or hunger. People who can't fall asleep might:

• relax with soft music or a warm bath.

• drink warm milk before bedtime. An amino acid in milk helps promote sleep.

• avoid vigorous exercise before bedtime.

• keep regular sleep hours to establish a pattern.

### Good Health Shows All Over!

• Adequate energy for daily activity
• Resistance to disease
• Normal rate of growth
• Skin that is firm and alive looking
• Bright, clear eyes
• Erect posture
• Desirable body weight
• Clean, shining hair that is free of dandruff
• Clean, cavity-free teeth
• Gums of good color
• Good muscle tone
• Ability to relax and sleep well
• Ability to adapt to change
• Willingness to assume responsibility
• Personal goals
• General happiness and positive attitudes
• Ability to cope with everyday stress

# Changes During Adolescence

As a teenager, your body is going through many changes. Many are physical. Others are emotional and social. These changes are normal processes of maturing. Recognizing and learning to handle these changes is part of good health.

Puberty marks the beginning of adolescence when many physical changes start to take place. Many of these changes are the development of sexual characteristics, such as the development of breasts in females and the enlargement of the male genitals. The genitals are the body's sex organs. Puberty begins when the sex glands begin to release hormones, or body chemicals. These hormones are responsible for many of the physical and emotional changes of adolescence. Not all body changes during adolescence are caused by hormones, however.

The following are some of the physical changes that take place in both females and males during adolescence:

- **Development of sweat glands**. This causes increased perspiration which, in turn, contributes to body odors.
- **Appearance of *acne***, or clogging of the skin pores, resulting in pimples and blackheads. Hormone changes that occur during adolescence may cause this condition.
- **Growth of body hair** on legs, underarms, and the pubic area. Pubic hair grows around and just above the genital area.
- **Appearance of additional permanent teeth**. Wisdom teeth appear and may cause pain if there isn't enough space in the mouth for them.
- **Adolescent growth spurt**. During the teenage years, both boys and girls achieve their adult height, and their bones continue to grow more dense. Girls usually have their teenage growth spurt between 12 and 13 years of age. For boys, it's somewhat later—between 16 and 17 years of age.

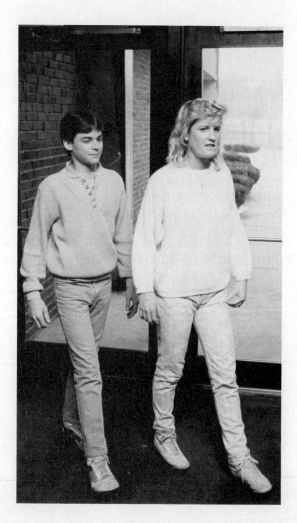

*Girls have their teenage growth spurt before boys do. By age 17 or 18, most boys reach their adult height.*

- **Strong appetites**. Because the body is growing rapidly, teenagers often feel hungry all the time.

The release of the female sex hormone, called estrogen, also causes these changes to gradually take place in the female body:

- **Development of breasts**. The breasts develop as a girl physically matures. They are a part of the life cycle. When a woman has a baby, they will provide breast milk as nourishment for the baby after childbirth.
- **Narrowing of the waistline and widening of the hips**. Again, these changes give a feminine body shape. Hips widen because fat is deposited there.
- **Maturing of the reproductive system**. The internal sex organs—ovaries and uterus—enlarge. The ovaries are the female sex organs where the eggs for reproduction are stored and where estrogen is produced. The ovaries are attached to the uterus by the fallopian tubes. The uterus is the organ that will enlarge to hold and protect the developing baby before birth. The vagina connects the uterus to the outside opening of the body, called the vaginal opening.

The menstrual cycle begins as the female body matures sexually. Each month, a bloody fluid is released from the uterus and expelled through the vagina and vaginal opening. This bloody tissue is formed in the uterine lining in preparation for pregnancy, but it is released about every 28 days, except during pregnancy. Menstruation continues through middle age until menopause when the process stops, and a woman can no longer become pregnant.

In some girls and women, menstruation may cause slight swelling of the breasts, cramps in the abdomen, headache, fatigue, and tension. When these symptoms become severe, the female might have premenstrual syndrome (PMS). A physician can recommend appropriate treatment to relieve discomfort and other symptoms.

Good personal hygiene is very important during menstruation. There is no reason to avoid bathing, swimming, and other forms of exercise. Mild exercise often helps relieve cramps.

The release of the male sex hormone, called testosterone, causes the following changes to gradually take place in the male body:

- **Growth of the larynx**, or voice box. The voice becomes deeper. Fairly often, while the vocal cords and voice are still in the process of changing, a boy's voice cracks and alternates between being high-pitched and being deep. This can be embarrassing to some individuals.
- **Appearance of facial and chest hair**. This hair changes gradually from soft fuzz to thick, darker hair. Males often choose to shave facial hair.
- **Broadening of the shoulders**. The shoulders grow wider than the hips, giving a masculine shape.
- **Development of muscle mass**. The male's body is able to develop more muscle mass than a female's body can.
- **Maturing of the reproductive system**. The external sex organs—testicles and penis—enlarge. The testicles are the male sex organs where testosterone is produced and where sperm for reproduction is made. The testicles are held in a bag of skin called the scrotum. Sperm move from the testicles through a tube and receive secretions from the seminal vesicles and the prostate gland. This forms the fluid called semen which leaves the body through the urethra. Ejaculation is when semen is discharged

from the body. When this happens while sleeping, it is called a wet dream. This is normal. Stimulation, which may be from a dream, causes more blood to flow into blood vessels of the penis. This makes the penis enlarge and become erect. A boy may have an erection without warning. This may be embarrassing, but it is normal.

# Hygiene and Personal Care

Along with diet, exercise, and rest, personal hygiene plays an important role in maintaining health. *Hygiene* includes the personal grooming and care of a person's skin, hair, teeth, eyes, nails, and ears. Good hygiene affects personal appearance, how people feel about themselves, and how others view them. Hygiene then influences physical, emotional, and social well-being.

## Skin Care

Cleansing the skin thoroughly with soap and water removes bacteria which can cause skin disease, as well as unpleasant body odors. A daily bath, shower, or sponge bath also helps a person look and feel better.

Proper cleansing means scrubbing the skin with warm water and soap. This opens the sweat and oil glands and helps remove dirt and oil from the pores. Cold water on the skin after cleansing closes the pores and protects them from dirt.

The best soap is largely a personal matter. Deodorant soaps have antibacterial agents in them. They have a tendency to dry skin, but they may help control acne. People with dry skin may prefer a super-fatted soap with added oils. There are also soaps for sensitive skins.

Special care should be taken to the feet when bathing. Carefully washing, especially between the toes, reduces bacteria and helps eliminate unpleasant odors. Thorough drying discourages athlete's foot. Athlete's foot is a condition that develops when a fungus grows in warm, moist areas of the foot. It causes itching and redness and spreads easily in locker rooms and showers. An antifungal powder helps cure this condition.

## BODY ODOR

Everyone perspires. Perspiration is a body fluid from the sweat glands that helps cool you down. Body odor comes from tiny organisms called bacteria which act on perspiration. Because the underarms have more sweat glands, body odor is often a problem under the arms.

In addition to daily bathing to remove bacteria, you can help control perspiration and body odor by using deodorants and antiperspirants. A deodorant helps mask odors, and an antiperspirant reduces the amount of perspiration. Many products have both properties. They should be applied as soon as the skin has thoroughly dried after bathing. Deodorants and antiperspirants shouldn't be applied to skin with open cuts or other irritations. And they can't substitute for daily cleansing.

The best product protects a person from odor and protects clothing from stains. It also agrees with the skin. If a rash develops from several different products, seek medical advice.

Besides underarm protection, some deodorants control other body odors, such as strong foot odors. Feminine hygiene products are also available to control odors from the menstrual cycle.

## ACNE

As indicated earlier in this chapter, acne is a very common teenage skin problem. It most often appears on the face, back, and shoulders.

*Frequent cleansing with soap and water helps
remove bacteria which contribute to acne.*

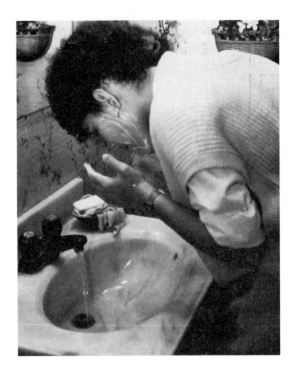

Acne is often caused by increased hormone production as the body matures. These hormones cause oil glands to produce excess oil. The oil, in turn, may cause pimples, whiteheads, and blackheads to form. Whiteheads are oils trapped in the pores. Blackheads are those oils which darken because they're exposed to air. Pimples form when bacteria gets into the clogged pore. Pimples or blackheads should never be squeezed or picked. This may cause an infection or scar. Acne usually clears up by adulthood.

Tension and stress contribute to acne problems. Just prior to or during the menstrual period, hormone changes may cause temporary acne.

Contrary to popular myth, acne is not caused by eating chocolate, fried foods, or soft drinks. So avoiding these foods won't clear up pimples. Neither inactivity nor sexual activity cause it. Facial saunas, vitamin E capsules, or vitamin E-rich creams won't cure acne either.

Frequent washing, along with a well-balanced diet, helps control acne. Cleansing with soap and water every morning and evening, perhaps more often, helps remove body oils and surface bacteria. Oily cosmetics, on the other hand, block the pores and cause skin eruptions when the oil becomes trapped. Makeup should be completely cleansed from the skin daily to help control acne. Applying an astringent on the skin after washing helps cut down on oiliness. You can also buy nonprescription medications that help some acne conditions. Plenty of rest and exercise, as well as a diet with adequate vitamin A, are also important in promoting healthy skin.

Some cases of acne can be helped by a dermatologist, or doctor who specializes in skin problems. A dermatologist may recommend medications for acne. Some medicine prescribed for acne can increase sun sensitivity. People taking these medications need sunscreens with more protection. You will learn about sunscreens in Chapter 5. The doctor or pharmacist can give advice. A pharmacist is the person at the drugstore who is trained and licensed to prepare and dispense medications and drugs prescribed by doctors.

## OTHER SKIN CONDITIONS

Other skin conditions also require special care:

- **Dry skin** has few oils. The objective for care of this type of skin then, is to keep body oils in. Most soaps dry skin out even more, so it's better to clean the face

## The Process of Tooth Decay

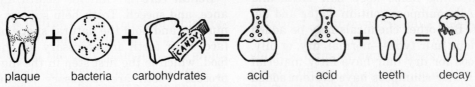

plaque + bacteria + carbohydrates = acid  acid + teeth = decay

proper way to brush. Using a soft bristled brush, angle the brush 45 degrees against the gumline. Gently vibrate the bristles, in a back-and-forth motion. Clean all tooth surfaces—inside, outside, and the tops of teeth. Also be sure to brush your tongue to remove remaining food and bacteria. This makes your whole mouth feel cleaner and fresher!

*Flossing* is the process of cleaning between the teeth and under the gumline with a special thread called dental floss. Flossing reaches places a toothbrush can't reach. Teeth should be flossed at least once a day when teeth are brushed. The picture on page **27** shows the right way to floss.

### FOOD AND DENTAL HEALTH

Wise food choices help ensure good dental health. A diet with adequate calcium and phosphorus is important because these nutrients become part of the tooth structure. Vitamin D helps the body absorb calcium from food. Vitamin C is a nutrient that is essential for healthy gums.

Eating patterns influence cavity formation. Carbohydrate in the form of simple sugars and starches are cariogenic, or decay producing. Every time you eat foods containing fermentable carbohydrates, acids made from plaque bacteria are produced for at least 20 minutes, and longer if food debris stays on teeth. Frequent snacking, including sipping sugary soft drinks all afternoon, can be very damaging to your teeth. So can sticky foods that stay on teeth.

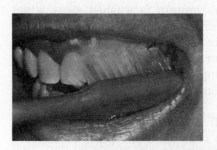

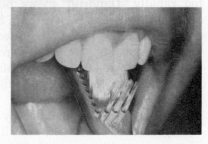

*The following method is one effective way of removing plaque:*
1. *Place the head of your toothbrush beside your teeth, with the bristle tips at a 45° angle against the gumline.*
2. *Move the brush back and forth in short (half-a-tooth-wide) strokes several times, using a gentle "scubbing" motion.*
3. *Brush the outer surfaces of each tooth, upper and lower, keeping the bristles angled against the gumline.*
4. *Use the same method on the inside surfaces of all the teeth.*
5. *Scrub the chewing surfaces of the teeth.*
6. *To clean the inside surfaces of the front teeth, tilt the brush vertically and make several gentle up-and-down strokes with the "toe" (the front part) of the brush.*
7. *Brushing your tongue will help freshen your breath and clean your mouth.*

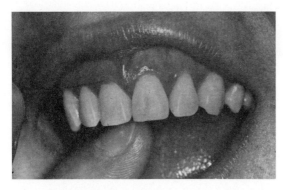

*When flossing, follow the instructions given to you by your dentist or dental hygienist. Here are some helpful suggestions:*
1. *Break off about 18 inches of floss, and wind most of it around one of your middle fingers.*
2. *Wind the remaining floss around the same finger of the opposite hand. This finger will "take up" the floss as it becomes soiled.*
3. *Hold the floss lightly between your thumbs and forefingers, with about an inch of floss between them. There should be no slack. Using a gentle sawing motion, guide the floss between your teeth. Never "snap" the floss into the gums.*
4. *When the floss reaches the gumline, curve it into a C-shape against one tooth. Gently slide it into the space between the gum and the tooth until you feel resistance.*
5. *Hold the floss tightly against the tooth. Gently scrape the side of the tooth moving the floss away from the gum.*
6. *Repeat this method on the rest of your teeth. Don't forget the back side of your last tooth.*

### CARE OF BRACES

Braces are used to correct misaligned, crooked, protruding, or overcrowded teeth. Such conditions can make chewing difficult. In addition, the risk of tooth decay, gum disease, and resulting tooth loss is greater because the teeth are harder to clean. By straightening teeth with braces, dental health, appearance, and self-image can be improved.

Braces are metal or plastic wires attached to the teeth by means of brackets. By tight-ening the wires and using rubber bands, the orthodontist gradually helps teeth move to proper alignment. An orthodontist is a dentist who specializes in straightening teeth. Sometimes a special mouthpiece, called a retainer, is used when braces are taken off to keep teeth from moving back into their old positions.

Faithful, thorough daily brushing and flossing is especially important for people who wear braces. Decay can develop easily when food debris is caught under the braces. A retainer also needs to be removed and cleaned daily, according to the orthodontist's directions.

### OTHER DENTAL CARE

Individuals who participate in contact sports, such as football and hockey, must protect their mouths. Inexpensive, plastic mouthguards are designed for this purpose.

## Eye Care

Personal care of the eyes involves preventing eyestrain and wearing corrective lenses, if necessary. Good hygiene can also prevent eye infections, and safety precautions can prevent eye injury.

### PREVENTING EYESTRAIN

Eyestrain causes headaches. With all the reading you do as a student, eyestrain can become a problem. Avoid eyestrain in these ways:
- Wear glasses or contact lenses if you need them.
- Read with adequate light.
- Keep a book about 15 inches away from your eyes as you read.
- Periodically, give your eyes a rest by focusing on an object far away.
- Watch television in a well-lighted room, and avoid long periods of viewing.
- If you work at a computer screen, follow the same guidelines as reading a book.

You can adjust the brightness and contrast of the screen for eye comfort, if necessary.

## VISION PROBLEMS

Normal vision is 20/20 vision. That means that you can stand 20 feet from an eye chart and read the top eight lines. People who are nearsighted can't see distant objects clearly, so they can't read all the letters on the eye chart. People who are farsighted have trouble seeing things close up. Both of these conditions can be corrected with eyeglasses or contact lenses. Vision should be checked once a year. Even if you already wear corrective lenses, your eyes should be checked to be sure the prescription is still right.

## CONTACT LENS CARE

Many people prefer contact lenses to correct their sight. Contact lenses need to be kept very clean to avoid infection. Follow these guidelines if you wear contact lenses:

- Use the appropriate cleaning procedures and chemicals for either soft or hard lenses.
- Wash your hands before handling lenses.
- Never use saliva to moisten lenses. The bacteria from your mouth could cause a serious infection.
- Don't wear lenses if you have an eye infection.
- Unless you wear extended-wear lenses, remove contact lenses before sleeping. Sleeping with hard lenses may increase dryness in the eyes and eventually scratch the cornea.

## OTHER EYE CARE

The soft tissue around the eye can easily become infected. For example, pink eye is a condition in which the white of the eye turns reddish, and the eye waters a lot. The roots of the eyelashes also can become infected,

forming a stye. Good health habits can protect eyes from infections:

- Don't touch your eyes with dirty hands.
- Use only your own towels and washcloths when washing your face.
- Girls should avoid makeup that causes irritation and never share eye makeup with another person.

Whether you have normal vision or you wear contact lenses or glasses, protect your eyes from accidents. Wear protective goggles for sports, such as racquetball. If you work in an industrial arts class, or have a hobby or job where chips of metal or wood fly or

*Protective equipment helps prevent injuries in many sports.*

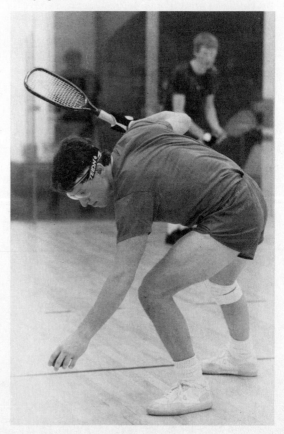

where strong chemicals are used, wear safety glasses.

Strong sun also can damage the eye. Wear good quality sunglasses which screen out ultraviolet rays. Sun-protective goggles are best for snow skiing. The glare from the snow and sun is hard on eyes.

## Nail Care

The state of a person's health may affect the growth and color of fingernails and toenails. Good nail grooming affects appearance and can even help prevent infection.

Good personal care of nails includes these practices:
- Clean fingernails with a soft brush or orangewood stick so dirt and bacteria don't build up. Bacteria under fingernails can contaminate the food that you handle.
- Trim fingernails with nail clippers and a file or emery board. Fingernails should be slightly rounded.
- Cut toenails straight across so they don't become ingrown. Ingrown toenails push into and cut the skin around the nail, often causing infection.
- Remove a loose cuticle around the edge of the fingernail so it doesn't tear. First soften it with oil or petroleum jelly. Then lift it away, and cut it carefully with manicure scissors.

The skin at the base of the nail is called the matrix. If a nail is torn off, it will grow again unless the matrix has been severely damaged. White spots on the nail are caused by bruises or other injuries. They grow out as the nail grows.

## Ear Care

Your ears require special care to help maintain normal hearing. Ears need cleaning to remove dirt and ear wax. Gently clean them with a cotton swab or wash cloth, never a pencil or sharp item. Don't push the swab past the outer edge of the ear canal. You may damage the inner ear.

Loud noises and music also can cause inner ear damage, which ultimately causes hearing loss. In Chapter 15, you'll learn more about the effects of noise.

## Posture

Good posture, or the way you carry yourself, promotes wellness. Good posture helps you move, stand, and sit more easily and makes you look better. Body organs, bones, and muscles develop and work properly with good posture. You can have good posture by following these guidelines:
- **Sitting.** Balance your weight evenly over your hips. Put your feet flat on the floor. Keep your back straight against the back of the chair.
- **Standing.** Stand so your weight is evenly balanced over the balls of your feet, forming an imaginary straight, vertical line down the side of your body from your ear lobes to your shoulder down to the outer edge of the anklebone.
- **Walking.** Balance your weight over the balls of your feet. Tuck in your abdomen, and comfortably hold your shoulders back. Let your arms hang easily at your side.

## Decisions for Wellness

Each day you make hundreds of choices that influence your health. You make decisions about food, exercise, rest, and hygiene. For example, will you snack on an apple or a candy bar? Will you play tennis or watch a game? Will you sleep eight hours or watch a late TV show? Each question may seem unimportant when considered alone. But all your decisions add up. Together they affect your health now and even years from now.

Using a step-by-step decision-making approach, you can make wise choices which match your goals for health.

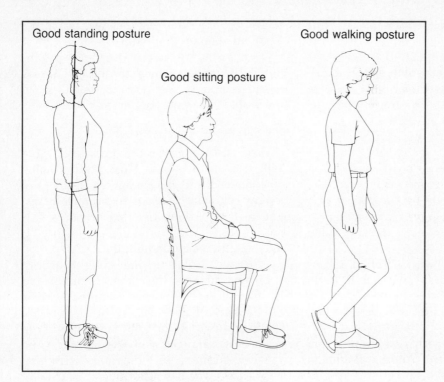

Good standing posture

Good sitting posture

Good walking posture

*The way you carry yourself tells other people at lot about you. Good posture also promotes your health.*

*Suppose you are ordering a fast-food meal. Which is the best beverage choice for you? Why?*

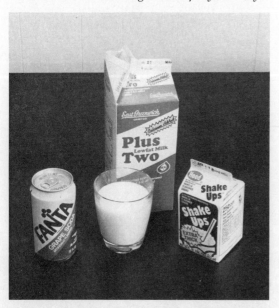

## Step 1. Set Goals

Goals are things you want to accomplish. Teenagers usually have many goals in mind, such as getting a job, completing their education, or buying a car. These are long-term goals. Being fit is a long-term goal, too. Most people want long, healthy lives. Fitness is also a short-term goal. You may need energy for tomorrow's game, or you may want to lose two pounds before next week's dance.

The best goals match your personal attitudes and priorities. Ask yourself, "What's important to me?" When health is important, it's easier to set fitness goals.

## Step 2. Know Yourself

Decisions are personal. What's best for your friend may not be right for you. For example, a skin-care product for your friend's oily skin may not be right if your skin is dry. An after-school milkshake may not be your best snack choice if you must struggle to control your body weight.

## Step 3. Consider Your Resources

Resources are things available to help meet your needs and reach your goals. Time, money, energy, and skills are resources. Good decisions match resources. For example, if your budget is tight, jogging is an inexpensive way to exercise.

## Step 4. Make a Plan

Usually you can reach the same goal in several ways. Before you make a decision, look at the possible choices. For example, to exercise, you can swim alone, play tennis with a friend, or join a school sports team.

## Step 5. Take Action

Follow your plan! Many times, people make excellent plans for achieving their health goals. Then they don't follow up on their plan. Inaction rarely helps people reach their desired goals.

## Step 6. Evaluate the Results

If you went through the decision-making steps, chances are you achieved your goals. But sometimes things don't turn out as planned. Perhaps uncontrollable circumstances got in the way. Maybe the effort wasn't worth the end result. Evaluation is to judge your decision and, if necessary, find another way to meet your goals for good health.

## Checklist for Good Health

- ✓ Balance your daily diet to include a variety of foods at each meal.
- ✓ Eat at regular intervals—don't skip breakfast or lunch.
- ✓ Drink six to eight glasses of water daily or the equivalent in beverages and soups.
- ✓ Maintain desirable weight for your age, sex, height, and body build.
- ✓ Exercise regularly.
- ✓ Allow time for relaxation and entertainment.
- ✓ Sleep seven to eight hours each night.
- ✓ Brush and floss teeth at least twice a day.
- ✓ Maintain good personal hygiene.
- ✓ Get regular medical and dental checkups.
- ✓ Avoid smoking and consumption of alcohol.
- ✓ Follow safety guidelines at home, school, work, and in the car.
- ✓ Maintain a positive attitude.
- ✓ Stay informed about health and about disease prevention.

*Reading current health magazines is one way to stay informed.*

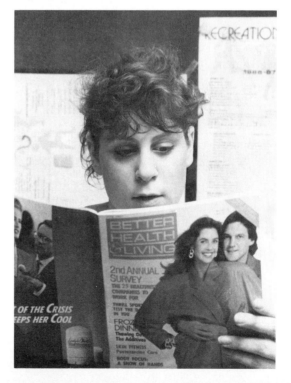

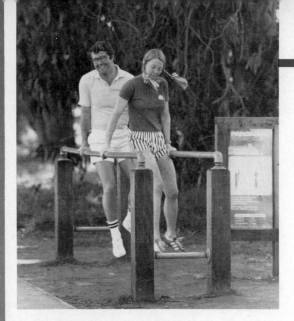

# FITNESS ON A BUDGET

Fitness is big business today. Athletic stores, department stores, and catalogs sell rowing machines, stationary exercise cycles, workout benches, weightlifting equipment, and many other types of exercise equipment. Shoe stores may specialize in athletic shoes with a different type for each activity—jogging, tennis, raquetball, and so on. Apparel is sold for every type of sport—sweat suits, leotards, jogging shorts and tops, leg warmers, tennis wear, ski wear, garments for cyclists, and sweat bands, among others. Videotape and record outlets sell a variety of exercise tapes and records. Health and fitness centers offer memberships so people can attend exercise classes and use workout equipment. Some hotels even have fitness centers available for a fee.

For some people, a fitness program can cost hundreds, even thousands, of dollars every year! But keeping in shape requires little, if any, extra expense. The choice is yours.

There are many ways for you to get fit on a budget:

- Jogging through your neighborhood requires only the investment in a good pair of running shoes. The rest is free.
- Communities and schools have outdoor tennis courts which you can often use free of charge. You can also get a good workout with a friend with a moderately-priced racket, tennis balls, and good tennis shoes.
- If you have a bicycle, use it! Cycling is excellent aerobic exercise.
- During warm weather, swimming can be an excellent way to keep in shape. Public and school pools are usually inexpensive to use.
- Calisthenics, such as push-ups, sit-ups, running in place, and leg lifts, can be done at home without special equipment or extra cost. All you need to have is motivation.
- Before you buy a book, tape, or record on fitness or exercise, check the library. Magazines reprint excerpts from popular books, too. And some television shows are created so that you can follow their exercise routines at home.
- Community organizations offer exercise classes at a much lower price than private fitness clubs. Some of these programs may be offered after hours in your school.
- Designer sportswear doesn't increase the benefits of exercise. For many sports, good footwear and loose-fitting clothing that washes easily will do just fine.

Don't let cost get in the way of your plan for fitness. The benefits of exercise are too important for your health.

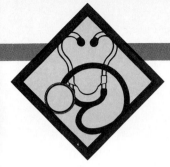

# CHAPTER CHECKUP

## Reviewing the Information

1. What are five signs of good health?
2. Name five physical changes that you might experience during puberty.
3. List the steps in decision making.
4. List the six categories of nutrients, and then name the major function of each category.
5. What are nutrient-dense foods? Give three examples.
6. What are empty-calorie foods? Give three examples.
7. Name the five food groups in the Daily Food Guide, and state food group recommendations for teenagers.
8. Why do athletes often need to drink more fluids?
9. What are five benefits of exercise?
10. Describe the four types of exercise and the physical function of each.
11. What are the three main components of a good exercise program?
12. Why does the body need rest and relaxation for wellness?
13. What causes body odor?
14. What causes acne?
15. How should a person treat dandruff?
16. Why is flossing important?
17. What causes tooth decay?
18. How can you help prevent eyestrain?
19. Name three health practices that protect your eyes from infection?
20. How does posture affect health?

## Thinking It Over

1. Using the formula on page **5**, calculate the number of calories you need each day.

2. Use the decision making process to make a decision related to your health. Write what you considered at each step.
3. Describe wellness in your own words.
4. Why is a varied diet so important?
5. Plan a balanced day's diet.
6. What nutrition guidelines should an athletic person follow?
7. How might you incorporate exercise into your own lifestyle?

## Taking Action

1. Visit a wellness center and talk to a staff member about their facilities and fitness tests. Write a summary of your findings.

2. Research wellness information. Prepare a resource list and share it with classmates.

3. Interview someone who is physically fit. Write about his or her wellness plan.
4. Make a poster with five health rules.
5. Analyze your food choices for a typical day using the Daily Food Guide or the RDA. If your diet falls short of the guide, what changes might you make?

# 2

# Emotional and Social Well-Being

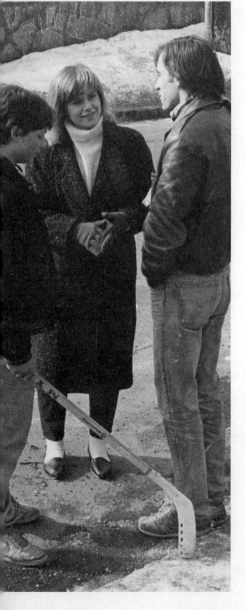

After reading this chapter, you should be able to:

• discuss how a positive self-concept affects behavior.

• discuss how emotions and social relationships can affect wellness.

• identify emotional and social characteristics related to good health.

• describe constructive ways to control emotions.

• describe positive ways to deal with others.

## Terms to Understand

| | |
|---|---|
| alienation | emotions |
| body language | peer pressure |
| communication | personality traits |
| defense mechanisms | self-concept |
| emotional maturity | |

Emotional and social health, along with physical health, contribute to a person's overall well-being and fitness. These three aspects of health are closely interrelated. In fact, the World Health Organization defines health as: "A state of complete physical, mental, and social well-being, and not merely the absence of disease or infirmity."

Personal needs must be met in order for people to be healthy. Physical needs are the most basic, and they must be met first for human survival. Beyond that, human beings need to have emotional and social needs satisfied for good health and for quality of life. The diagram on this page shows the personal needs which must be met.

Your *emotions,* or your feelings, and your social relationships have more impact on your health, happiness, and success than you may realize. Think of these situations. Before you go for a job interview or a meeting with your principal, does your stomach feel queasy, and do your palms sweat? Or do you even break out in a rash? How might your body feel after you've had a drawn-out, serious argument with your best friend? These examples suggest the close connection there is between a person's body, emotions, and social relationships. These factors cannot be separated.

Researchers have found that people who have good mental health early in life tend to have good physical health later in life. Researchers are trying to find out just how health is affected by people's thoughts and emotions and why some people stay well while others get sick under the same conditions. Researchers do know that the brain interprets a person's experiences and that the body responds chemically to emotions. These changes affect physical health and well-being.

Emotional and social well-being affect all aspects of life. Your performance at school and at work, your athletic abilities, your

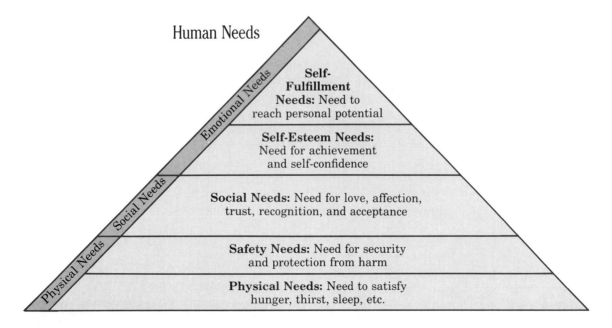

Human Needs

**Self-Fulfillment Needs:** Need to reach personal potential

**Self-Esteem Needs:** Need for achievement and self-confidence

**Social Needs:** Need for love, affection, trust, recognition, and acceptance

**Safety Needs:** Need for security and protection from harm

**Physical Needs:** Need to satisfy hunger, thirst, sleep, etc.

*Emotional Needs*
*Social Needs*
*Physical Needs*

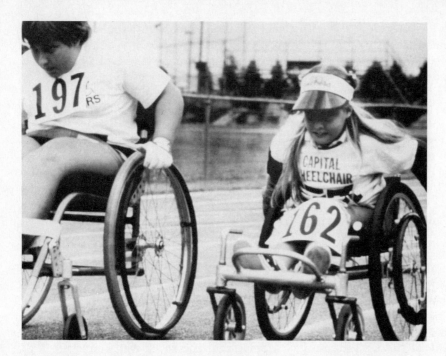

*These people are functioning at a high degree of emotional, social, and physical wellness.*

creative abilities, and your enjoyment of life are linked to your total health, or wellness. By learning who you are, by understanding your emotions, and by knowing how to relate positively to others, you promote your own total well-being.

## Personal Identity

Your identity is who you are. Your name, family background, nationality, and group affiliations are part of your identity. Your personality and self-concept also define who you are.

No one else is exactly like you. And you can't find out who you are by looking at someone else. Everyone develops in a different way, at his or her own rate. Different experiences, abilities, and attitudes shape different personal identities. Most important, each person can make a unique contribution to the school, family, community, and world.

## Personality

Your personality traits make up part of your personal identity. *Personality traits* are mental, rather than physical, characteristics which set one person apart from others. These traits determine how a person interacts with others. Your emotions, behavior, strengths and weaknesses, and how you think all are part of your personality. Personality is influenced by environment and, to some extent, heredity. Heredity includes those characteristics acquired biologically from parents. Heredity determines basic intellectual capacity. Some people also feel heredity affects one's general disposition.

Your environment is everything in your surroundings, including your family, friends, teachers, home, and community. Each of these factors has had an impact on your personality. Your personality shows in your behavior. For example, you learned which of your behaviors were good or bad by observing reactions of family and friends to what you did. Then you adjusted your behavior, often to get their approval. You also learned appropriate behavior by watching others and following their examples. Through your experiences and observations you developed a standard of behavior which is part of your personality.

The way you act and the way you respond to people are influenced by your personality. For example, some people are outgoing, while others are quiet. Some people are bubbly, while others are serious. Some are flexible, while others are inflexible. One type of personality trait is not necessarily better than another.

Personality traits evolve, or develop and change, throughout the life cycle. For example, as people become more emotionally and socially mature, they may become more assertive and outgoing. Other people take deliberate action to make personality changes. A person who tends to be very quiet may want to use self-help skills to become more outgoing. Other personality changes happen after a very stressful event, such as the death of someone close or a serious illness. People may teach themselves to be more patient and relaxed after learning that their stressful lifestyles are contributing to their own health problems, such as heart disease.

Sometimes people prejudge the personalities of others inaccurately and perhaps unfairly. They may stereotype, or judge, them only on physical attributes. To stereotype is to believe that people with certain characteristics all think or act alike. People may stereotype others according to their body type, religion, nationality, or where they live. These beliefs lead to misjudgments and often keep people from responding to one another in positive ways. For example, popularity is often linked to good looks or athletic ability because people assume people with these physical traits have good personalities. That isn't always true.

## Self-Concept

*Self-concept* is the image people have of themselves now and who they will be in the future. A positive self-concept means that people feel good about themselves. People with a positive self-concept usually relate well to others. A person's physical characteristics, attitudes, abilities, and experiences contribute to self-concept.

### PHYSICAL CHARACTERISTICS

The way people perceive or feel about their bodies is part of their self-concept. People who know they are healthy and physically fit often feel and act with confidence because they know they look their best. Often they know they have the energy and stamina to be successful, too.

Self-concept is often linked to body type. Magazine ads and television often make people with sleek, slim bodies seem glamorous and appealing. Because of this our society, as a whole, places high value on these physical qualities. As a result, many people judge themselves according to society's definition of physical attractiveness, even though they may be attractive in their own right.

Regardless of height or body build, people who take care of themselves make the most of their physical characteristics. Good nutrition, exercise, hygiene, and rest all contribute to feeling good about oneself.

### PRIORITIES AND ATTITUDES

People's priorities and attitudes help define their self-concept. Priorities are what are important to you. Attitudes are your personal views on issues or things. For example, health may be an important priority to you. If so, you likely have good attitudes

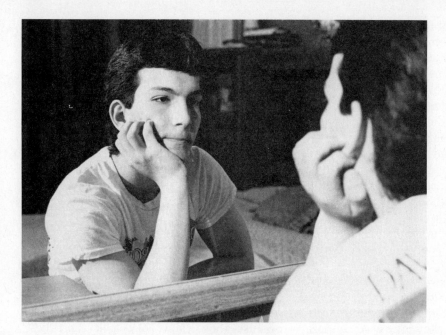

*Build a positive self-concept! Look in the mirror. Give yourself some compliments. Start with obvious good features: "I like your eyes," "You have a nice smile," or "You look healthy." Move on to your less obvious traits: "I like your honesty," "You're friendly to others," or "You gave a good class presentation today." Try this often until it becomes easy. How does this make you feel?*

toward exercise, nutrition, hygiene, and rest. Knowledge of good health practices helps direct your attitudes toward decisions and lifestyles which promote wellness.

Priorities and attitudes are shaped by your experiences. Family, friends, religion, and culture are among the factors which influence your view of life. Attitudes change as you grow older and more mature and have more personal experiences.

## ABILITIES

Most people do some things well and other things less skillfully. No individual can be good at everything, including you. A person's abilities contribute to his or her personal identity. For example, if you know you paint well, you might see yourself as an artist. Those people who haven't identified their abilities may not recognize their own self-worth.

What abilities do you have? Identify and develop new abilities by trying many things.

Keep a list of your strengths and build on them. Focus on what you can do, not what you can't do.

## Giving Yourself Credit

Do you worry so much about your shortcomings that you're afraid to take risks and try new responsibilities? You may not be giving yourself enough credit! Build your self-confidence and your self-concept by recognizing the things you do well.

Practice accepting credit from others when you deserve it. Don't feel foolish when other people praise you. How do you accept compliments like these?

- "You did a very good job."
- "You look nice today."
- "You really helped me. I couldn't have done it without you."
- "That was a good grade you got on that test."

## EXPERIENCES

Almost every experience in life affects an individual's self-concept. Interaction with others is important. Good or rewarding experiences, such as being respected, promote a positive self-concept. Being ignored promotes a negative self-concept. Experiences which help people achieve their personal goals give satisfaction and help define their identity.

How a person approaches life is affected by self-concept. The activities people choose to do each day influence the way they view the world and themselves. For example, an athlete who trains five hours a day has a different self-concept than a person who watches five hours of television each day.

## Emotions

As stated earlier, your emotions are your feelings. Everyone has emotions. These feel-ings are part of your personal identity, and they add color to your personality. Emotions are a natural human response.

You can see and feel the outward and physical signs of emotions. The gasp of surprise at an unexpected gift, the perspiration which accompanies anxiety, the widened eyes of fear, and the blush of embarrassment are familiar. Emotions affect your physical and mental health in many less obvious ways, too. Emotions influence the way you act around others and often how well you achieve your goals.

Some emotions are associated with the body's hormonal changes during adolescence. Excitement, happiness, and enjoyment come from things that appeal to you. Love and compassion are emotions which accompany relationships with others. Anger, fear, depression, anxiety, alienation, grief and guilt can be stressful emotions that

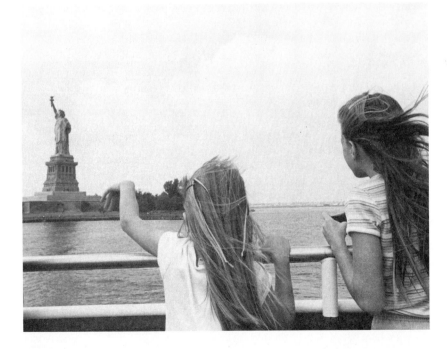

*You are the sum total of all you see, do, and feel. What experiences are important in your life?*

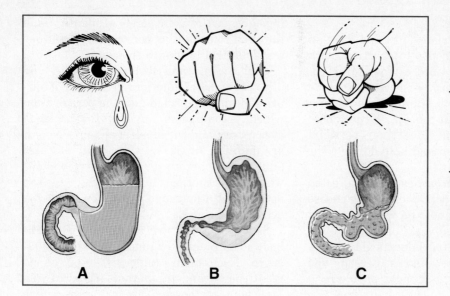

*Emotions can affect digestion. A) When a person feels depressed, the stomach stops producing digestive juices and stops digesting food. B) When a person is aggressive or resentful, the stomach produces digestive juices and gets ready to digest food. C) When a person is angry, food reaches the small intestine before it is ready, causing indigestion.*

A　　　　B　　　　C

that people must learn to handle to stay healthy.

Sometimes emotions are hard to identify, and people recognize them as something different. An upset stomach may be caused by tension, not disease. A person who says, "Playing tennis is boring" might really feel that he or she is not good enough to play tennis with you.

When people say they have mixed emotions, they recognize many different feelings about the same event. For example, you may be happy to graduate but be sad about leaving your school friends. Mixed emotions can make decision making difficult, especially when goals are unclear.

Emotions are neither healthy nor unhealthy. Instead, they are an expression of you. Recognizing and understanding emotions can help you express and deal with them in a healthful, positive way.

## Emotional Well-Being

Emotional health is difficult to define because each person is unique. Emotionally healthy people, however, feel comfortable with themselves. They feel right about others. And they can meet the demands of life.

Although no one has all these characteristics, emotionally healthy people are:
- accepting of themselves.
- self-confident.
- positive about their self-image.
- willing to take risks.
- optimistic.
- sensitive to others' feelings and needs.
- respectful and accepting of others.
- satisfied with life.
- able to laugh at themselves.
- friendly.
- able to interact well with others.
- able to accept and give love.
- sincere.
- flexible and able to change.
- open-minded.
- able to recognize and accept personal limitations and abilities.
- able to cope with success and failure.
- helpful.

*Have you ever heard, "Laughter is the best medicine"? People who know how to laugh live less stressful lives.*

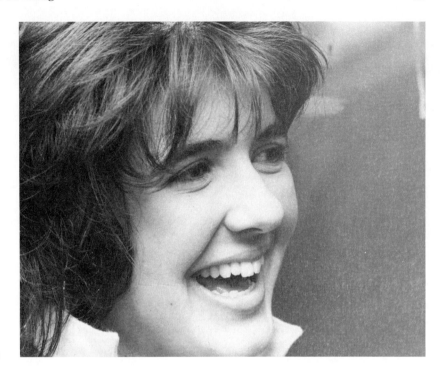

- able to channel emotions, such as frustration, disappointment, anger, and hostility, in an acceptable way.
- relaxed.
- able to set personal goals and work toward them.
- not suffering from unreasonable fears.
- guided by their personal standards of behavior.
- able to enjoy being alone.
- willing to accept responsibility.
- able to face problems rather than avoid them.
- able to handle moderate levels of stress.

## Dealing with Emotions

Sometimes, emotions overcome a person's ability to think objectively or behave appropriately. Emotions may hinder a person's ability to complete tasks, to relate to others, to achieve personal goals, and to feel person-

ally fulfilled. People may need to learn to manage their emotions and to express them in constructive ways.

### ANGER

Anger can build up from many small frustrations and irritations or may result from one single maddening event. It's neither a good nor bad emotion. But the way anger is expressed may have a positive or negative result.

Learn to work off anger. It's a sign of maturity. Every time you get angry, your body reacts. Anger may speed up your heart rate and breathing rate. If you are often angry and let your anger smolder, you are just setting yourself up for one or more emotion-caused reactions.

What are constructive ways for you to handle anger?

- Express anger in a non-violent way.

- Do some constructive physical activity right away as an outlet for anger. Practice some basketball shots, take a vigorous walk, or do a household task.
- Express your anger by talking or writing it out. You might write your feelings in a journal or tell a friend how angry you feel and why. This gives you the chance to think about your feelings and see if being angry is justified.
- Wait a while before you confront a friend you're angry with. Many times anger subsides when you have time to put it in perspective. Being too upset might result in more anger instead of a constructive settlement. But settle disagreements as soon as you've calmed down. Then you don't carry negative feelings with you forever.
- If you're angry with someone, settle the argument through discussion. Don't verbally attack the person.
- Cry if you need to. Often when you are angry, you're also hurt.

### FEAR

Fear is a normal reaction to a perceived threat. It is nature's way of alerting you to danger. Your body prepares to respond as your heart beats faster and more blood and oxygen go to your muscles. If the danger is real, you seek safety or protection.

Some fears have no basis in reality, and they may be destructive. For example, concerns about failure and rejection often make adolescents afraid to try new experiences or to meet new people. These fears may come from insecurity and low self-esteem. Low self-esteem indicates a lack of confidence in and respect for oneself.

Learn to face your fears head-on and evaluate them. Are they realistic or unrealistic? Then work to overcome unrealistic fear by taking some personal risks. You may even find others share your same fears. For example, you may be avoiding meeting someone because you fear he or she may reject you, while all the time that person fears that you'll reject him or her!

### ANXIETY

Nearly everyone feels anxious from time to time. Being nervous or tense are two signs of anxiety.

Sometimes anxiety can help you perform well. For example, before competing in a sports event or giving a speech or music concert, a little nervous tension can get your adrenaline flowing. Adrenaline is a body chemical that increases heartbeat, increases breathing rate, and suppresses the digestive process. Adrenaline helps prepare the body for action.

Anxiety can cause problems and even an inability to function properly, however. It may cause embarrassment, panic, worry, and distraction. People who are overly anxious can develop stomachaches, headaches, sleeplessness, and other physical problems. Some people learn to handle anxiety with simple coping techniques. When anxiety gets out of hand, counseling and medications may be needed. In Chapter 3, you'll learn more about severe anxiety and its effects on health.

If you feel anxious before competing, performing, or attempting something new, try to cope by using these easy relaxation strategies:

- Prepare yourself well for the event. For example, write out your speech and practice ahead. Or train adequately for athletic competitions.
- Get plenty of rest beforehand.
- When tension builds, concentrate on your breathing. Take three deep breaths and let them out slowly, letting your body relax as you exhale.

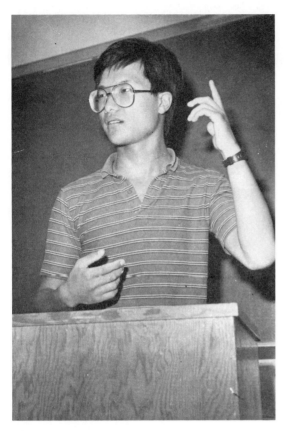

*Public speaking is an activity that makes most people anxious.*

- Close your eyes and imagine that you are successfully and confidently handling the event. This is like a "dry run" in your mind. Thinking you are successful will help you be successful!

## DEPRESSION

Life is full of "ups" and "downs," and depression is truly down. People who are depressed might feel a mild sadness or just feel a little low. Or they might experience severe feelings of hopelessness, anxiety, or withdrawal.

Almost everyone experiences mild depression from time to time. Perhaps nothing seems to go right, or they blame themselves for everything that goes wrong. They may feel helpless or ineffective. These aren't good feelings. Depression among teenagers is often the result of low self-esteem, lack of self-confidence, feelings of guilt, and lack of control. Loneliness, pressure, breaking up with a boyfriend or girlfriend, having a friend move away, or feeling out of touch with their families are also situations which often cause teens to be depressed.

Depression often interferes with a person's ability to do everyday tasks. It may result in these characteristics: appetite changes, prolonged loss of energy, headaches, irritability, feelings of emptiness, and feeling that nothing will ever go right.

Severe and prolonged depression is very serious because it may lead to thoughts of death and suicide. Anyone who feels this way should get professional help immediately from someone trained to counsel people with emotional problems.

You can help yourself avoid or get over feelings of mild depression.

- Avoid sitting or lying around dwelling on your feelings.
- Get out of bed. Get dressed. Follow your usual routine.
- Do something you enjoy. Be good to yourself. Perhaps take time for a hobby or walk with a friend.
- Join friends for a swim, play tennis, or wash the car. Rigorous physical activity produces body chemicals which work as antidepressants.
- Relax and rest. Relieve tension by letting your muscles become very loose. Being overtired can contribute to depression, too.
- Don't shut your friends or family out. Let your emotions out. Talk and share

your feelings with someone who can listen, understand, and give support.

- Look toward the future when you feel down. Don't dwell on past events, especially failures. Make plans. Set goals. Take control of your life.

## BAD MOODS

As a teenager, your body and your life are changing in many ways. Your body is maturing. Your relationship with your parents is changing. You may be making new friends, but losing old friendships. People expect more of you as you become increasingly independent. You may feel more easily hurt for no apparent reason by what other people say or do. Your feelings may baffle even you at times.

It doesn't make much sense to let the things other people say or do put you in a bad mood. Yet people let the opinions and

*Being in a bad mood doesn't accomplish anything. What might you do to feel better when you're in a bad mood?*

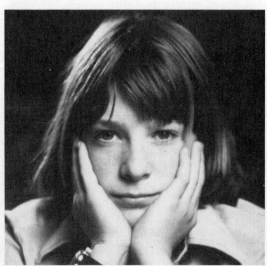

actions of others affect their feelings. Feeling inferior, angry, tense, depressed, or jealous often comes when other people have hurt you, even if they hurt you unintentionally. Or perhaps things didn't go as planned so you're in a "bad mood."

People react in different ways when they're in a "bad mood." Some retreat from the world. Others feel like lashing out at anyone who comes near. When you're in a bad mood, you probably are not pleasant to be with. As you become an adult, opinions and actions of others won't bother you as much.

Coping with a bad mood can be like curing mild depression. Consider the same suggestions listed on page **43**. And take time to figure out what the problem really is. Then plan to change it.

## GUILT

Guilt comes from feeling you did something that wasn't right or from feeling personally responsible when something goes wrong. Sometimes guilt feelings can help you live up to your conscience. If, for example, you told a lie, you might admit your mistake. Then you feel better.

Many times, however, people blame themselves when things aren't really their fault. Perhaps they jump to conclusions without talking to others or gathering all the facts. Communication is often the best way to relieve guilt or avoid it in the first place.

Guilt can become a source of severe emotional distress. Professional advice is necessary when a person can't function because of overwhelming guilt feelings.

## FRUSTRATION

Frustration is feeling unable to control something. When you are frustrated you get discouraged and feel ineffective.

Have you ever felt frustrated when you

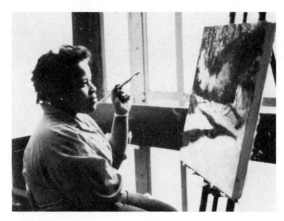

*Many people relax and release tension through artistic expression.*

couldn't understand something in class no matter how hard you tried? Or have you felt frustration because a friend, a brother, or a sister couldn't do a task as you explained it? Everyone feels frustrated occasionally.

Frustration can lead to anxiety and tension. But these feelings won't relieve frustration or accomplish anything else. When situations that cause frustration are out of your control, learn to tolerate them. Accept people and things you can't change. Avoid frustrating circumstances. For example, carry your own school lunch if a long cafeteria lunch line frustrates you. Plan and lay out your clothes the night before if deciding what to wear first thing in the morning is frustrating. Take time to talk with your parents if you feel frustrated because they don't seem to understand your needs.

### ALIENATION

Do you ever feel left out of things? Perhaps you feel that others don't want you around, or maybe you set yourself apart from everyone else. *Alienation* is feeling cut off from others.

During adolescence, alienation can be a real concern. As teenagers strive to become independent and develop their own identity, they may feel that others, including parents, don't understand them. They may feel alone with their problems and the rapid changes in their lives. They may withdraw, or isolate, themselves from others and from outside activities. Without knowing it, their actions and words may alienate others. For example, people who act conceited may find that others don't enjoy being with them.

Alienation and withdrawal can lead to loneliness, which further distorts their understanding of the real situation. Feeling that there's no one to turn to is unhealthy. People need other people for good emotional health. Being with others instead of isolating oneself makes it easier to adjust to the changes of adolescence.

People don't need to feel alienated. When they start talking with others, they often find that they share common feelings and problems. Parents are often more understanding than teenagers think. Many adults experienced similar feelings when they were young.

## Emotional Maturity

Maturity is reaching the level of development that is appropriate for one's age. Each person matures physically, socially, and emotionally at a different rate. No one can control the biological clock which affects a person's physical maturity. Becoming emotionally mature is within a person's control, however.

*Emotional maturity* is when a person learns to control and express emotions and attitudes in positive ways. It includes taking responsibility for one's own feelings rather than blaming others. Emotional maturity also means understanding and accepting oneself.

## Words Express Attitudes

Listen for these positive phrases:

- I can.
- You may be right.
- It's possible.
- Let's get started.
- We can do it.
- I feel great!
- Let's try.
- What a good idea!
- Go for it!

Watch out for these negative phrases:

- I can't.
- It's been tried before.
- It won't work.
- That's a terrible idea.
- I never could.
- You make me feel bad.
- No way!
- I doubt it.
- Impossible.

Emotionally mature people approach life with positive attitudes. In fact, successful people tend to be positive thinkers. You can often identify positive people by the things they say. The chart on this page gives phrases that suggest positive and negative attitudes.

If you want to approach life in a positive way, consider these guidelines:

- Think positive thoughts about yourself. Be confident.
- Set realistic personal goals, and expect to reach them.
- Expect good things to happen in your life.
- Expect to be healthy and happy.
- Make a habit of finding positive, not negative, traits in your friends and teachers. Don't gossip about them.
- Give compliments readily and sincerely, but don't be insincere and give compliments you don't really mean.
- Receive compliments graciously.

- Welcome new experiences as opportunities for enjoyment and learning.
- Avoid being oversensitive. Don't carry a chip on your shoulder or hold a grudge.
- Use facts, not emotions, when you evaluate situations.
- When you feel you have been unfairly treated, briefly explain your feelings to the offender. Be tactful and calm as you talk.
- Be friendly, helpful, and courteous to others.
- When some unpleasant experience occurs, handle it as best you can. Then adopt the attitude that "This, too, will pass."
- If you have hurt or offended someone, sincerely apologize. Then move on with new goals to try to develop a positive relationship.
- Make a personal commitment to consciously approach your life with a positive attitude.

## Defense Mechanisms

*Defense mechanisms* are the responses and behavior people use when their emotional well-being is threatened. Defense mechanisms enable people to protect the way they feel about themselves when they face the situations that threaten their self-concept. Defense mechanisms are normal reactions. Sometimes they are beneficial; sometimes they are harmful.

Sometimes defense mechanisms help people maintain a healthy self-concept. These responses can keep people from feeling overwhelmed by distress, anxiety, tension, and lowered self-concept.

Defense mechanisms can also be harmful by keeping people from facing reality, accepting responsibility, taking risks, or changing negative personality traits. When they are used, defense mechanisms actually keep people from discovering their own identity or solving their daily problems.

These defense mechanisms are common:

- **Rationalization**. This is making excuses to explain away behavior. For example, a student might say, "The teacher forgot to assign the chapter so I didn't know the answers."
- **Repression**. This is forgetting something ever happened in order to avoid pain. For example, a teenager who was the driver in a car accident in which his or her best friend was killed may have no memory of the accident.
- **Denial**. This is refusing to admit that something is true. Refusing to admit or talk about a drug or alcohol problem is denial.
- **Reversal**. This is acting or thinking directly opposite of how you really feel or want to behave. For example, a person who is really sad deep down becomes a class clown.
- **Projection**. This is putting the blame on someone else. For example, someone might say to a parent, "I would have more friends if you'd only give me a car."
- **Sublimation**. This is acting out one's feelings in a different but safe place or manner. For example, a person may shout loudly at a sports event because he or she really feels angry with his or her parents.
- **Displacement**. This is directing feelings of anger, hurt, or aggression toward another target that may be considered "safe." For example, someone may hit the dog when a friend disappoints him or her. The dog won't talk back!
- **Identification**. This is acting like a role model. For example, teenagers may dress, talk, and act like their favorite movie stars or school heroes instead of expressing their own identities.

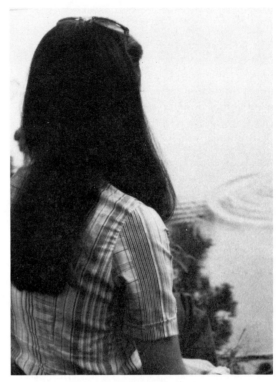

*What defense mechanism might this girl be using?*

- **Daydreaming**. This is letting one's mind wander away from problems, and instead, imagining oneself in a more ideal situation. Fantasy can be used in a positive way. People might face a problem and use fantasy to visualize how the situation can be resolved with success.
- **Compensation**. This is focusing on positive attitudes instead of real or imagined shortcomings. For example, would-be athletes might try out to be team managers when they don't think they can compete as athletes.

Silence, bragging, and criticizing others are other defense mechanisms. They may cause others to dislike being with you.

# Relationships with Others

Emotional well-being and personal identity are closely linked to relationships with others. Personality, self-image, and self-esteem are shaped by interactions with others. For example, by praising and accepting people, you help build their self-confidence. Constant criticism, on the other hand, may lead people to withdraw from others. When emotional needs aren't met, people might not get along well with others. Positive social experiences help build a good self-image, which, in turn, can contribute to good emotional and physical health.

## Social Well-Being

Your family is the first social network you had. While you have relationships with many people—friends, teachers, neighbors—your relationship with your family will probably be the strongest and most important in your life. Within the family, people learn appropriate social behavior, and they learn to be sensitive to the needs of other people. Supportive family members create an environment of trust, affection, and acceptance. They help children develop personal responsibility. They also recognize the unique contribution each individual makes.

Friends become more important as people get older. You may think only of people your own age as friends, but you can be friends with an elderly neighbor, a teacher, or a young child, too. Friendships may change, but people who learn to be good friends as teenagers will always make friends wherever they go. To have a friend, you must be a friend. Characteristics of good friends are listed on this page.

Social well-being is built on feelings of acceptance, responsibility, recognition, trust, and affection. Close friendships, satisfying work relationships, and loving relationships within the family contribute to social well-being.

The signs of good social health are the ability to:
- make and keep friends of both sexes.
- work and play cooperatively.
- enjoy other people.
- accept rules of the group.
- share with others.
- be considerate of others.
- be helpful.
- control emotions in relationships with others.
- take part in a variety of activities with others.
- maintain a personal moral code in social relationships.

### TRUST

Trust is being able to rely on people. Knowing that family and friends will give consistent support, love, and attention builds trust. Not betraying or rejecting another person also builds trust. Dishonesty destroys trust. Teens build trust by acting in responsible ways. Trust allows people to

## Friends Are People Who ...

- value each other.
- share.
- like and respect each other.
- praise one another.
- are loyal.
- help each other.
- listen and understand.
- usually have things in common.
- advise each other honestly.
- keep confidences.

feel safe and secure in the world around them. Feeling safe and secure is a basic human need. Trust is built over a long period of time.

## RESPONSIBILITY

Being responsible to oneself and others promotes social well-being. Accepting responsibility and following through on that responsibility help you feel valued and needed. Responsibility also shows your trustworthiness and personal commitment. Positive experience help prepare adolescents for the responsibilities of adulthood.

## RECOGNITION

Recognition is important for a person's sense of self-worth and self-confidence. You need recognition and so do your friends and family.

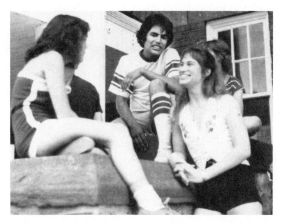

*Everyone needs to feel accepted by people he or she respects.*

*Everyone needs to feel special from time to time. What might you do to recognize someone you care about?*

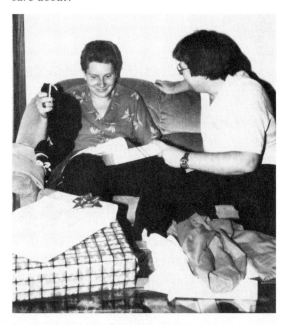

Recognition may be formal, such as an award for achievement, or it might be a casual thanks or praise for a job well done. Gifts are thoughtful ways to recognize people. There are other simple ways you can offer recognition to someone else.

- Acknowledge them. Don't ignore them.
- Introduce people who do not know one another.
- Encourage everyone to participate in conversations or activities.
- Recognize when someone does a favor for you. Maybe you can return the thoughtfulness by doing him or her a favor.
- Give friends and relatives a quick phone call just to say, "Hi."

## ACCEPTANCE

Everyone needs to feel that he or she belongs. That's a basic human need. Being accepted by family and friends is important, especially to teenagers. Joining organizations and doing things informally with friends, helps fill this need. You can also help others feel accepted by recognizing them and including them in what you do.

## AFFECTION

People not only need acceptance, they also need to give and receive affection throughout life. Responding to the needs of each other builds love and affection. You need to share affection within your family. Some people take their family's affection for granted, but family members support and nurture each other. To nurture is to care for someone in a loving and emotionally-supportive way. Friends can also play a role in filling this need.

# Problems in Social Relationships

Sometimes people have problems in dealing with social relationships. A difference of opinion may cause a conflict. Other times people may put pressure on others to do things they really don't feel right about.

## CONFLICT

Conflict can happen in any situation where there are different beliefs or when people haven't communicated their beliefs. Conflict may occur when people make judgments about others that aren't accurate.

You can expect to have some conflict in life. Conflict helps people explore issues, share ideas, clear the air, or encourage change. It provides an opportunity to grow. In fact, conflict is part of human relationships. It's also part of growing up. Teenagers undergo many conflicts with their parents as they learn to become independent.

A conflict between two or more persons may be a disagreement. The differences can be quite simple. One person might want to go to a movie while the other prefers to watch a game. In simple arguments, there are choices. One side can give in, each can agree to go separate ways, or there can be a compromise. In a compromise each side changes its position a little to meet on a "middle ground." Then both sides feel good.

Sometimes conflicts are dealt with in combative ways, such as hostile arguments. This usually doesn't result in solutions where everyone feels satisfied. Instead, anxiety, anger, or frustration is created.

Conflict is best approached in a constructive manner. Consider this approach:

- Identify the true causes or issues involved. Sometimes people don't know why they disagree.
- Identify your goals related to the conflict. What would you like to happen? How would you like your relationship with the other person to end up?
- Look at all the alternatives and then take a position which matches your goals. Be politely assertive as you state your position.
- When you feel torn between two positions, apply the decision-making process you learned in Chapter 1.

Success in dealing with conflict with others comes from your ability to adapt and from your respect for the other person's position. Being open-minded when it comes to the other person's views helps avoid conflicts. Using decision-making techniques in advance can help avoid many conflicts in the first place.

## OVERCOMING SHYNESS

Shy people have difficulty communicating. As a result, they often have a hard time forming relationships. They may be uncomfortable in social situations because they don't feel they have anything to say or perhaps they feel insecure.

Experts believe that people learn to be shy and that people also can learn to overcome shyness. These are some ways to overcome your own shyness.

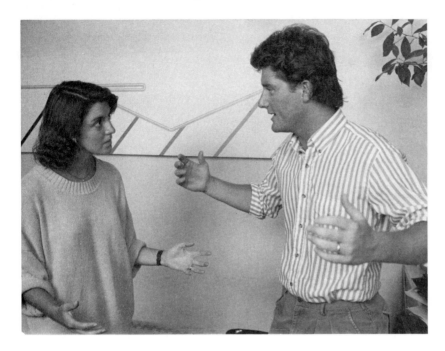

*Talking together is often the best way to resolve a conflict.*

- Learn to be a good listener. Show other people that you care about what they're saying.
- Ask people about their hobbies, job, and interests. Or ask for an opinion or a recommendation for a movie, a book, or a restaurant.
- Learn to relax when you're around other people.
- Look directly at the person speaking and smile.
- Learn to value your own self-worth.

**SOCIAL AND PEER PRESSURE**

Social pressure means that people try to persuade others to act in certain ways. Often social pressure is difficult to resist.

Encouraging someone to wear a seat belt is positive social pressure. That's because the goal contributes to the person's safety and well-being. Not all social pressure is positive. For example, sometimes there is social pressure to smoke or drink alcohol. Neither promote health.

*Peer pressure* is social pressure when people are influenced by others their own age to behave in a certain way. Usually, people follow their peers so they will be accepted. It's hard to resist peer pressure because everyone needs to belong. Agreeing with friends and doing what they do is easier than making independent decisions.

Following peer pressure may keep you from achieving your goals, maintaining your personal standards, or enjoying your own interests. The goals, interests, and standards of your friends may be different from yours even though you like each other. Peer pressure is easier to resist when you have a positive self-image and clear goals. Then you can decide when doing certain things is in your best interest.

## Communication

Communication skills are important to your relationships with family and friends. *Communication* is both sending and receiving information. Talking and listening together are communication. Sometimes you send and receive messages from other people, even without speaking a word. Slamming a door, smiling, putting your hands on your hips, and dressing in certain styles all communicate your message to others. These nonverbal communications are called *body language.*

Sending and receiving accurate messages is essential to good communication. However, the message you think you heard or received may not have been the one the other person meant to send. This can create misunderstanding or conflict. For example, a person who refuses your invitation or doesn't say "hello" might not be a snob. He or she instead may feel insecure or shy. Or perhaps that person didn't hear or understand what you said.

### COMMUNICATING WITH FRIENDS

A good friend helps a person build a positive self-concept. The way you communicate reinforces a friend's own self-esteem and self-worth. It also helps build a trusting, supportive relationship. For example, you can support your friends by telling them that you are glad to see them. You can praise their behavior and their appearance, congratulate them for their success, listen to their problems, encourage them, and show appreciation for their friendship. Neg-

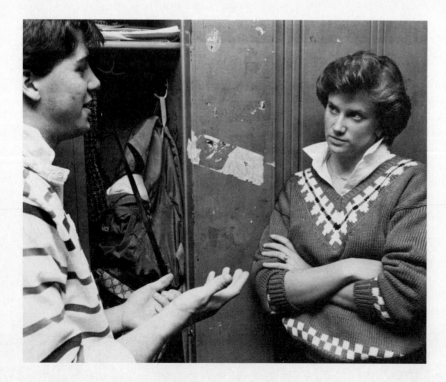

*What does this body language tell you?*

## Do You Really Communicate?

Phrases that encourage communication:

- Tell me about _____.
- Are you saying that _____?
- Do you mean that _____?
- Did I understand that _____?
- Please explain how _____.
- Help me understand _____.

Phrases that stifle communication:

- That's stupid!
- I don't believe that!
- I don't want to talk about it!
- You don't know how I feel!
- Nobody your age can understand this!
- You don't know!

ative communications, such as criticizing, interrupting, or ignoring them, are destructive to a relationship.

### COMMUNICATING WITH YOUR FAMILY

Communication within a family is important for emotional and social health. Open communication within the family helps heal emotional wounds from the outside world. Talking together helps people sort through the personal goals, decisions, and conflicts which are part of life.

Just as you need their input and support, members of your family need to communicate with you and know you care about them. Express how much you appreciate their help. Don't take them for granted. Praise them for their accomplishments. Ask them for help when you need it, and give help when they need it. Respect their feel-

ings and needs. As you go on to become more independent, assure them that they are still important in your life.

## Social Maturity

Socially mature people get along with others even when they have differences of opinion. They recognize that they can't be the center of attention all the time. They also can recognize the needs of others and offer support and friendship. Their expectations about relationships with others are also realistic and not overly demanding.

Emotional and social health are intertwined. Self-confident, emotionally mature people are more likely to also be socially mature.

## Wellness—It's Your Responsibility

What's your level of overall wellness? It's time to look at yourself and take a wellness inventory such as the one on page **54**. Identifying and evaluating your attitudes and behavior are the first steps in making responsible and knowledgeable health decisions for yourself.

How did you rate on "The Wellness Inventory"? Did you score high in one area and low in another? Remember that the healthiest and most successful people have good scores for physical, emotional, and social health. Look at your answers again to see what changes could promote your health.

Change is never easy, but it results in growth. A secret to success is to change what can be changed. Set some goals for yourself. Then use the decision-making process described in Chapter 1 to take action.

Your health is your responsibility. No one else can make choices and follow habits that keep you well. Develop a positive attitude toward healthy living. Actively involve yourself in your own good health!

## The Wellness Inventory

On a separate sheet of paper, indicate each statement that is true for you. Count how many statements are true for you in each area and refer to the scoring directions below.

### Physical Health
- I seldom feel tired or rundown.
- I get at least 8 hours of sleep per night.
- I regularly use dental floss and a soft toothbrush.
- I do not use tobacco.
- I keep within 5 pounds of my ideal weight.
- I use stairs instead of escalators or elevators whenever possible.
- I do at least 20 minutes of aerobic exercise at least three times a week.
- I eat breakfast every day.
- I do not use alcohol or nonmedicinal drugs.
- I take at least 10 minutes each day to relax completely.
- I limit my dietary intake of refined sugar and salt.
- I eat a balanced diet that includes a variety of foods.

### Mental Health
- I ask for help when I need it.
- I am happy most of the time.
- Sometimes I like to be alone.
- I can name three things I do well.
- I feel okay about crying and allow myself to do so.
- I give others sincere compliments.
- I can accept compliments.
- I listen to and think about constructive criticism.
- I am able to say no to people without feeling guilty.
- I can be satisfied with my effort if I have done my best.
- I express my thoughts and feelings to others.
- I have at least one hobby or interest I pursue and enjoy.

### Social Health
- I meet people easily.
- I am comfortable entering into conversation with new acquaintances.
- I continue to participate in an activity even though I don't get my way in an argument.
- I have at least one or two close friends.
- When working in a group, I can accept other people's ideas and suggestions.
- I can say no to my friends if they are doing something I do not want to do.
- I can accept the differences in my friends and classmates.
- I usually have success making friends with females my age.
- I usually have success making friends with males my age.
- I am comfortable carrying on a conversation with an adult.
- If I have a problem with someone, I try to work it out.
- I avoid gossiping about people.

*Scoring:* The highest possible score for each area is 12. If your total score is 10 to 12 in any area, your level of health in that area is *very good*. A score of 7 to 9 is *good*, 4 to 6 is *fair*, and below 4 indicates a general area you may *need to be working on*.

# FORMULA FOR SUCCESS

What do you want to be successful at? Sports, music, acting, writing, building, cooking? Being successful at anything requires good health—physical, emotional, and social.

Athletes know that success depends on more than physical abilities. Having the competitive edge takes mental concentration, self-discipline, and emotional strength. Team members also must get along with others. A successful athlete also knows how to accept the coach's advice.

As a figure skater and bronze medal winner at the U.S. Olympic Festival, Angelo D'Agostino has learned the formula for success.

Angelo begins his success story: "Five years ago, I had mastered the physical side of skating. But I couldn't handle the emotional pressure of being judged, and my performance suffered. Luckily my coach recognized my problem and found someone to help me."

Angelo says, "Good skating is 90 percent mental and 10 percent physical." Learning to concentrate, to use your imagination, and to relax isn't just for skaters but for anyone who wants to get somewhere in life. According to Angelo, "These skills certainly helped me take control and make progress in competitions."

Building on one's strengths and interests and minimizing the limitations are also important to success. Angelo had always been the second shortest boy in his class. That ruled out a lot of sports, but he liked skating. His slender body would help him be agile on ice. Angelo also recognized that his family was one of his strongest assets. They were willing to support his long hours of training. He also knew that his self-discipline and stubborn personality would help him stick to training.

Setting realistic goals, making a plan to reach them, then putting the plan into action is part of the success formula. Angelo knows this: "Goal setting has become my way of life. I think we're all a little like guided missiles. If we don't program ourselves, we may self-destruct. Then we never reach the target that was right for us."

What are Angelo's goals? In the near future, he wants to be a U.S. World Team Member for the Olympics. Then he looks forward to a successful career in ice shows, perhaps sportscasting, and later, coaching.

Angelo follows a careful plan to achieve these goals. Currently he skates six hours a day. He develops his upper body strength with special exercises off the ice. He eats four nutritious meals a day and avoids empty-calorie snack foods. When he gets too busy and misses a meal, he says that his performance suffers. He schedules relaxation and private time—listening to music surrounded by the Colorado mountains. Yet he takes time for friendships with nonskaters. He also makes certain he gets about eight hours of sleep each night.

Angelo has a message for other teenagers: "Take care of your body, your mind, and your relationships. Set goals and put your whole heart into them. We all need a sense of personal direction. Make choices that match your goals. You always have a choice, even if it's to make no choice at all. You'll enjoy the good feelings you get as you reach each step along the way to your goals. Success really feels good!"

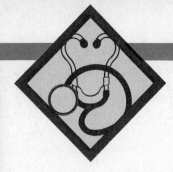

# CHAPTER CHECKUP

## Reviewing the Information

1. What human needs should be met for good health and quality of life?
2. What determines one's personality?
3. What are five personality traits?
4. What factors contribute to a person's self-concept?
5. What are ten characteristics of someone who is emotionally healthy?
6. List three positive ways to handle your anger.
7. What is fear? How does your body react to fear?
8. How does anxiety affect the body?
9. How can a person control anxiety?
10. Describe four ways a person might control feelings of depression.
11. What does it mean to feel alienated. How does this affect a person's social well-being?
12. What does it mean to be emotionally mature?
13. What are five positive ways to approach life?
14. Why do people use defense mechanisms?
15. Describe three defense mechanisms.
16. What are five social needs that contribute to health and self-esteem?
17. What does it mean to compromise when you disagree with someone?
18. Explain the ways that people communicate with one another.

## Thinking It Over

1. List five positive personality traits.
2. List five ways you might improve or reinforce your self-concept.
3. Suppose you woke up in a bad mood. How might you control these feelings?
4. Give two examples showing how your emotions have affected a relationship.
5. How might you resolve a conflict in a positive way?
6. Describe an experience you've had with peer pressure and how you handled it.
7. Why is communication so important to emotional and social well-being?

## Taking Action

 1. Research the personality and accomplishments of a famous person. What personality traits helped make the person successful?

 2. With another student, write a skit showing a positive and a negative defense mechanism for a common situation. Present the skit in class.

 3. Choose a personality trait of yours that you would like to change. Write a personal plan to help make that change. Put your plan into action.

 4. Visit the school counselor or library to find reliable self-help books about emotional and social health. Read one book, and report back to class.

# Health Risks

3

After reading this chapter, you should be able to:

• identify the health hazards of substance abuse.

• discuss the consequences of obesity and underweight.

• plan a healthful way to achieve and maintain desirable weight.

• identify how stress affects health.

• discuss ways to manage stress.

## Terms to Understand

| | |
|---|---|
| anorexia nervosa | obesity |
| bulimia | passive smoking |
| fad diet | stress |
| intoxication | substance abuse |
| leukoplakia | support group |
| nicotine | |

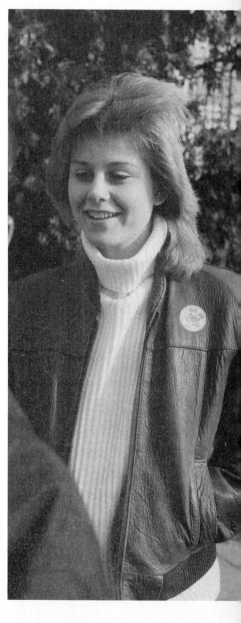

Every day you make choices. Some decisions aren't really that important, like what you'll wear to school tomorrow. But many other decisions significantly affect your health now, even years from now.

By following habits of good nutrition, exercise, hygiene, and rest, you make choices that promote wellness. Some decisions, such as using tobacco, alcohol, and illegal drugs, create serious health risks for you and for others. Poor eating habits that result in obesity or being underweight and stressful lifestyles also pose health risks.

## Substance Abuse

*Substance abuse* is using alcohol, drugs, or tobacco in ways that don't promote physical, emotional, and social health. Substance abuse often results in physical and mental health problems, such as malnutrition, depression, ulcers, long-term disease, permanent brain damage, even death. It can destroy family and social relationships with deceit and mistrust. Ultimately it also may have a negative impact on a person's self concept and success in life.

## Tobacco

Tobacco in any form is a threat to health and life. In recent years, there has been a decline in the number of smokers. But smoking among women, particularly teenage girls, is rising. And the average smoker is smoking more heavily. In spite of repeated warnings, millions of people continue to smoke.

### EFFECTS OF SMOKING

Cigarette smoke contains three main components—carbon monoxide, nicotine, and tar. There is no safe cigarette. Even low-tar, low-nicotine cigarettes contain harmful amounts of these chemicals. The average smoker inhales 79,000 times per year, taking in concentrated amounts of these chemicals with each breath.

Carbon monoxide, which is the same gas emitted from cars, takes the place of oxygen in the blood when it's breathed in. It makes a smoker short of breath and causes the heart to beat harder to get the oxygen the body needs.

Tobacco tars contain cancer-causing substances which are deposited and build up in the lungs. Tar contributes to lung diseases and also discolors teeth.

*Nicotine* is a dangerous stimulant. It is absorbed from the lungs into the bloodstream. It travels to all parts of the body, but mainly it affects the cardiovascular and nervous systems. Nicotine speeds the heartbeat and constricts, or narrows, the blood vessels so the heart works harder. Nicotine

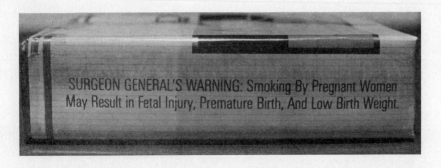

SURGEON GENERAL'S WARNING: Smoking By Pregnant Women May Result in Fetal Injury, Premature Birth, And Low Birth Weight.

*Even with warnings, people continue to smoke. Why do you think they do?*

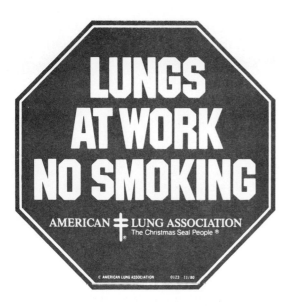

affects the nerves by causing trembling and irritability. Nicotine is also addictive, or habit forming. People who use it develop a physical and psychological, or mental, need for it. That's part of the reason it's often so difficult to quit smoking.

These are some of the health risks related to smoking:

- Cigarette smoking is responsible for 83 percent of all cases of lung cancer, as well as cancers of the mouth and throat. Even pipe and cigar smokers, who usually don't inhale smoke, have a high incidence of lip and mouth cancers.
- Cigarette smoking kills about 16,000 people every year with lung disease. Emphysema and bronchitis are the most common smoking-related lung diseases.
- Smoking contributes to heart disease and high blood pressure. About one-fourth of heart attacks are caused by smoking.
- Smoking affects pregnancy. Mothers who smoke are more likely to have problems with their pregnancies.

*The American Lung Association cautions people about the health risks of smoking.*

- Smokers are more prone to stomach ulcers and repeated colds. Ulcers are open sores in the digestive tract.

## PASSIVE SMOKING

*Passive smoking*, or second-hand smoke, occurs when nonsmokers breathe in smoke from cigarettes, pipes, or cigars. They inhale the same nicotine, tar, and carbon monoxide that smokers do.

Passive smoking exposes people to the same health risks that smokers have, including breathing problems, headaches, and eye irritations. Nonsmoking spouses, children of smokers, and co-workers are exposed to the dangers of second-hand smoke.

Today nonsmokers are beginning to recognize their rights. They are beginning to speak out if they're bothered by smoke. You can ask to be seated in nonsmoking areas in airplanes, many restaurants, offices, buses, trains, and hotels. Or you can politely ask others not to smoke in your presence.

Smokers have a responsibility to be considerate of nonsmokers. They should ask others before lighting up, avoid smoking near small children, pregnant women, or people with breathing problems, avoid smoking in tight quarters, and step outside to smoke.

## SMOKELESS TOBACCO

The use of smokeless tobacco, in the form of chewing tobacco or snuff, is just as harmful to health as smoking. People who chew tobacco or use snuff take in nicotine through the mucous membranes of the mouth. Snuff, which is tobacco rolled into a wad, is placed between the gum and cheek where nicotine is absorbed.

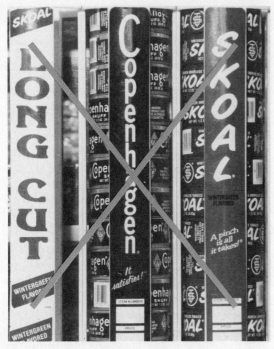

*The use of smokeless tobacco is on the rise, especially among young males. With baseball players as role models, it's often seen as glamorous and masculine. It's neither—it's unhealthy.*

Using chewing tobacco or snuff results in nicotine addiction. Many users are tempted to switch to cigarettes for quicker and larger amounts of nicotine. Also, smokeless tobacco users have a high risk of developing *leukoplakia*, or white raised sores in the mouth, from constant tobacco irritation. These sores can become cancerous. Smokeless tobacco also causes bad breath, discolors teeth, and damages teeth and gums.

## QUITTING THE SMOKING HABIT

The only solution to the health and safety hazards of smoking is to quit. Quitting a habit isn't easy. It takes self-discipline, time, effort, even discomfort to change behavior.

For some, it also takes willpower to avoid substituting eating too much food for smoking.

People who successfully quit smoking must first recognize when and why they smoke, then they can devise their own plan to quit. The following are some guidelines they may consider. People who use smokeless tobacco can follow similar guidelines to help "kick" the habit.

- Substitute exercise for smoking.
- Drink water to resist the urge for a cigarette. Avoid beverages such as coffee or alcohol that seem to go with smoking.
- Breathe deeply for relaxation when craving a cigarette, then think of something else.
- Eat a low-calorie snack instead.
- Remove cigarettes, ashtrays, and other reminders from the area.
- Set daily goals to quit, and give personal rewards that are healthy.

Smokers don't have to kick the habit alone. Stop-smoking programs are sponsored by the American Cancer Society, American Heart Association, American Lung Association, and many private support agencies.

You can help friends in their efforts to quit smoking by supporting their decision. Express confidence in their ability to quit, and inquire periodically about how they're doing. Don't tempt them with a cigarette or other forms of tobacco.

Ex-smokers claim many benefits of kicking the smoking habit such as:

- improved senses of taste and smell.
- ability to breathe more deeply.
- extra money that had been spent for smoking materials.
- no discoloration on teeth.
- fresh breath.
- increased physical stamina for activities and daily life.

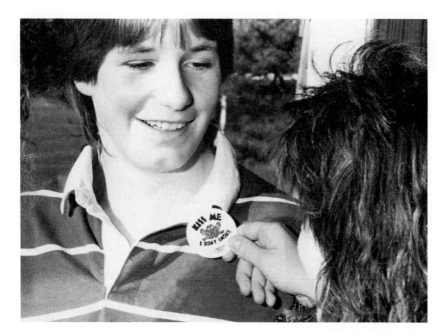

*Nonsmokers live longer, healthier, and happier lives than smokers.*

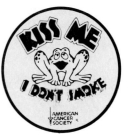

• longer and healthier future to look forward to because the risks of cancer, heart disease, and respiratory diseases are reduced.

## Alcohol

In spite of the minimum drinking age of 21 in most states, approximately 20 million teenagers drink alcohol. Why? Adults and teenagers give similar reasons, such as to forget about their problems, to relax, to relieve stress, to help them socialize, or to stimulate their appetite. Teenagers also express other reasons, such as being accepted by the crowd, showing independence, portraying a sophisticated image, and gaining courage.

The pressure to drink is often intense. But wise teenagers know the risks involved in drinking, and they find other, more healthful ways to meet their personal needs. They don't drink just because of what others say, do, or think.

### Say "No" to Drinking

Many teenagers say "no" to drinking. If someone offers you an alcoholic drink, you can say "no" casually but firmly. You don't have to give a reason or make excuses. But if you want to, you can say:

• I just don't want it.
• I don't need it.
• I'd rather remember this evening.
• I want to enjoy your company sober.
• I'm driving.
• You're too important to me to risk your safety if I drink and drive.
• I'm too important to risk my safety by drinking and driving.
• I don't need the calories.
• It's against my training rules.
• It's against the law.
• I like being in control of myself.
• It makes me sick to my stomach.
• I don't like the way it tastes.
• I have more fun without it.

## EFFECTS OF ALCOHOL

Alcohol is the intoxicating ingredient in beverages, such as beer, wine, and hard liquors. *Intoxication* means being drunk.

Alcohol passes through the digestive tract like food does, but it enters the bloodstream faster. It's absorbed directly from the stomach and the small intestines without being digested, or broken down. That's why the effect is so fast.

The main effect of alcohol is on the nervous system, although it goes to all organs of the body. Initially alcohol appears to stimulate and excite people, but this isn't really so. The apparent stimulation is actually the relaxing of inhibitions, and people do or say things they might not otherwise.

Alcohol, in fact, depresses or reduces brain function and nerve activity. So it causes memory lapses, poor judgment, lack of self-control, drowsiness, and poor muscle coordination, including slurred speech and clumsiness.

Alcohol consumption affects the body in other ways, too:

- Lack of coordination often causes people to fall and injure themselves.
- Dehydration is a common problem when alcohol causes the kidneys to produce more urine. Dehydration is the excessive loss of body fluids.
- Alcohol contains calories. Moderate drinking can contribute to weight gain.
- The liver processes, or breaks down, alcohol. But excess drinking can cause serious liver damage which, in turn, results in life-threatening conditions. The liver is a body organ essential to life. It regulates blood composition, and it is necessary for proper nutrient absorption.
- Malnutrition, or poor nutrition, occurs when the liver can't properly process nutrients or when people substitute alcohol for nutritious foods.

- Too much alcohol consumption can damage parts of the brain. Heavy drinkers may black out or hallucinate. To black out means to experience temporary memory loss. To hallucinate means to imagine seeing things that aren't really there.
- Moderate to heavy drinking during pregnancy can cause birth defects.
- Too much drinking increases the risk of health problems, such as heart disease, cancer, and ulcers. These diseases may cause early death.
- Drinking causes some people to have exaggerated moods which may cause abusive behavior. Severe depression or mental confusion caused by drinking can have a negative effect on the emotional health of the individual and the person's family.

The effects of consuming alcohol can be noticed after just one drink. By drinking more alcohol, the effects intensify to the point of intoxication. The chart on page **63** shows the stages of intoxication.

The body processes alcohol at a rate of about one drink per one and one-half hours. As the alcohol is processed, the effects wear off. When the body is free of the effects of alcohol, the person is said to be sober. Nothing can make the body process alcohol faster. A cold shower, black coffee, or fresh air will not make a person sober any faster.

The aftereffects of alcohol, or hangover, continue for several hours after a person gets sober. This usually includes a headache, dry mouth, and upset stomach.

## DRINKING AND DRIVING

Drinking and driving don't mix. Every year, 5,000 teen traffic deaths are attributed to drinking. Another 130,000 teens are injured. And thousands of people on foot, on bicycles, or in other cars are the innocent victims.

| Stages of Intoxication | |
|---|---|
| 1. Relaxation | Happy and friendly |
| | Slowed, deliberate movements |
| 2. Confusion | Stumbling gait |
| | Slurred speech |
| | Disoriented about time, place, and people |
| 3. Stupor | Unable to stand or walk |
| | Speech incoherent |
| | Periodically nods off |
| | Poor judgment or reason |
| 4. Coma | Completely unresponsive |
| | Death may occur |

Alcohol consumption has these dangerous effects on driving:

- It slows reflexes. Drivers can't respond quickly to road conditions.
- It reduces ability to judge speed, turns, distances, and driving ability.
- It reduces inhibitions. Drivers are more likely to take risks.
- It causes drowsiness and inability to concentrate. Drivers don't keep their minds on their driving, or perhaps they even fall asleep at the wheel.
- It causes forgetfulness. Drivers may forget to signal or forget about cars in other lanes.

Be a friend, and don't let your friends drink and drive. Don't ride with someone who's been drinking. You might need to take their keys away and find them a ride. To get somewhere, call someone to pick you up, walk, take a bus, or call a taxi. Stay where you are until you can find a safe ride.

The public is more aware of the dangers of drunk driving. Organizations such as M.A.D.D., Mothers Against Drunk Driving, and S.A.D.D., Students Against Driving Drunk, are making the public aware of its dangers. As a result of increased public pressure, laws for driving while intoxicated (D.W.I.) and driving under the influence (D.U.I.) are getting stricter.

## ALCOHOLISM

Excessive drinking over time leads to an illness called alcoholism which is a physical and pyschological addiction. Alcoholism may be different from problem drinking. An alcoholic has lost control over drinking, while a problem drinker may be in control if he or she wants to be. Alcoholics often can't control stress in any other way or can't keep from drinking.

Alcoholism often runs in families. There may be an inherited tendency toward alcoholism, or alcohol abuse may be a behavior children watch and learn at home. Children with alcoholic parents have a higher risk of becoming alcoholics themselves. A child with one alcoholic parent has a 50 percent chance. A child with two alcoholic parents has a 93 percent chance.

Alcoholism cannot be cured, but it can be successfully treated and controlled. Early detection followed by treatment in community facilities are the best approaches. The support of family and friends is also very important.

There are many medically-supervised government and private alcohol treatment facilities. If you know someone who has an alcohol problem, encourage him or her to get help. But don't be judgmental or critical. Be supportive instead.

School officials and employers recognize the value of rehabilitation rather than punishment, so they support alcoholic treatment programs for students and employees who have drinking problems. Most health insurance policies pay for at least part of the cost.

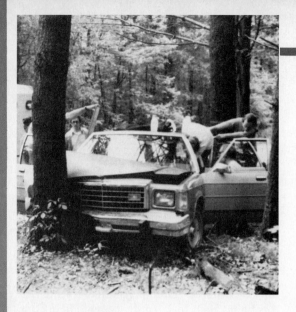

# S.A.D.D.— STUDENTS AGAINST DRIVING DRUNK

In 1981, two of Coach Robert Anastas' high school athletes died in traffic accidents. Both were victims of drunk driving. Robert Anastas and many others, including students, at Wayland High School in Wayland, Massachusetts were outraged by the unnecessary and tragic waste of those lives. They started Students Against Driving Drunk (S.A.D.D.) to help teens, their families, schools, and communities work together to save lives by fighting drunkenness on the road.

The statistics relating teenagers to drunk driving are exceedingly high:

- Drunk driving is the number one killer of Americans who are under the age of thirty.
- Eighty-seven percent of all high school students in the United States have a drink by the time they graduate.

- Five thousand teenagers die every year in alcohol-related vehicular accidents.

Thousands of young people are killing themselves and others because of irresponsible drinking. Bob Anastas believes there are four major problems that contribute to teen drinking and driving:

- Peer pressure
- Teenagers' desire to preserve their image to their parents. As a result, they might not call for a ride because they don't want to get in trouble.
- A sense that accidents happen to someone else, not to them

---

S.A.D.D.
P.O. Box 800
Marlboro, MA 01752
Tel: 617-481-3568

Dear Parents,

As an educator and a parent of three teenage boys, I understand your concerns about the use and abuse of alcohol and other drugs by our children. My experience has led me to believe that as determined as we are to provide for our children a drug free environment; statistics have proven that our efforts to date have fallen on deaf ears.

This is not to say that we must not continue to work toward this end, but must begin to react to the present reality. As our children grow, it seems we become less and less a part of their intimate world. We hear such things as; "Don't worry." "I know what I'm doing." "It's my business." "My world is different from yours." No wonder many of us are shocked when we find out that our children have been using illegal substances.

I am convinced that parents and their children by working together, and by recognizing how death has been camouflaged through lack of communication can eliminate this needless slaughter on our highways.

The SADD "Contract for Life" is meant to act as a safe guard against death. I believe, that if our children realize that they can and should call us if they are ever faced with a drinking-driving situation; that this does not condone the illegal use of alcohol on their part. It does, however, show that our love for our children and their love for us is strong enough to combat any obstacle that may force them to challenge death.

Our children are precious; believe in them, as they believe in you.

Sincerely,

Robert Anastas
Founder & Executive Director

**FRIENDS DON'T LET FRIENDS DRIVE DRUNK**

• Lack of communication with parents and other responsible adults

Part of S.A.D.D.'s program is educational. It also stresses teenage involvement and responsibility. It's a program for teenagers run by teenagers. S.A.D.D. encourages family communication, learning to say "no," talking about teenage problems, and responsible partying.

As part of the program, teenagers and their parents sign a Contract for Life, which is really a contract of love. It's a way to open the door to communication between parents and teenagers. In the contract students promise to call home at any hour if there is no one sober to drive them home. And parents promise to come get them at any hour or place, without asking questions or arguing at the time. They leave the door open to talk later.

Since 1981, S.A.D.D. chapters have sprung up on over 100 high-school campuses. A new program is now offered to junior-high schools. By reaching thousands of kids of all ages, S.A.D.D. hopes to continue to get them away from alcohol and eliminate the number one killer of young people—drunk driving!

# CONTRACT FOR LIFE

**A Contract for Life
Between Parent and Teenager**

**Teenager**    I agree to call you for advice and/or transportation at any hour, from any place, if I am ever in a situation where I have been drinking or a friend or date who is driving me has been drinking.

_____
Signature

**Parent**    I agree to come and get you at any hour, any place, no questions asked and no argument at that time, or I will pay for a taxi to bring you home safely. I expect we would discuss this issue at a later time.

I agree to seek safe, sober transportation home if I am ever in a situation where I have had too much to drink or a friend who is driving me has had too much to drink.

_____
Signature

_____
Date

S.A.D.D. does not condone drinking by those below the legal drinking age. S.A.D.D. encourages all young people to obey the laws of their state, including laws relating to the legal drinking age.

Distributed by S.A.D.D., "Students Against Driving Drunk"

SADD and the SADD logo are registered with the United States Patent and Trademark Office. All rights reserved by S.A.D.D.— Students Against Driving Drunk, Inc., a Massachusetts non-profit corporation.

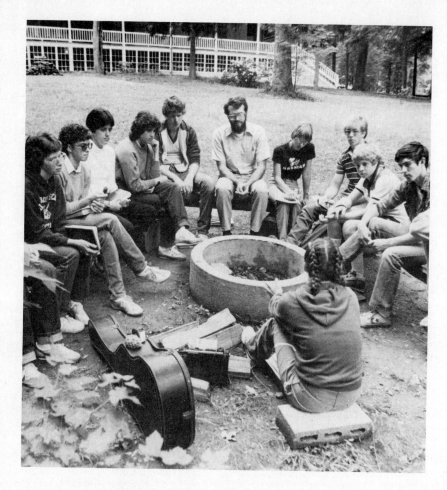

*Support groups, such as this, help people cope with the emotional aspects of alcoholism.*

Alcoholics Anonymous (AA) is a support group of former alcoholics. A *support group* is a group of people with similar concerns or problems who join together to help one another. AA members support each other in their struggle to remain sober. They pledge each day not to drink. Through abstinence, they regain control over their lives and feelings of self-respect. In most communities AA chapters are listed in the phone book.

Alcoholism can have devastating effects on family life, especially when there's no one to discuss the problems with. Alateen is an organization for teenagers who live with an alcoholic. At Alateen meetings, members discuss family and personal problems openly and honestly. They don't criticize or feel sorry for each other. Rather, they constructively offer suggestions for solving problems. Facing and dealing with the problems of alcoholic parents helps teens to live their own lives. They see that they aren't the cause of their parents' drinking.

Other agencies give information on alcohol, referrals, and support for alcoholics. They include the National Council on Alcoholism and Al-Anon, which help spouses, friends, and relatives of alcoholics.

# Drugs

The proper and legal use of many drugs is both beneficial and justified in health care. Doctors have long prescribed drugs to control and cure disease and to relieve pain from injury and illness. The use of drugs in today's health care is one reason why people live longer, healthier lives.

Drugs aren't always used for the purposes or in the way intended, however. Drug abuse is the use of chemical substances for non-medicinal, nonlegitimate reasons. The scientific fact is that the improper use of drugs is dangerous!

Drug abuse can take different forms. Overdosing on diet pills to lose weight fast or taking steriods to build muscles is drug misuse. So are using medicine prescribed for someone else or using a prescribed medication long after overcoming the condition for which it was prescribed. Usually, drug abuse refers to using illegal drugs to alter a person's mental state, often to change someone's mood or emotions.

## WHY DRUGS?

Many Americans believe that medications are quick cures for everything. Advertisements on television, on radio, and in magazines show medications that relieve problems easily and quickly. Legally or illegally, people have learned to take drugs for many purposes—reduce appetite, induce sleep, relieve pain, alter moods, improve appearance, and relax.

Mixed messages about drugs are confusing to teenagers. Parents say, "Don't take drugs." But they may overuse medications or alcohol when they're under stress. Doctors say, "Drugs are unsafe and unhealthy." But movies and TV glamorize their use.

The abuse of drugs in the United States has reached alarming proportions. The availability of drugs and the present attitude about their ready use has had a strong influence on America's youth.

People begin abusing drugs for a variety of reasons: peer pressure, boredom, loneliness, curiosity, relief from anxiety, low self-esteem, or for the adventure. Whatever the reason, the desired effect of drugs is only temporary and the end result can be devastating.

Using drugs is a very unhealthy way to try to resolve problems. Drug abuse doesn't change situations a person is running from. When the drug's effects wear off, problems are still there. In fact, drug abuse often makes problems worse.

*Using drugs doesn't solve problems. Instead, it creates them.*

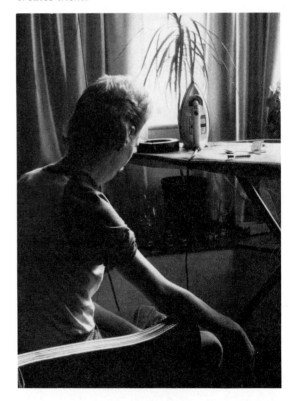

## EFFECTS OF PSYCHOACTIVE DRUGS

Commonly abused drugs are often referred to as psychoactive or mind-altering drugs because they affect the nervous system. They can be physically and psychologically addicting. Drug abuse is a health risk that can cause death.

Psychoactive drugs fit into categories based on how they affect the mind:

- **Stimulants**, such as cocaine and amphetamines, speed up the nervous system, initially giving the false feeling of extra energy, a "high," or euphoria. That's partly because they make the heart and lungs work harder. They may cause hallucinations and serious damage to the heart or lungs.
- **Depressants**, such as tranquilizers and barbituates, slow down body systems, initially giving a feeling of relaxation. But they also cause confusion and loss of coordination. They can slow the body too much causing a coma or death.
- **Hallucinogens**, such as LSD and PCP, give a temporary distortion of mental images. They may cause panicky feelings, confusion, and dangerous physical effects. Some cause convulsions, coma, and death.
- **Cannabis**, such as marijuana and hashish, changes moods and perceptions, causing confusion. It may cause damage to the lungs because it's usually smoked.
- **Narcotics**, such as heroin, morphine, codeine, and opium, relieve pain. They're usually injected through shared needles, so there is a high risk of infection and transmission of such diseases as AIDS. These drugs cause loss of appetite which may lead to malnutrition. They cause apathy, loss of judgment and self control, and overall lack of energy. An overdose may cause convulsions or death.
- **Deliriants** are fumes of chemicals used at home or industrially, such as lighter fluids and paint thinner. They produce a brief sensation of euphoria when inhaled. Deliriants can cause mental confusion, permanent brain, lung, and liver damage, and even death.

Stimulants, depressants, and narcotics are sometimes used as medicines in carefully controlled amounts. Hallucinogens and cannabis are illegal. Abuse of all drugs endangers health.

Alcohol, nicotine from tobacco, and caffeine are also considered drugs. You have learned about alcohol and nicotine. Caffeine is a mild stimulant found in coffee, tea, cola, and chocolate. For most healthy people, moderate amounts of caffeine aren't harmful. But pregnant women and people with heart and stomach problems should avoid caffeine.

Drug abuse can have progressive physical effects on the body. Over time, the body adjusts by building up a tolerance to the drug's presence. When the body develops a tolerance, it takes larger and larger doses to pro-

*Regular or caffeine-free? Today consumers have a choice about the beverages they buy.*

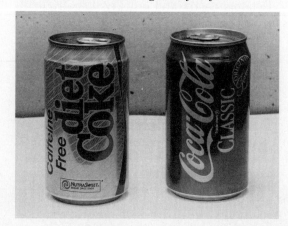

duce the same desired effect. Eventually, the body becomes physically dependent on the drug just to function. This is a physical addiction.

Once physical addiction has developed, withdrawal symptoms occur when the body is deprived of the drug, even for a short time. Withdrawal symptoms include tremors (the "shakes"), nausea, convulsions, and hallucinations. Sudden and complete withdrawal, called cold turkey, can be painful and may result in death.

Using two or more drugs or mixing drugs and alcohol can be deadly combinations. This may be fatal when the body can't handle all these chemicals at one time. Depressants and alcohol, for example, can result in brain damage and death.

Some drugs cause psychological addiction. People depend on them for social and emotional reasons.

Drugs are destructive in other ways. Like alcohol abuse, drug abuse can cause vehicular accidents, injuring and killing the driver and innocent victims. Studies done with marijuana showed that its use delays reaction time and causes poor concentration, indicating that marijuana use and driving can be a deadly combination.

Drug abuse also destroys relationships with family and friends and causes personal isolation and often paranoia. A person suffering from paranoia is excessively suspicious and distrustful of others and may misinterpret other people's behavior toward him or her.

Moreover, a drug habit is expensive. And possessing street drugs is unlawful, often resulting in arrest and imprisonment.

## HELP FOR DRUG USERS

Drug abusers usually deny that they have a problem. But sometimes you can see common signs. Drug users may steal or assault

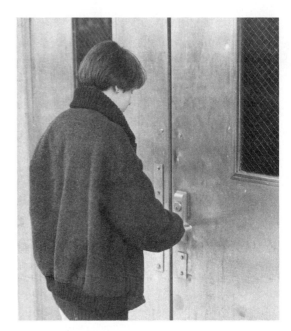

*Teenagers with drug problems can get help from local drop-in centers for drug abuse.*

people to get money for drugs. Perhaps they miss a lot of school because they're high on drugs. Their behavior may be erratic, strange, or very different than normal. Or maybe their grades suddenly go down, and they don't seem to care about school at all. These signs may signal drug use although they might be caused by other physical, emotional, or social problems as well.

What would you do if you knew someone who had a drug problem? Don't criticize, threaten, or feel sorry for the person. Rather, confront the individual in an objective but caring way. Suggest he or she get help from a counselor, doctor, or community drug treatment center. Know that this person might not want your help.

Some professionals are trained to help people get over drug dependencies. In rehabilitation programs, drug abusers receive counseling, medical care, and personal support to overcome their drug problem. They also receive assistance in dealing with the personal problems that underlie drug use.

## Avoiding Substance Abuse

Most teenagers, if left alone, wouldn't choose to participate in substance abuse. Studies show that teenagers, for the most part, don't like the taste of alcohol, don't want to risk arrest, would rather not lie to their parents, and prefer to spend their money on other things.

Peer pressure, which you learned about in Chapter 2, can be a strong influence on behavior. Sometimes teenagers do things because "everybody else is doing it," not because they really want to. Some kids feel forced to do things to feel accepted. Often this is why people initially experiment with tobacco, alcohol, or drugs. Experimentation often leads to abuse.

When you consider the dangers of drugs, alcohol, and tobacco, would you say that a real friend would encourage you to join in? You have a right to make your own decisions. In reality, substance abuse won't bring popularity, true friendship, or a grown-up image.

There are many healthful alternatives to drugs and alcohol for coping with everyday problems or for making people feel good about themselves. For example, many people describe the feelings they get from aerobic exercise as a natural "high." And good physical, emotional, and social health also gives you a natural "high"!

## Weight Problems

Obesity is a serious health risk in the United States. *Obesity* is defined as being 20 percent or more over desirable weight. About 25 percent of the American population is considered obese. Many more are overweight, or 10 percent over their best

weight. Others are underweight, or 10 percent under their desirable weight.

## Health Risks of Being Obese or Underweight

Maintaining desirable weight promotes physical, emotional, and social well-being. Both obesity and being underweight are health risks. See-saw dieting, the practice of repeatedly losing and gaining and losing weight, is also a physical strain.

Obesity has many health risks. Excess body weight puts a heavy workload on the heart which has to pump blood to the entire body. Extra stress is put on bones, muscles, and joints which must carry excess body weight. The risk of diseases that shorten life expectancy, such as heart disease, high blood pressure, diabetes, cancer, and liver disease, goes up with excess weight.

Being underweight also poses health risks. When being underweight is caused by poor food habits, people might miss nutrients essential for good health. They may have little strength, tire easily, and become ill more often.

Body weight can contribute to a person's self-concept. Obese or underweight people might not feel good about their appearance, especially in a society that views a well-proportioned body as an important asset. A poor self concept has a negative effect on emotional and social health.

## Causes of Obesity and Being Underweight

Gaining or losing weight is a matter of calorie balance. Obesity comes from eating more calories than the body uses for its activities. Underweight comes from eating less. People who maintain weight use just as many as they consume.

Sedentary lifestyles contribute to obesity. People who don't get much exercise don't burn many calories. The excess calories are stored as body fat. The reverse is also true. People who are extremely active may burn more calories in exercise than they consume in a single day.

Body weight is influenced by metabolic rate, or how fast the body burns calories for its basic functions, such as heartbeat, breathing, and keeping warm. People whose metabolic rate is slower than normal have a tendency to put on weight easily.

Emotions contribute to the incidence of obesity and underweight. Feelings affect how much, what, when, why, and where people eat. People often eat when they're bored, tense, anxious, or depressed. Others lose their appetites when they have the same feelings.

Ignorance of food and nutrition contributes to weight problems. Some people eat high-calorie diets without knowing it. Others don't know how to choose nutritious, but lower-calorie foods.

## Your Desirable Weight

What is your most desirable weight? Each person has a weight that's best for his or her inherited body type. Some people are naturally lean with a small frame. Others are stocky with a medium or large frame. And others tend to have a rounder shape.

These are ways you can determine if you are overweight, underweight, or at your own best weight:

- **Height-weight tables** suggest the desirable weight for height and body frame. You must use a chart appropriate for teenagers. Other charts are made for adults.
- A **mirror test** is a look at yourself. A lean body is firm without bulges or rolls of body fat. You should have some fat, however, to pad your bones.
- A **skinfold test** determines how much body fat you have and if you have too much or too little. It measures the layer

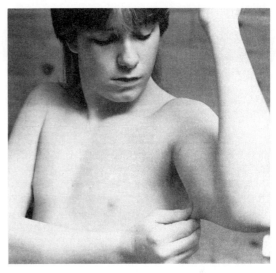

*To measure body fat, do this pinch test. Hold your arm out to one side. With your thumb and index finger, pinch the back of your arm. Gently pull the skin away from the muscle so you are pinching only skin and fat. A thickness of ½ to 1 inch is considered normal. Repeat the pinch test on your thigh and waist. Was the measurement about the same?*

of fat under your skin. You can approximate this measure with a pinch test.

Weight can indicate obesity, overweight, or underweight. But body composition, or the amount of body fat in relation to lean muscle, is the health issue. Many muscle-bound athletes weigh more than the chart suggests, but their body's fat layer is normal. Others fall within the normal weight range, but they have relatively little muscle compared to body fat; this is hidden obesity.

Determine your body composition using the chart on page **72**. Over 20 percent body fat for teenage boys and over 30 percent for teenage girls is too much. Under 7 percent fat for teenage boys and under 17 percent for girls is too little.

# Weight-Loss Gimmicks

For some people, losing weight is agonizingly slow. For other people, gaining weight rather than losing weight, is the problem. Because our society moves at a fast pace, people have learned to expect fast results.

It's not surprising that many people turn to weight-loss gimmicks which promise fast, miraculous weight loss. Who could resist a plan that offered weight losses of a pound per day "while eating fettucine and cheesecake"?

## Determining Desirable Body Weight

A height weight chart is often used to determine desirable weight. This chart is meant for adults. For good health a teenager should weigh somewhat less.

| Women | | | | Men | | | |
|---|---|---|---|---|---|---|---|
| Height (without shoes) | Weight in pounds | | | Height (without shoes) | Weight in pounds | | |
| | Small Frame | Medium Frame | Large Frame | | Small Frame | Medium Frame | Large Frame |
| 4'10" | 102–111 | 109–121 | 118–131 | 5' 2" | 128–134 | 131–141 | 138–150 |
| 4'11" | 103–113 | 111–123 | 120–134 | 5' 3" | 130–136 | 133–143 | 140–153 |
| 5' 0" | 104–115 | 113–126 | 122–137 | 5' 4" | 132–138 | 135–145 | 142–156 |
| 5' 1" | 106–118 | 115–129 | 125–140 | 5' 5" | 134–140 | 137–148 | 144–160 |
| 5' 2" | 108–121 | 118–132 | 128–143 | 5' 6" | 136–142 | 139–151 | 146–164 |
| 5' 3" | 111–124 | 121–135 | 131–147 | 5' 7" | 138–145 | 142–154 | 149–168 |
| 5' 4" | 114–127 | 124–138 | 134–151 | 5' 8" | 140–148 | 145–157 | 152–172 |
| 5' 5" | 117–130 | 127–141 | 137–155 | 5' 9" | 142–151 | 148–160 | 155–176 |
| 5' 6" | 120–133 | 130–144 | 140–159 | 5'10" | 144–154 | 151–163 | 158–180 |
| 5' 7" | 123–136 | 133–147 | 143–163 | 5'11" | 146–157 | 154–166 | 161–184 |
| 5' 8" | 126–139 | 136–150 | 146–167 | 6' 0" | 149–160 | 157–170 | 164–188 |
| 5' 9" | 129–142 | 139–153 | 149–170 | 6' 1" | 152–164 | 160–174 | 168–192 |
| 5'10" | 132–145 | 142–156 | 152–173 | 6' 2" | 155–168 | 164–178 | 172–197 |
| 5'11" | 135–148 | 145–159 | 155–176 | 6' 3" | 158–172 | 167–182 | 176–202 |
| 6' 0" | 138–151 | 148–162 | 158–179 | 6' 4" | 162–176 | 171–187 | 181–207 |

Determine your frame size by measuring your wrist.

Female's wrist measure: —less than 6 inches is a small frame
—between 6 and 6½ inches is a medium frame
—more than 6½ inches is a large frame

Male's wrist measure: —less than 6 inches is a small frame
—between 6 and 7 inches is a medium frame
—more than 7 inches is a large frame

*Source: The Metropolitan Life Insurance Company's Desirable Weight table, 1983.*

## What's Your Body Composition?

Determine your body composition by connecting the dots on this test.

*For females:*

Put a dot at your hip measurement and another at your height on the chart below. Draw a straight line to connect these two dots.

*For males:*

Put a dot at your weight and another at your waist measurement on the chart below. Draw a straight line to connect these two dots.

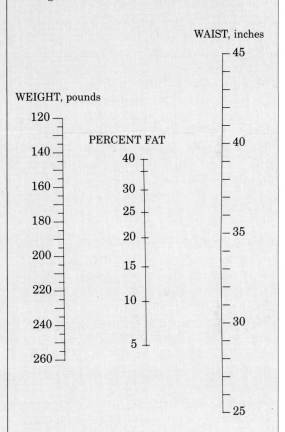

HIP, inches    PERCENT FAT    HEIGHT, inches

WEIGHT, pounds

PERCENT FAT

WAIST, inches

Where does your line cross the percent fat scale?

☐ a. 30% of more

☐ b. 17–29%

☐ c. less than 17%

Where does your line cross the percent fat scale?

☐ a. 20% or more

☐ b. 7–19%

☐ c. less than 7%

For the majority of people, gimmicks for weight loss or gain are unsuccessful. If weight goals are achieved, they are rarely maintained. These gimmicks tend to have these common characteristics:

- **Unrealistic weight loss claims**. Two to three pounds a week is realistic. Any more is unrealistic.
- **Testimonial advertising** rather than scientific facts. Individuals tell how much weight they lost on the diet. Remember that people are paid for what they say.
- **Endorsements by quacks**, or people without adequate health care training
- **Claims that the diet works for anyone**. No diet is effective for everyone.

Two gimmicks often used to promote weight goals are fad diets and over-the-counter diet pills.

## FAD DIETS

*Fad diets* are diets which are popular for only a short time. For weight control, there are fasting diets, liquid diets, high-protein diets, high-carbohydrate diets, one-food diets, and many more. All claim that theirs is the easy answer.

Do fad diets work? Most fad diets don't result in the advertised weight change, at least not for very long. Initial weight loss is primarily water loss, quickly regained after dieting is over.

Following fad diets can be more harmful than healthful. Many are nutritionally unsound, especially for long periods of time, because they don't include adequate amounts of foods from the Daily Food Guide. They don't have all the nutrients needed for health, energy, and growth. They often cause muscle weakness and fatigue and interfere with the body's normal functions. The chart on page **75**, "The Myth of 'Miracle'

Diets," describes various fad diets and the health risks they pose.

Most quick weight-loss schemes don't establish sound eating habits that help people maintain weight goals.

If you're in doubt about the soundness of a diet plan, consult a qualified health professional for advice. The only safe and certain weight loss diet is nutritionally balanced with reduced calories and increased calorie expenditure through exercise.

## DIET PILLS

Some people look to diet pills as the quick, easy way to lose weight. Womens' magazines in particular advertise pills that are "the ultimate cure for fat" or "the fastest, easiest weight loss ever." But experts consider diet pills of little value in weight control for most people.

Most diet pills are classified as appetite suppressants. Those purchased without a prescription contain one or more mild stimulants, such as caffeine. While studies have not found these pills to be harmful to most people, there is no scientific proof of any benefit. In fact, people who take appetite suppressant pills often regain weight faster than dieters who only temporarily change food habits. For people with high blood pressure, these diet pills can be very dangerous.

In some cases, doctors prescribe diet pills with appetite suppressants such as amphetamines. Amphetamines can be addictive, and their abuse can be harmful. The ability to depress appetites only lasts a few weeks so they too may be ineffective.

Some people inappropriately use laxatives and diuretics to promote weight loss. Used properly, laxatives loosen the bowels and relieve constipation, and diuretics increase urine production so some water weight might be temporarily lost. But neither of these

## The Myth of "Miracle" Diets

Many so-called "miracle" diets are health hazards. They can do serious damage to your body. Most lack nutrients you need every day. Here are some typical "miracle" diet methods to stay away from:

- **Low-carbohydrate, high-protein diets** are based on the myth that carbohydrates should be avoided because they are fattening. There are many variations of this diet, each with a different name. None of them supply enough of the carbohydrate you need for energy. They can make you feel sick and weak and give you headaches or other symptoms. In addition, some of these diets are high in fat. They can lead to serious health problems, such as heart or kidney disease.

- **Liquid formula diets** involve a powdered preparation that is mixed with water or another beverage and taken in place of all meals and snacks. These diets are intended to be used for only a few weeks and do not result in new eating habits. Some formulas claim to supply complete nutrition. But since scientists are still learning about nutrition, it is impossible to know whether that is true. Other formulas supply nothing but protein. They offer only about 200 to 400 calories a day, which is dangerously low. These diets can cause illness and even death.

- **One-food diets** are based on eating only one food or combination of foods, such as bananas and milk, seafood, vegetables and fruit, or yogurt. They are monotonous and do not even begin to provide all the nutrients the body needs every day.

- **Fasting**—going completely without food for several days or even longer—is the worst "diet" of all. The results range from severe depression to sudden death.

methods promotes loss of body fat. Used improperly, they may cause dehydration, weakness, and less absorption of nutrients into the body.

Diet candies are also used for weight loss. They are bulk fillers that swell the stomach. Diet candies cut down on appetite because they give the feeling of being full. They do nothing to change poor eating habits.

## A Healthful Way to Diet

Instead of fad diets and diet pills, there are many healthful ways to lose or gain weight. These are some guidelines:

- People who need to gain or lose more than 10 pounds should check with a doctor first. A doctor, nurse, or dietitian can help plan a safe weight control program.
- A diet for weight loss or gain should be nutritionally balanced with adequate servings from the Daily Food Guide.
- A pound of body fat equals 3,500 calories. A person loses by cutting back calories in the diet or by burning more calories in exercise. He or she gains by adding calories to the diet.
- A healthful diet is planned to provide a weight change of no more than one to three pounds a week.
- To succeed, the diet should match the individual's likes, needs, and lifestyle.
- An effective weight control strategy teaches people to change eating habits permanently so weight goals are maintained.

Successful weight reduction or gain is only the first step in achieving weight goals. Maintaining a desirable, healthy weight throughout life is the true goal.

There are many organizations and support groups for weight reduction. These groups encourage weight loss, provide information and guidance, and boost morale.

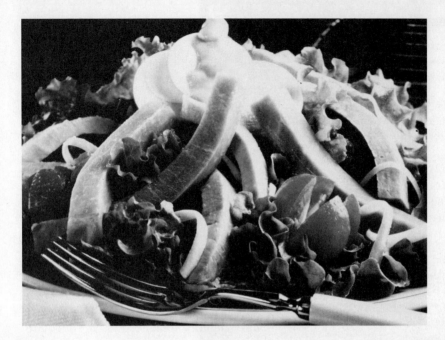

*A balanced diet of low-calorie foods from the four food groups is the best diet for weight loss. What food group does each food belong in?*

## Stress

Any change in life, for the better or worse, makes demands on physical and emotional resources. The changes your body undergoes to meet these demands may be stressful. *Stress* is the strain put on your body by the way you react to change.

The causes or sources of stress that put emotional demands on you are called stressors. Some stressors are small, such as exams, or perhaps a long spell of bad weather. They are small irritations that go away quickly. Others, such as changing schools, a prolonged family illness, the death of someone close, the loss of family income, or a family divorce, are major changes that have a long, often lasting impact.

Adjustments at each point in life contribute to stress as well. Your teenage years, for example, can be very stressful to you and your family because your body and lifestyle goes through so many changes, and you

have so many decisions to make. The test on page **77** helps identify changes that cause stress during adolescence and often later in life, too.

Not all stress is bad. Actually, moderate amounts of stress can have a positive effect on your life. For example, a little stress before a test may help you think better, try harder, and do well.

Often when we talk of stress, we refer to its negative impact on health. Stress can be dangerous when it isn't managed effectively. That's when illness or accidents happen. For your health and safety, identify your sources of stress and change what you can. When situations can't change, learn to manage stress in your life.

### Stress and Health

If something is stressful for you, your body will react emotionally and physically. This series of emotional and physical changes, in

## The Adolescent Life-Change Event Scale

| Rank | Event | Unit |
|---|---|---|
| 1. | A parent dying | 98 |
| 2. | Brother or sister dying | 95 |
| 3. | Close friend dying | 92 |
| 4. | Parents getting divorced or separated | 86 |
| 5. | Failing one or more subjects in school | 86 |
| 6. | Being arrested by the police | 85 |
| 7. | Flunking a grade in school | 84 |
| 8. | Family member having trouble with alcohol | 79 |
| 9. | Getting into drugs or alcohol | 77 |
| 10. | Losing a favorite pet | 77 |
| 11. | Parent or relative in your family getting very sick | 77 |
| 12. | Losing a job | 74 |
| 13. | Breaking up with a girlfriend or boyfriend | 74 |
| 14. | Quitting school | 73 |
| 15. | A close girlfriend getting pregnant | 69 |
| 16. | Parent losing a job | 69 |
| 17. | Getting very sick or badly hurt | 64 |
| 18. | Hassling with parents | 64 |
| 19. | Trouble with teacher or principal | 63 |
| 20. | Having problems with acne, weight, height | 63 |
| 21. | Attending a new school | 57 |
| 22. | Moving to a new home | 51 |
| 23. | Change in physical appearance (braces, eyeglasses) | 47 |
| 24. | Hassling with a brother or sister | 46 |
| 25. | Starting menstrual periods (for girls) | 45 |
| 26. | Having someone new move in with your family (grandparent, adopted brother or sister, or other) | 35 |
| 27. | Starting a job | 34 |
| 28. | Mother getting pregnant | 31 |
| 29. | Starting to date | 31 |
| 30. | Making new friends | 27 |
| 31. | Brother or sister getting married | 26 |

*Scoring.* Add the points for each event that you have experienced over the past year. Of those people with over 300 points during a year, 80% will get sick. With a point total of between 150 and 299, people have a 50% chance of getting sick, and people with less than a 150-point total have a 30% chance of getting sick.

The important point is that you can significantly decrease your chances of serious illness by decreasing the amount of stress in your life. You can control much of the change that occurs.

In addition, by anticipating changes and planning for them, you better prepare yourself to handle stress.

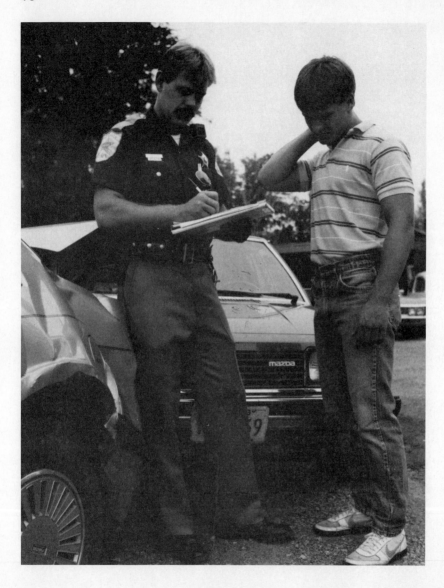

*When people are under stress, they often perspire, and their muscles tense up. People under stress are more prone to accidents, too.*

response to a stressor, is called a stress reaction.

Have you ever felt butterflies in your stomach or your heart pound before you spoke in class or performed before an audience? Have you felt your muscles get tense when you were really angry? Or have you felt tired even after getting plenty of sleep because you were worried about a test? These are all stress reactions. Stress may also result in headaches, shakiness, cold hands, a knotted feeling in the stomach, rapid breathing, or a squeaky voice.

When you're under stress, your body prepares to swing into action to protect you. Body activities, such as breathing and heart rates, speed up so you take in more oxygen. Your digestion slows down. Muscles tense up so you can move quickly. You perspire so your body can cool down.

Stress reactions go away when the stress does. You may change the conditions causing stress, avoid them, or just endure it. If stress isn't relieved, however, the stress reactions may continue and worsen. Then the likelihood of health risks increases.

Constant, unrelieved stress can lead to health problems and accidents. Some people respond to stress by eating, which in turn causes overweight. High stress levels also cause ongoing, serious conditions. These include high blood pressure, ulcers, heart attacks, severe headaches, and other ongoing illness. People constantly under high levels of stress are also more prone to accidents because their attention is focused on their problems instead of the situation at hand.

Stress is closely linked to mental health. Often it causes psychosomatic, or mind-body, illnesses. Diarrhea, constipation, and physical pain are conditions that can be caused by stress. When people learn to control stress, these conditions usually disappear. Stress may also lead to mental illness.

The way you react to potentially stressful situations depends on many factors, including culture, income, religion, experiences, health, and personality. Personalities are sometimes grouped into two different categories—type A and B—depending on the way they handle stress. Type A personalities tend to be competitive, hurried, impatient, and controlling. Type B personalities tend to be more relaxed and more flexible. Those with type A characteristics are more likely at risk for stress-related diseases.

## Managing Stress

Good management helps people reduce or avoid high stress levels. These personal management techniques help reduce stress:

- Manage time wisely. Set objectives, then plan what you need to do. Planning ahead relieves the worry of uncertainty.
- Learn to say "no." Don't take on more than you can reasonably handle.
- Find the most efficient method of doing things and then pace yourself to accomplish your tasks.
- Take one step at a time. If you worry about all the work you have to do, the job may seem impossible.

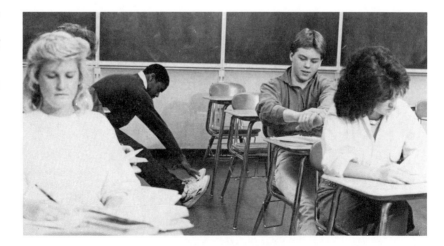

*Every hour, take five minutes to stretch and revive yourself when you're studying. This helps relieve the stress you may feel.*

- Delegate work to others. Don't try to do everything yourself.
- Avoid trying to do too much at one time.
- Reward yourself for a job well-done, and take time to experience your success.

Sometimes stress is unavoidable. Learn to recognize what causes stress in your life, and find positive ways to cope. You might handle stress in these ways:

- Take stress breaks. If studying or work is stressful, stop and do something different for five minutes.
- Learn to relax. Breathe deeply—taking in air through your nose and letting it out through your mouth, taking a full ten seconds for each full breath.
- Exercise. Swim, run, walk, or do what you enjoy for at least thirty minutes three times per week to relieve stress.
- Talk it out. Express your feelings to a friend, teacher, or family member rather than wait until your feelings build up to the point of exploding.
- Learn to laugh at simple irritations or embarrassments. It's healthier than being angry or upset.
- Think positively and realistically. Don't spend your energy worrying over things you can't change.
- Avoid caffeine. It can cause jittery nerves and can contribute to stress.
- Eat a nutritious diet. Being well nourished promotes a healthy nervous system. Healthy people cope with stress better.
- Sleep seven to eight hours daily. You can handle stressful situations better if you're rested.

*Laxatives are ineffective in promoting weight loss. The body still absorbs most of the nutrients that supply calories.*

# Uncontrolled Stress

Some people are unwilling or unable to manage and cope with stress. Eating disorders, violent behavior, and suicide can result from uncontrolled stress.

### EATING DISORDERS

Stress may show itself in distorted eating habits. These conditions are self-destructive, life threatening emotional disorders. Anorexia nervosa and bulimia are two such eating disorders. *Anorexia nervosa* is self-imposed starvation. And *bulimia* is when someone periodically eats large amounts of foods, then vomits or uses laxatives or diuretics to get rid of the food. This is called

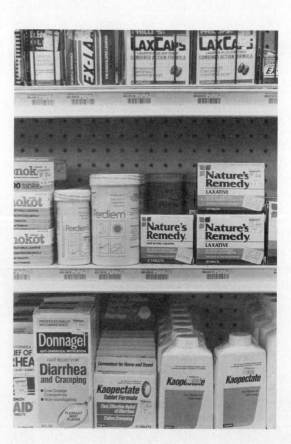

binging and purging. A person can have either condition or a combination of both.

Health professionals aren't sure of the causes of eating disorders. But these are characteristic traits:

- high, perhaps unrealistic standards of achievement
- need for extreme control over life
- low self-esteem
- parents or other caregivers who are controlling
- distorted desire to be attractive
- fear of growing up or getting fat

Typically, anorexics are obsessed with food, body weight, and exercise. They have a fear of becoming fat which doesn't disappear even with extreme weight loss. They often weigh themselves and follow eating rituals, such as cutting food into tiny pieces or eating very slowly. Anorexics are often compulsive about exercising so they burn as many calories as possible. Anorexia is seen more frequently in females than in males.

Anorexics often lose at least 25 percent of their body weight. They may eat little or nothing, yet deny being hungry. Even at 70 pounds they may claim they feel fine and "want to drop just a few more pounds." They may lose scalp hair. Instead, fine hair may grow over the body. For females, menstrual periods often stop. By starving themselves, anorexics miss the nutrients necessary for health. One to two percent of anorexics die, often due to heart irregularities or suicide.

Bulimia is more common than anorexia. People at high risk are those whose work demands strict weight control, such as models, dancers, jockeys, and actors.

Bulimics eat and purge enormous amounts of food. They may do this in a futile attempt to meet needs for security, ego, acceptance, and attention.

Bulimia has serious health consequences. Frequent purging leads to dehydration,

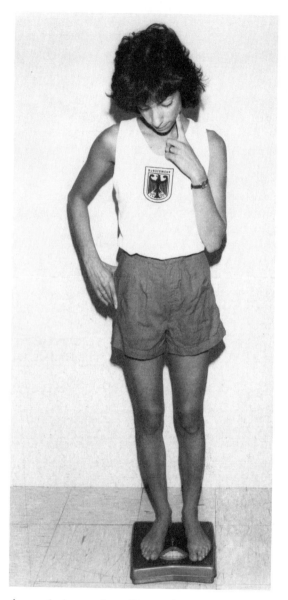

*Anorexia is a serious disease that requires medical treatment.*

chemical imbalance in the body which affects the heart, damage to kidneys from excessive diuretics, stomach rupture from repeated vomiting, decayed teeth from the acid in vomit, internal bleeding from the stress of vomiting, and difficulty swallowing and retaining food because the stomach muscles are conditioned to automatically cause vomiting.

These eating disorders affect all aspects of an individual's life. Besides physical health, anorexia and bulimia cause problems with relationships, schoolwork, growth and development, and sleep.

Getting people with eating disorders to admit their problem to themselves and to get treatment is hard. Often they have such a distorted view of their bodies that they don't consider themselves dangerously thin or unhealthy. Possibly they may be too embarrassed about the problem to seek outside help. Or they may think they can resolve it themselves.

The most successful treatment for eating disorders is a combination of psychiatric counseling and medical care for the person and his or her family. Treatment facilities just for eating disorders are staffed by trained doctors. Group therapy and self-help groups are often effective. The Association of Anorexia Nervosa and Associated Diseases has chapters on college campuses in most states.

Recovering from an eating disorder can be long and slow. Some things you can do to support a recovering friend are:
- Communicate your concern and desire to help.
- Don't discuss food, body weight, or calories.
- Avoid commenting about his or her personal appearance.
- Build self-esteem through comments about the person's natural talents and abilities.
- Learn about and support the person's professional treatment.

## VIOLENCE

Uncontrolled stress is sometimes acted out in violent, forceful behavior. The intent is to hurt someone or damage something. It may come from frustration, anger, or an inability to resolve conflict in a constructive way. Child or spouse abuse, for example, is a negative and destructive stress reaction.

Violence has obvious affects on health. It causes injury, even death. It also destroys personal relationships and can bring out feelings of self hatred.

## SUICIDE

Suicide is the deliberate taking of one's own life. Often the victims are unable to adjust to life's stresses. Suicide is most common among males, the elderly, and those who are alone.

While the overall suicide rate in the United States hasn't changed recently, the rate among adolescents and young adults has tripled in the past 25 years. Suicide is the second leading cause of death among teenagers. Even worse, official statistics are misleadingly low because as many as one-half of all suicides are incorrectly reported as accidental deaths.

Most teen suicides are associated with severe depression. Depression is characterized by feelings of sadness and low self-esteem. Depression is often associated with the inability to manage stress.

Why some depressed people commit suicide and others don't is not understood. There are no universal clues. Often a stressful event, such as punishment, loss of someone close, or a personal defeat triggers a suicide attempt. Suicide is usually preceded by a specific plan and a warning to others. If these warnings are detected, a suicide attempt may be averted. Sometimes rebellious teenage behavior is difficult to separate from serious emotional problems.

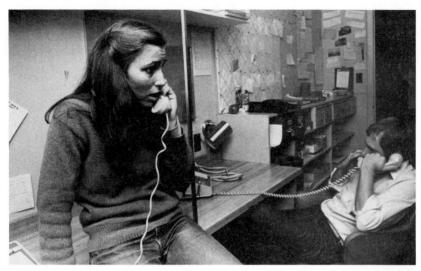

*Suicide "hot lines" in many communities give help to troubled teens.*

If you suspect someone is contemplating suicide, follow these guidelines:

- Listen and try to understand. Be accepting without agreeing.
- Don't leave the person alone.
- Take the threat seriously. Eight out of every ten people who commit suicide have talked about it.
- Act decisively. Contact a teacher, health professional, or another adult for immediate help.
- Follow through, and do what you say for your friend, such as calling to check on him or her.

Depressed, suicidal people can be effectively treated by qualified health professionals, such as psychiatrists. Psychiatrists are physicians who specialize in mental health. Therapy usually includes stress management, counseling to find and treat the causes of problems, and support of family and friends.

Telephone "hot lines" in most larger communities help emotionally-troubled and suicidal people. Trained people know what to say to someone in trouble, and they find immediate help.

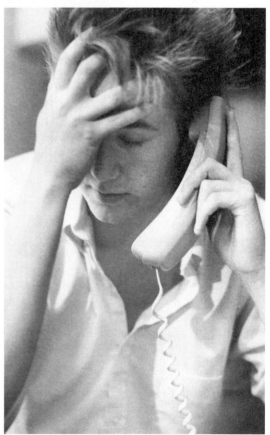

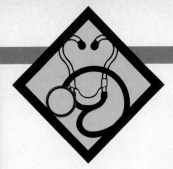

# CHAPTER CHECKUP

## Reviewing the Information

1. How can tobacco affect health?
2. What is passive smoking?
3. What three suggestions could you give friends to help them quit smoking?
4. Name and describe the stages of alcohol intoxication.
5. What are the health risks related to alcohol abuse?
6. How does drinking affect driving?
7. What support groups help people with an alcohol problem?
8. List three types of commonly abused drugs and a health hazard of each.
9. Describe physical and psychological dependence on drugs.
10. Besides the physical effects, why are drugs harmful?
11. What are the health hazards of obesity? Being underweight?
12. What are three causes of obesity?
13. How could you determine your desirable weight?
14. Tell how you could spot weight-loss gimmicks.
15. Describe three types of fad diets and the health risks each poses.
16. What is a stress reaction?
17. List five health problems that can be caused by stress.
18. List five ways to reduce stress.
19. Define anorexia and bulimia.
20. Where could a suicidal person get help?

## Thinking It Over

1. How might you discourage a younger brother, sister, or friend from smoking?
2. How might you effectively say "no" to alcohol or other abusive substances?
3. Why do people say that drinking and driving don't mix?
4. What could you do if others at a party started to drink alcohol, and you had no one to drive you home?
5. What makes an effective weight-loss diet?
6. List three causes of stress in your life and what you could do to reduce it.
7. What are the serious health implications of eating disorders?

## Taking Action

 1. Read about traffic accidents in your local newspaper. How many are alcohol related?

 2. Compile a list from the phone book of treatment facilities in your community for alcohol and drug abuse, smoking, obesity, stress, and eating disorders.

 3. Cut out ads for weight-loss gimmicks from a few popular magazines. Bring them to class and evaluate the truthfulness of the claims.

4. Call several restaurants in your local community. Compile a list of those with nonsmoking sections.
5. Find out about stress or suicide "hot lines" in your community.

# Health Care Systems

After reading this chapter, you should be able to:

- identify various health services.

- choose reliable resources to help maintain your health.

- explain the role of health insurance.

- describe government agencies that assist communities and individuals in health promotion.

- identify health services in your community.

## Terms to Understand

diagnostic tests

health maintenance organization

insurance

Medicare

private practice

specialist

surgery

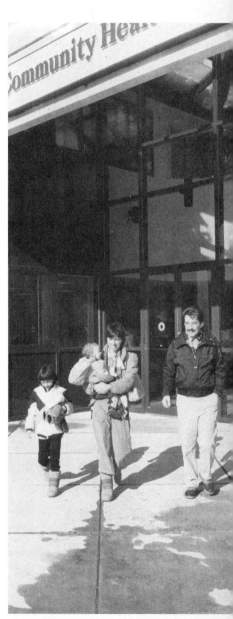

Your health and your family's health are very important. For this reason, a vast network of services is available to help you and your family attain and maintain good health. Private services, government agencies, commercial businesses, and community organizations all offer valuable health services. The health network in the United States is among the best in the world!

Today health professionals do more than cure disease and heal injuries. Health promotion, or staying well, has become the primary focus of good health care.

Taking care of your body is like taking care of a car. In both cases, preventive maintenance is smart so neither the body nor the car breaks down. Repair work is more costly than maintenance work, and it's inconvenient. Sometimes neither the car nor your body can be fixed to run perfectly again.

By following good health habits, being knowledgeable about your body, and getting regular physical examinations, you help prevent disease and injury from occurring and thus help yourself keep well. It then can be said that you are practicing preventive health care and thus taking personal responsibility for your own good health.

## Health Care Services

The physical, emotional, and social aspects of wellness are served through a network of health care services. Many different professionals in the health field provide care in a variety of settings.

## Health Care Team

The team of specially-trained professionals who work to meet your health needs must meet very high standards. Many, including physicians, dentists, and nurses, must pass state licensing tests before they can provide health care. Nursing, medicine, and dentistry are the most common professions in health care.

*Many members of the health care team work together to save a life.*

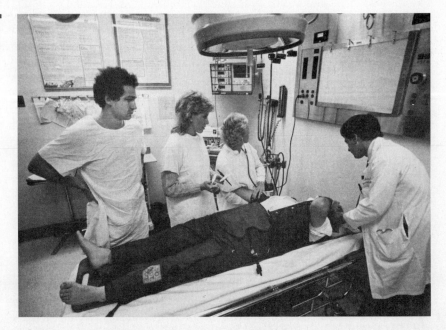

## PRIMARY HEALTH CARE

The health professional who treats a wide range of health conditions is in primary health care. These physicians and nurses are generalists. They're the health care providers you see for checkups and you call when you're sick. Primary-care physicians include:

- internists who care for adults.
- pediatricians who care for babies, children, and teenagers.
- family practitioners who care for people of all ages.

A physician may be an M.D., which is a Doctor of Medicine, or a D.O., which is a Doctor of Osteopathy. They perform many of the same functions, and today they have similar training.

Nurses also can give primary health care. Highly-educated nurse-practitioners can treat routine diseases and provide health promotion services. They are usually in practice with a physician.

A new trend in medicine is holistic health care which treats the whole person—physically and mentally. Some of this treatment is provided by legitimate physicians. Often, however, the approach to treatment is quackery. The feature on page **91** discusses medical quackery.

## Doctors Have Many Specialties

| Specialist | Specialty |
|---|---|
| Allergist | Asthma, hay fever, and other allergies |
| Anesthesiologist | Drugs that induce sleep or ease pain during surgery |
| Cardiologist | Heart and blood vessels |
| Dentist | Teeth |
| Dermatologist | Skin |
| Endocrinologist | Glands |
| Forensics | Medicine and the law |
| Gastroenterologist | Stomach and intestines |
| Gynecologist | Female reproductive system |
| Neurologist | Nervous system |
| Obstetrician | Pregnancy and delivery |
| Ophthamologist | Diseases of the eye |
| Orthodontist | Poorly structured teeth |
| Orthopedist | Bones and joints |
| Otolaryngologist | Nose, ear, and throat |
| Otologist | Ears |
| Pathologist | Laboratory diagnoses |
| Periodontist | Gums |
| Plastic surgeon | Skin and soft tissue deformities |
| Proctologist | Lower intestines and rectal area |
| Psychiatrist | Mental health |
| Radiologist | X-rays |
| Surgeon | Surgery (operations) |
| Thoracic surgeon | Surgery on the chest and lungs |
| Urologist | Urinary system and male reproductive system |
| Vascular surgeon | Surgery on the heart and blood vessels |

## SPECIALISTS

How many different health professionals have you been to? The health care field has many divisions of specialty today. A general practitioner may refer patients to another physician, called a specialist, for specific care. A *specialist* is a health professional who practices in one field of health care.

Specialists originally train as generalists and then continue their education to further study one specific aspect of medicine. Specialists master a narrow medical field and keep up on the latest research in that field. They are highly skilled and knowledgeable in their area of expertise.

There are specialists for every body system and for many age groups. Two specialists that most children and teenagers have seen are those who provide eye care and those who provide dental care. The chart on page **87** lists many other medical specialties. Non-physicians also provide limited but specialized care.

**Ophthalmology.** Eye care requires special equipment and professionals who specialize in that field. An ophthalmologist is a medical doctor who specializes in eye care. Ophthalmologists can treat eye diseases, prescribe medicines, and perform eye surgery. They also prescribe and fit eyeglasses and contact lenses.

Routine eye exams are an important part of health care. Whether you have abnormal vision or not, you should have your eyes checked every year. A typical eye exam includes:

- reading an eye chart to test vision.
- examining the internal parts of the eye with a lightscope.
- measuring pressure in the eyeball.

*Different eye charts have been developed to test different audiences. The chart with all E's tests people who can't recognize alphabet letters. A young child's eyesight is often tested with pictures of animals.*

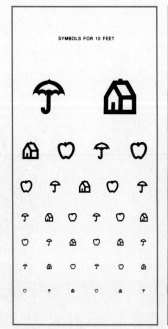

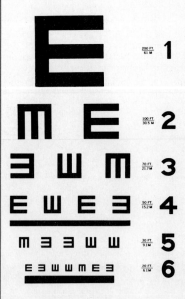

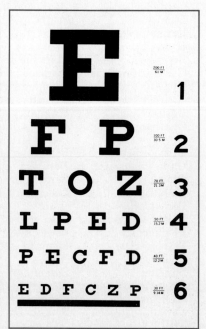

If eyes are found to be abnormal, they need to be treated as soon as possible. Blindness can result if you ignore certain eye problems. Poor eyesight can cause eye strain, headaches, and accidents. It can affect your school work, too.

**Dentistry.** Dentists are professionals who treat conditions and diseases of the teeth, gums, and mouth. Their work includes:

- filling cavities.
- making dentures, or false teeth.
- pulling teeth.
- preventive care such as X-rays and cleaning. X-rays are internal pictures of the body. An X-ray photograph looks much like the negative for an ordinary photograph.

Dentists with additional training specialize in oral surgery, straightening teeth, or children's dentistry.

To keep your teeth and gums healthy, people should see the dentist twice a year. A routine dental visit includes a thorough exam and cleaning. You learned about dental care in Chapter 1.

**Non-Physician Specialists.** Some specialists don't have the same medical training as physicians do. They receive less training and are limited in the services they may legitimately perform. Some use the title "doctor," however. For example:

- podiatrists treat minor foot ailments such as corns, bunions, and deformities.
- chiropractors manipulate the spine in an attempt to relieve the pain of back and neck injuries.
- optometrists test the eyes and fit corrective lenses. Optometrists do not deal with eye diseases and cannot perform surgery or prescribe medicine as ophthamologists do.
- opticians measure and grind eyeglasses according to a prescription.

These non-physician professionals can detect and treat many health conditions. Their work cannot substitute for the highly-skilled care a physician provides for treating disease and serious injury.

# Health Care Delivery

Doctors and other health professionals offer their services in different ways. Some have their own offices, and others work as a group to deliver health care.

### PRIVATE PRACTICE

Many health professionals who are in business for themselves are self-employed in a *private practice*. They have offices where they see patients. And they have privileges to care for patients in certain hospitals. Doctors in private practice set their own rules about hours, services, and charges.

### GROUP PRACTICE

Group practice is when several health professionals work together to provide medical care. This is similar to a private practice, but doctors share resources such as facilities, equipment, and personnel. This is a cost saving since medical offices are very expensive to operate.

A clinic is a type of group practice. Clinics usually have both primary-care physicians and specialists on staff. In this way, many different conditions can be examined and treated in the same place. Clinics charge according to the services provided.

A group practice or clinic might specialize in one area of health care. Pediatric, adolescent health, and sports medicine clinics are three examples. Others specialize in psychiatry, or mental health.

### HEALTH MAINTENANCE ORGANIZATION

A *health maintenance organization*, or HMO, is a prepaid group health plan. For a fixed monthly fee, an HMO provides complete health care to families and individuals.

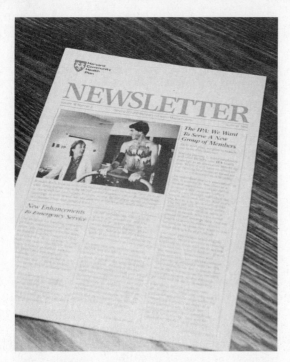

*Many HMO's provide newsletters as part of their health education program and services.*

The monthly fee covers all medical services in the HMO office. There is no charge for an office visit, or the cost is minimal.

The goal of an HMO is to keep members healthy. They provide services when people are ill, but they also offer health promotion services. Regular checkups are encouraged because they are part of the prepaid service. Many also offer wellness classes and health club benefits.

In an HMO, members must be cared for by the doctors and other professionals on staff. Outside doctors aren't part of the HMO program, so members have little choice of the doctor who will care for them. However, like a clinic, specialists and laboratories for medical tests are part of the health care services.

HMOs were created to help keep health costs down. The preventive care provided helps people avoid conditions which may be costly. And HMO doctors receive salaries from membership fees instead of payment for each visit.

## HOSPITALS

Some accidents and illnesses are too serious to be cared for at home or in a doctor's office. They require hospitalization. For example, a teenager might be hospitalized following a car accident or for a serious infection.

Hospitals provide around-the-clock, specialized care for sick and injured people. Nurses are always available. The attending doctor usually visits once a day. Many other specialized professionals are involved in patient care. These professionals are described in Chapter 16, which is about health careers.

Most surgeries are performed by medical specialists in the hospital. *Surgery* is cutting into the body to remove or repair an unhealthy or injured body part. Following major surgery, such as heart or stomach surgery, recovery in the hospital may last seven to ten days. Less serious surgeries, such as many plastic surgeries, require only a two- to three-day stay.

Minor surgical procedures, such as removing a mole or having a wisdom tooth pulled, can be performed in a doctor's office or special non-hospital facility. This is called outpatient, or ambulatory surgery. Ambulatory means being able to walk. You walk in before surgery and walk out later, without staying overnight. Outpatient surgery is usually cheaper and, depending on the type of anesthesia, sometimes safer. An anesthetic is a drug or gas that induces sleep or causes partial or total loss of pain. It may also dull the other senses.

# MEDICAL QUACKERY

Quackery or the practice of offering unproven methods of medical treatment, has been around for ages. Where there is illness, someone is always ready to take advantage. With false promises and costly "cures," quacks peddle their wares.

In the past, quacks, also called charletons, conmen, and hucksters, took their medicine shows on the road. Many times the quack looked like a circus performer.

Today many quacks appear to offer legitimate medical services. They often have attractive offices, professional attire, technologically advanced medical equipment, certificates on their walls, and perhaps credentials after their names. Many advertise treatments and other products in magazines. All these things give the impression of legitimacy. But it just isn't as it seems. They often have no medical training from recognized colleges. Instead they may buy a degree from a business that sounds like a college. The initials after their name often stand for a degree that is unrelated to medicine.

Quackery flourishes today as a multibillion dollar business. Why?
- People hope to cure diseases or conditions that can't yet be cured.
- They're afraid of death or pain.
- They're ignorant of what causes and cures disease.
- They want easy remedies.

Don't people have a right to seek whatever medical treatment they choose? Certainly, but they also have a right to be honestly informed of the benefits and effects of all treatments.

Claims made by quacks are often untrue. To some people they may appear more attractive than anything the traditional medical establishment can offer. By the time people realize the uselessness of quackery, it may be too late for proper medical treatment. They also may have spent a great deal of money.

Cancer and arthritis, attract the most quacks. Because not all medically recognized treatments for these diseases are successful, quacks have stepped in, often at a very high price. They offer meditation, pills, diets, and devices as miracle cures.

These treatments are among the medical quackery promoted today:
- Laetrile, promoted as an anti-cancer medicine. Made from apricot pits, laetrile has small amounts of a potentially harmful chemical called cyanide.
- Fountain-of-youth age reversers, which are large doses of vitamin E. Large doses, of vitamins are a waste of money and can be harmful to health.
- Bust developer, or sponge ball to grip. It can only firm muscles.
- Metabolic steriods to build muscles and increase physical performance. Steroids can stunt adolescent growth, and damage the reproductive system.
- Hair analysis to detect nutritional deficiencies. Hair can't be easily tested. Urine and blood tests are more accurate.

The best way to combat quackery is through education. Informed people don't turn to quacks. They recognize a hoax by asking questions such as those listed on page **92**. A responsible health consumer also may report medical quackery to the U.S. Food and Drug Administration.

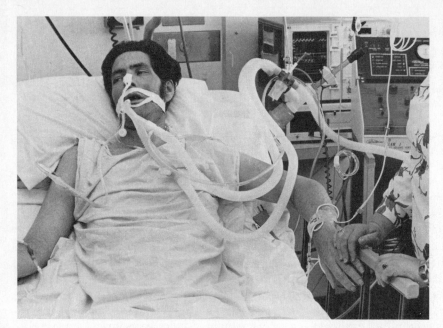

*The intensive care unit (ICU) of the hospital is where critically ill and injured patients are cared for. The professionals working there are highly skilled, and visiting hours are very restrictive.*

Besides hospitals, skilled care is provided in nursing homes. Nursing homes provide short- or long-term care after sick or injured people are released from a hospital.

## Using Health Services

Finding the right health service is like buying anything. You go shopping. From among the services available, you pick and choose what is best for you. First you must identify your needs, then ask a lot of questions. Learn as much as possible about the health care services available so you can make wise decisions. That way you can match appropriate professional help with your health needs.

## Choosing a Doctor

Many qualified health professionals serve the public. The best doctor for you is someone you respect and feel comfortable with. Convenience of health care is an important consideration, too.

The time to choose a doctor is when you're well. That way you can make a well thought-out decision. If you wait until you're ill or at a hospital emergency room, there's little opportunity for choice. For example, parents are advised to choose a doctor for their baby before the baby is born.

Where do you start looking? To find a specialist or a doctor when you are moving to a new town, ask for a referral from your present doctor. Talk with friends about their doctors. Or call a local hospital or medical society for a doctor's name. The phone directory should be the last place you look.

You might make an office visit to interview one or more doctors before you make your decision. Consider these points:

- How crowded is the waiting room? How long must you wait to be seen?
- Are the office employees pleasant and concerned about you?
- Is the examining room equipment modern and clean?

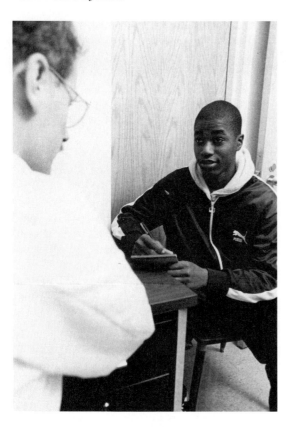

*As a patient, you have a right to speak to a doctor about your health status and medical care.*

- Is the doctor's office conveniently located for you?

Look for the certificate of training which usually hangs in the doctor's office. He or she should be educated to provide the services you need.

For a serious illness, doctors should encourage you to get a second opinion on the best treatment. It's part of learning everything you can in order to make a smart decision. A second opinion from a specialist is particularly helpful.

Sometimes people need medical care when they're away from home. If you think this might happen, prepare before you go. Have your doctor choose a physician in the area where you are going and communicate all the necessary information to that office. If you need unexpected treatment, find a local doctor in one of these ways:

- Call your doctor at home for a local referral.
- Ask your local acquaintances or the hotel personnel.
- Contact the local medical society.
- Go to a hospital emergency room.

Always ask the out-of-town doctor to send information about your illness or injury to your doctor at home for follow-up care.

## Visiting the Doctor

People visit a doctor for several reasons. They may feel ill and require treatment or a cure. They may want an opinion about vague or suspicious symptoms. Or they may feel fine and just want a routine exam or health advice. All of these are legitimate reasons to visit a doctor. They show personal responsibility for health care. Putting off

- Does the doctor welcome questions?
- Can the doctor explain things in terms you can understand?
- Does the doctor take enough time with you, or do you feel rushed?
- What is the cost of an office visit? Is there a charge for phone questions to the doctor? How must you pay for your visits? Now? Billed later? Will the office submit the insurance forms for payment or are you expected to pay, then get reimbursed?
- Who will care for you during the doctor's vacations?
- What are the office hours?
- What hospital does the doctor work in? You would be admitted to that hospital if you were under his or her care.

doctor's visits, on the other hand, doesn't make good health sense.

### ROUTINE CHECKUPS

Routine checkups about once a year help keep you healthy. The physician may diagnose conditions that can be cured or controlled. If you play a sport or have school health insurance, you may be required to have an annual exam. This gives you and your parents reassurance that you're well. Children and adults need regular checkups, as well.

In a routine examination for a teenager, the physician usually:
• checks your weight and measures for normal growth.

*As part of a checkup, a physician looks to see if the ear passage is clear.*

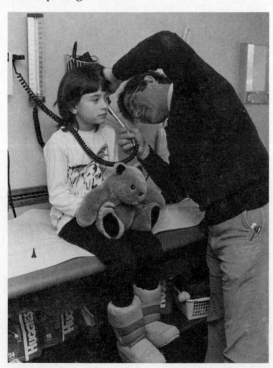

• listens to your heart and lungs with a stethoscope for irregularities.
• feels your abdomen for lumps and enlarged organs.
• checks the nervous system by testing balance, coordination, and reflexes.
• checks your neck and groin for enlarged glands.
• looks into your eyes, ears, and throat for abnormalities. Special instruments are used to see into the inner ear and into the inner eye.
• takes your blood pressure.

In their later teenage years, girls should begin regular checkups with a gynecologist. Gynecologists are medical doctors who specialize in the care of the female reproductive system. An annual exam includes a breast exam, an internal exam of the female reproductive organs, and a Pap smear. A Pap smear is a sample of scraped cells taken from the base of the uterus to test for disease. Examinations are handled in a way that helps maintain a girl's modesty.

### DIAGNOSTIC TESTS

Diagnostic tests are part of many doctor's visits. *Diagnostic tests* help identify health conditions or diseases. They may either confirm or disprove the physician's diagnosis. Common diagnostic tests include a blood pressure reading, urinalysis, blood tests, and X-rays.

Blood pressure measures blood circulation. A reading of 120/80 is normal for most healthy people. A higher reading may signal a health condition which needs treatment. You will learn more about blood pressure in Chapter 7.

A urine sample may be taken for analysis. This is called urinalysis. This test can reveal early stages of an infection, how well the kidneys work, and other health problems. A patient is given privacy to provide the sample.

A blood sample is taken, usually from a vein in the arm, by a medical technician. After just a little pressure with a cotton ball, the puncture site stops bleeding. This sample can tell many things about the body's chemistry, including whether there's enough iron in the blood. Nutritional deficiencies as well as many other health problems can be detected this way.

The doctor may request X-rays. This could show a broken bone, dislocated joint, or infection in the chest. Because of the concern about radiation exposure from X-rays, they're ordered only when the doctor suspects a problem which needs confirmation. You should request a lead apron to protect other parts of the body from the X-rays.

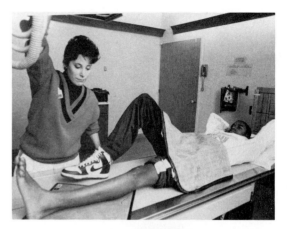

## TALKING TO A DOCTOR

To make a doctor's visit most beneficial and ensure quality health care, good communication is essential. Doctors need to know how patients care for themselves and how they feel. Patients have the right and the need to know about their physical condition. They also need to know the correct way to treat an illness or injury.

People often feel intimidated by doctors. Doctors are people just like your friends, neighbors, and relatives. Respect them, but don't be afraid of them. Speak up. Ask questions, and listen carefully. Answer questions completely and honestly, for sometimes things you don't think are important may be very helpful to the physician's understanding of your problem. Your appointment entitles you to the time and full attention of your doctor.

Prepare for your conversations with your doctor.

- Before you visit, make a list of your symptoms. See the chart, "Be Ready to Tell the Doctor..." on this page.
- Tell your doctor everything about your condition. If this is embarrassing, prac-

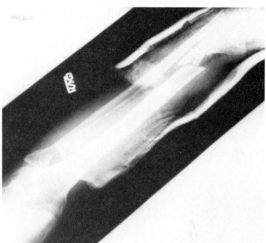

*An X-ray is taken when a broken bone is suspected. Can you see the fracture in the X-ray of the injured leg?*

### Be Ready to Tell the Doctor ...

My symptoms are _____.

They are brought on by _____.

They get worse when I _____.

They go away when I _____.

I have treated myself with _____.

tice aloud in front of a mirror until you feel comfortable saying the words. Talk about any emotional problems, too. Many times physical ailments are related to your feelings.

- If the doctor uses medical terms you don't understand, just ask for an explanation.
- Be sure you understand by repeating back what the doctor says about your condition and treatment. You have a right to know if a treatment will be painful. Bring a pen and paper to take notes.
- If it will help, ask a parent or another adult to go with you for support.
- If the doctor prescribes a medicine, ask about side effects or special requirements for taking the medicine. Side effects are the undesired effects a medicine might have, in addition to the desired effects. For example, a medicine for a sore throat may also cause a rash.
- Take the medicine as prescribed, for the length of time indicated, unless side-effects occur.

Remember that you're a consumer of health care. If you're not pleased with your doctor, speak up. You have a right to competent, informed care.

## Maintaining Health Records

Records help health care providers give immediate and appropriate care. They also make doctors aware of conditions that might appear because of a family history of certain health conditions.

Your medical and family history is an important part of your health records. The first visit with a doctor will include detailed questions about your personal and family health. For example, you'll be asked what childhood diseases you have had, previous medical care, diseases of blood relatives, and your personal habits. The doctor will also

ask questions about the changes in your body which come with adolescence. This information helps the doctor diagnose any conditions more accurately and treat you properly.

The doctor's office keeps records of all office visits and treatments. In this way, patients receive consistent care. The doctor can also track any conditions to see if problems are appearing. If you change doctors, ask that these records be transferred with you.

If you're under the age of consent (18 in most states), signed medical releases should be kept at school, with the doctor, and in the family health records. In this way, you can be treated in an emergency without waiting for your parents to get to the scene. The chart below shows a sample form.

Each family should keep a family and individual health history updated at home.

---

### Sample Medical Release for a Child

I, _____, Parent or Legal Guardian of _____, a minor child, hereby authorize any medical or surgical treatment which may be necessary in an emergency, and in my absence, for the well-being of the above mentioned minor. I agree to hold the physician or hospital treating the above mentioned minor, harmless.

_____ has the following allergies: _____ and has the following medical conditions: _____.

Hospitalization Insurance:
Name of Company _____
Policy Number _____
Group Number _____
Dated _____ Signed _____
                    Parent or Legal Guardian

# Family Health Record

Family Name _____  Date of Health Record _____

Father's Occupation _____  Mother's Occupation _____

| Family Member | Birthplace and Date | Physician's Name, Address and Phone | Serious Illnesses with Date & Treatment | Immunizations* with Dates | Allergies |
|---|---|---|---|---|---|
|  |  |  |  |  |  |

## Insurance Policies

| Family Member | Policy Number | Company | Type |
|---|---|---|---|
|  |  |  |  |

## Family Medical History

| Father's Family | | Mother's Family | |
|---|---|---|---|
| Relation | Disease | Relation | Disease |
|  |  |  |  |

*Immunizations
1 DPT (Diphtheria/Pertussis/Tetanus)
2 DPT booster
3 Polio
4 TB (Tuberculosis)
5 Rubella
6 German Measles
7 Mumps
8 Other

The purpose is to have accurate information to share with health professionals. This helps physicians diagnose health conditions faster and more accurately. It also helps you make decisions and practice lifestyles that might prevent diseases common among your immediate family and blood relatives. Page **97** shows a typical family health record.

## Preparing for a Hospital Stay

When doctors recommend hospitalization for surgery, diagnostic tests, or treatments, there are some things patients should know.

Before agreeing to surgery, patients should find out as much as they can to avoid unnecessary surgery or surprises. A second opinion and alternatives should be explored. The doctor should also explain the procedures, the benefits and risks, how long the hospital stay might be, how long the recovery will be, and what the doctor and hospital fees will be. Even minor surgery has some risks, so it's best to consider it carefully.

When people know in advance, they can plan for a hospital stay. If you're a patient, take only personal items that you will use, such as a robe, slippers, and your toiletries. The hospital provides everything else. Depending on how well you expect to feel, you might bring magazines, schoolwork, or other things you can do in bed.

As in a doctor's office, patients have the right to be informed about all hospital procedures. As a patient or caregiver, ask questions about everything that you don't understand. Participate in decisions about hospital care. Answer all questions fully and truthfully so you get the best possible care.

Parents must give written consent for all hospital procedures performed for teenagers and children. Adults give consent, too, when they are patients. Being informed about your condition lets you know what you are agreeing to.

## Health Insurance

*Insurance* is a system of protecting people from financial loss or high costs. Individuals

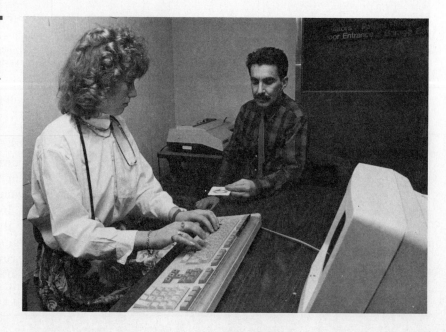

*Carry your identification card for your medical insurance at all times. You'll need to present it for doctors' visits and trips to the emergency room.*

or groups agree to pay certain sums for a guarantee that their costs or the cost of their loss will be paid, at least in part, from the fund when the need arises. The purpose of health insurance is to protect people against the high cost of health care.

## Private Insurance

Health insurance is provided by over 1500 private companies. A quick look in the phone directory will show how many insurance companies there are.

### TYPES OF COVERAGE

There are several kinds of health insurance coverage. Adequate protection means that you are covered in each of the following areas:

- Basic hospitalization. This covers the often expensive stay in a hospital. The room, food, operating room, X-rays, laboratory tests, and many other hospital services are covered.
- Basic medical/surgical. This covers doctors' fees that result from hospitalization. Sometimes this also includes doctor's visits after being released from the hospital, too.
- Major medical. This is often called catastrophic insurance. It pays for services for long-term illnesses and for injuries incurred after the basic hospitalization and medical/surgical policies stop.

Although you may have health insurance, the total amount of most medical bills isn't always covered. The amount paid depends on the insurance and how much the doctor and the hospital charge.

Most insurance companies pay fixed amounts of money for services. For example, the insurance company may pay $125 per day for a hospital room and $38 per day for your doctor to visit you there. If the hospital charges $132 per day for a room and the doctor charges $40 per day for a visit, you have to pay the difference out of your pocket.

Most medical insurance pays for your medical bills only when you become ill or badly injured. Routine checkups and preventive care are not covered, but diagnostic tests often are. Also, some insurance policies pay for hospitalization for only a limited number of days. After that point has been reached, usually 60 days, only a major medical policy will pay for services. Few people expect they'll need this kind of insurance, so they don't buy a policy. But it offers good protection for the unexpected.

Besides health insurance, other types of insurance are health-related. These also offer protection for consumers.

- Disability insurance pays for lost income when illness or injury make someone unable to work at a paying job. Many companies provide this for their top-level employees.
- Dental insurance pays for the costs of dental care. Many policies cover costs for preventive care such as cleaning teeth. Coverage for problems such as fillings, braces, and other dental work depend on the policy.
- Life insurance pays a lump sum upon death to designated individuals. Life insurance is usually used to pay funeral expenses and support the deceased's family for a short time.

### BUYING INSURANCE

Insurance companies charge a monthly fee called a premium for providing insurance protection. The amount of the premium differs among people. In general, people who are older, frequently ill, or have dangerous jobs pay higher premiums. Also, the more coverage the policy provides, the higher the premium. Group insurance is cheaper than individual policies. Group insurance covers

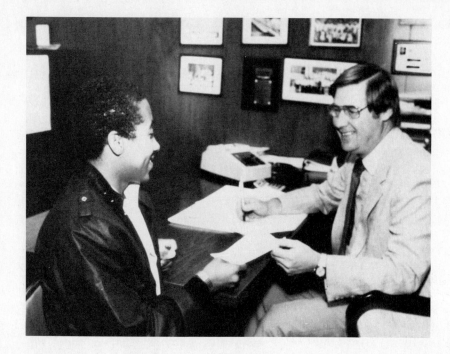

*Ask many questions
as you shop for
medical insurance.*

all employees of a company or all members of an organization. As a benefit, some companies pay part or all of the premium.

Insurance policies vary greatly in their coverage and premiums. So it's smart to shop around.

A wise consumer asks many questions of an insurance agent. These questions should include:

- What does the policy cover?
- Does the policy cover preventive care, such as checkups?
- How much of most typical hospital and doctor charges does it pay, or is there a percentage of the cost I must pay?
- What is the amount of the premium? Will it decrease if I don't file any claims? Will it go up if I do?
- How are claims submitted? Is it complicated? How long would I wait for payment? Or will the insurance pay the health care provider directly?

- Who can cancel the policy once it's started—the insurance company, only me, or my employer if this is a company policy?
- If I'm no longer employed, can I continue a company policy?

## Government Programs

The government also helps protect citizens from high health costs with two programs—Medicare and Medicaid.

### MEDICARE

*Medicare* is a health insurance program for people over 65 years of age and for certain disabled people. It is supported by social security funds, which workers in the United States pay into. Because it's run by the federal government, it provides the same benefits to everyone who is covered.

Like any insurance plan, people pay monthly premiums which are automatically deducted from the paycheck—or social security check. Then when eligible people have hospital or doctor bills, Medicare pays.

Medicare doesn't cover all costs, however. It pays for a specified number of days in a hospital or skilled nursing home, and it covers about 80 percent of some doctor bills. Some medical services and supplies are also covered. The federal government regulates what bills are paid by Medicare. Since this kind of insurance doesn't cover all costs, many people choose to have additional insurance, called a supplemental policy.

## MEDICAID

Medicaid is an assistance program to pay the medical bills of low-income people. It's not really an insurance program because people don't pay premiums. Instead, it is financed by the federal and state governments from tax funds. Each state administers its own program, so the eligibility requirements and benefits vary from state to state.

Medicaid pays for almost all medical bills. In some states it even pays for eyeglasses, dentist bills, and medicine. This program is coordinated through community welfare departments.

*People may apply for Medicaid at the local welfare office. Medicare is granted through the Social Security office.*

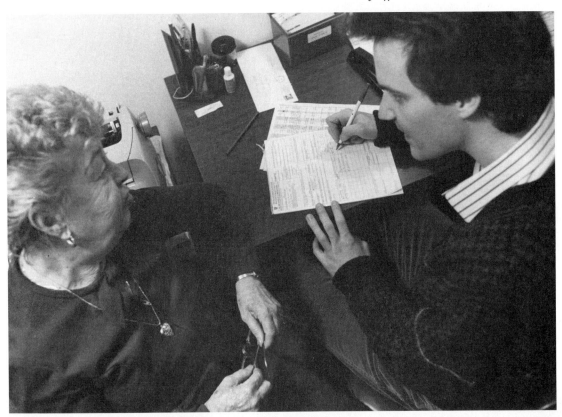

# Health Organizations

Besides doctors' offices, hospitals, and other health care facilities, a network of organizations provides additional health support for the public. Private organizations, government services, and international agencies work together to promote health, cure disease, and treat injuries. They also offer emotional and social support for people in need.

## Private Health Organizations

In many communities, private charitable and social organizations offer health services. Many of these organizations are supported with private funds from people like you. They also depend on volunteer help. Perhaps you have participated in a fundraising event for a health charity, such as a fun run or a bike-a-thon.

Many voluntary health organizations are organized on a national level, but most of their services are local. They sponsor medical research, offer educational programs, provide helpful literature, and assist people and their families with health problems. Many of these organizations are listed on this page.

Sometimes local organizations are established in response to a specific need. In one poor community, a group of people formed an organization to provide shoes to children. In an elderly community, a fleet of taxicabs, specially equipped for wheelchairs, was financed by a group. In a large, crowded metropolitan area, an overnight haven was established for abused children to escape the violence of their homes. Are there services like these in your community?

You and your friends may enjoy helping people in your community by giving volunteer time and support to an organization. Chapter 16 gives more information on volunteer opportunities for teenagers.

## Volunteer Agencies That Help the Public

The American Cancer Society
The American Diabetes Association
The American Foundation for the Blind
The American Heart Association
The American Lung Association
The American Red Cross
The Arthritis Foundation
Association for Retarded Citizens
The Cystic Fibrosis Foundation
The Epilepsy Foundation of America
The Kidney Foundation
The Leukemia Society of America
The Multiple Sclerosis Foundation
Muscular Dystrophy Association
The National Council on Alcoholism
The National Foundation for the Blind
The National Foundation—March of Dimes
The National Hemophilia Foundation
The United Cerebral Palsy Association

## Government Health Services

Federal, state, and local governments provide health care services to citizens. Many health services of the federal government are offered through the Department of Health and Human Services. The Public Health Service (PHS) with six agencies is one division of that department:

• The National Institute of Health finances and conducts research on the causes and cures for diseases.
• The Health Services Administration provides family planning, and maternal and child health services.
• The Health Resources Administration provides community training for health workers in the community.

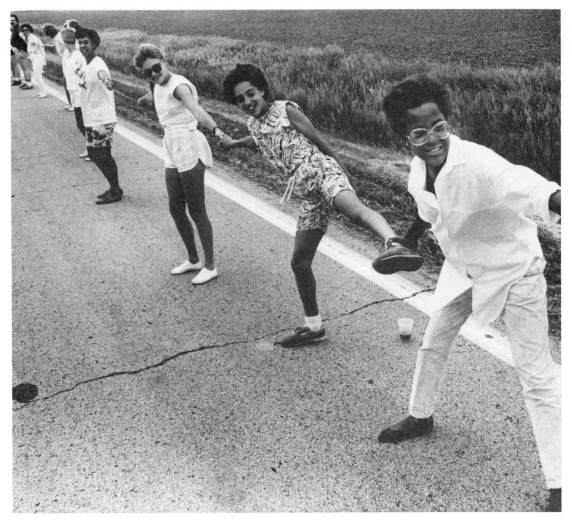

*In 1986, Americans from coast to coast held hands to raise money to feed hungry people.*

- The Food and Drug Administration enforces laws to keep food, drugs, and cosmetics safe.
- The Center for Disease Control provides programs to prevent and control the spread of disease.
- Alcohol, Drug Abuse, and Mental Health Administration works to control and prevent alcoholism, drug abuse, and mental illness.

Each state has a board of health which regulates and advises local health services and cooperates with federal agencies. They also provide direct services, such as care for mentally and physically impaired people.

Every county has a public health department which works to guarantee that public facilities are healthy and safe. The county health department also coordinates community health clinics, health fairs, and education programs. They help maintain data on health within the community. Sometimes they provide free health screening, or examinations. In Chapter 15, you'll learn more about the services the public health department provides.

Other departments of the government also protect the health and safety of citizens. For example, the Department of Agriculture provides nutrition programs and also establishes food safety standards. The Consumer Product Safety Commission establishes regulations for product safety. The Environmental Protection Agency regulates industry so air and water stay clean.

## International Health Agencies

The World Health Organization (WHO), an agency of the United Nations, is the most prominent international health organization. The purpose of WHO is cooperation among countries in promoting the health of their populations. One hundred and fifty nations, including the United States, belong to WHO, which has its headquarters in Switzerland.

WHO has done much over the years to control disease and to promote health, including:

- gathering information and conducting research about health problems.
- controlling the spread of disease.
- providing doctors, other health professionals, supplies, and medicines to underdeveloped countries.
- establishing high standards for food and medical companies to follow.

Many voluntary agencies, including the International Red Cross, also provide health services throughout the world.

## Professional Associations

Associations of health professionals promote quality health care. Doctors, nurses, and other health care providers belong to associations, such as The American Medical Association, The American Nurses Association, or the American Public Health Association. The associations' goals include maintaining high standards of patient care. They also help educate the public on health promotion and treatment.

## Health Information

Accurate information about health practices, services, and products helps you and your family make smart, responsible health decisions. As a health consumer, accurate information is your right.

Where do you look for health information? Everywhere people are talking about health. Teen magazines, newspapers, TV, and radio all carry stories and advertisements which tell how to stay healthy. Self-help books, which are often best sellers, also give health advice. Many times the information seems contradictory, so it's confusing. It's difficult to know what information you can trust.

To judge the information, ask these questions:

- Does it make sense? Does it seem accurate? Is it backed by scientific research? Unless the information seems reasonably possible and accurate, don't follow it, no matter how much you want to believe it.
- Who is providing the information or promoting the product? Is the person qualified to provide this information? Medical doctors and registered nurses are among the experts you can trust. However, some people who call themselves doctors have no medical training.

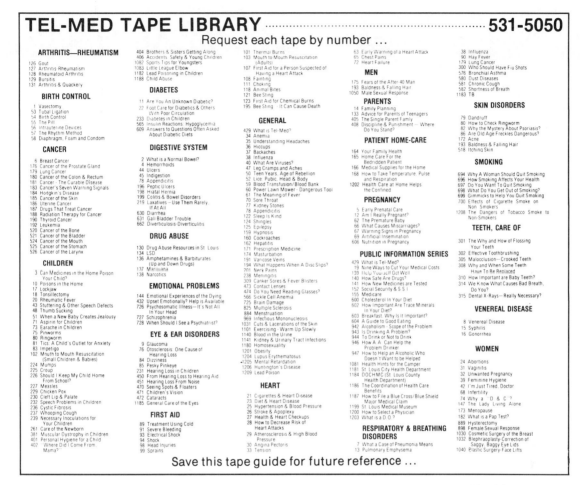

- Is the person or article trying to sell you something? If so, the message may be biased, or prejudiced.
- Is the person using emotion or facts to give advice or sell a product? Smart decisions are based on facts.
- Where was an article or ad shown? Reputable sources usually review materials before printing them.
- How new is the service or advice? Tried and true methods that have stood the test of time are usually more reliable.

*Tel-Med is a reliable source of health information on many different health and medical topics. Call your local tel-med operator, ask for a topic, and listen to the tape.*

If you're uncertain about how good a service is or how accurate the advice is, ask a known expert. Reliable information can come from your doctor, school nurse, or home economics or health teacher. You might also call a community organization listed earlier in this chapter.

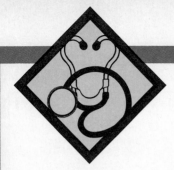

# CHAPTER CHECKUP

## Reviewing the Information

1. What is health promotion? Preventive health care?
2. Name three types of physicians who offer primary health care, and describe the patients they see.
3. List the names of eight medical specialists and their fields of specialty.
4. What's included in a routine eye exam?
5. What are two types of health care delivery?
6. List six questions to consider when choosing a doctor.
7. Why are routine checkups important?
8. Describe two diagnostic tests done routinely in a medical examination.
9. What are two suggestions for talking with your doctor?
10. What are four kinds of information that are included in a health record?
11. Tell what is the purpose of health insurance.
12. Briefly describe Medicare and Medicaid.
13. Describe four types of health-related insurance.
14. Name five private organizations that promote public health.
15. Name three agencies in the Public Health Service, and tell what each does to protect consumer health.
16. How does the World Health Organization contribute to health care?
17. Identify three reliable sources of health information.

## Thinking It Over

1. Explain the differences between a family practitioner and a specialist.
2. What specialists might treat you if a car accident caused broken bones, cuts on your face, and broken teeth?
3. Why is choosing your doctor before a medical emergency a good idea?
4. Compare the advantages and disadvantages of belonging to an HMO.
5. What steps would you follow to find a physician for your general needs?
6. What information about yourself might belong in your family health record?
7. How might you judge the reliability of a magazine article about health care?

## Taking Action

 1. Write to a volunteer health organization and request a list of its services. Report back to the class.

 2. Contact the county public health department to learn more about one of its services. Write a report about what you learned.

3. Look in your local phone book. Write down the medical specialties available in your community.
4. Call two insurance companies to learn about health insurance. Compare the costs and benefits of similar policies.
5. If you have not seen an eye doctor or dentist in the last year, make appointments to do so in the next month.

# Safety for the Family

5

After reading this chapter, you should be able to:

• identify common causes of accidents.

• describe safety practices to avoid accidents.

• describe the procedures for maintaining food safety at home.

• explain proper precautions for weather exposure.

• explain how to avoid personal assault.

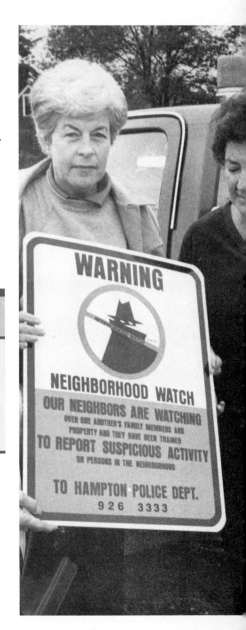

## Terms to Understand

| | |
|---|---|
| assault | smoke inhalation |
| flammable | sun protection factor |
| heat index | windchill factor |
| poisons | |

Accidents—at home, school, work, and recreational activities—account for over 90,000 deaths yearly in the United States. That figure is astounding, especially since most accidents are preventable!

Some people seem prone to accidents. People who are tired or sick may not pay attention to what's happening around them. Hurried people often take shortcuts instead of following safety precautions. Others might not know safety rules.

You and your family can live safely and minimize your risks of accidents and other personal hazards. The conscious choices about what you do, where you go, and how you do things affect your safety.

There are safe and unsafe ways to do everything. If something can't be done safely, don't do it. If your girlfriend drives her motorscooter too fast, don't ride with her. If your brother asks you to take out a boat with him when a thunderstorm is threatening, don't do it. For your safety and theirs, say "no."

## Safety at Home

Home feels like a safe, secure place. But over 20,000 people die at home every year from accidents. Fires, falls, poisonings, and lawn mower accidents are the most common home accidents. Many people injure their backs at home. Others get sick or die from food-related incidents.

Prevent accidents in your home by preparing for the unexpected. Watch for hazards and prevent accidents from happening to your family. Be prepared to act quickly and wisely in a home emergency.

## Fires and Burns

Home fires happen all too often. People get burned, lose valuable possessions, even lose their lives in home fires.

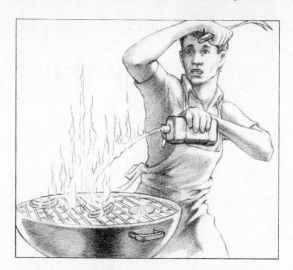

*Never squirt fire starter or other flammable liquids on hot coals or a smoldering fire. The fire can ignite the stream of liquid and cause the can to explode in your hands!*

### FIRE AND BURN PREVENTION

Stoves, appliances, fireplaces, outdoor grills, and smoking have the potential for causing fires and burns. Although fires can start anywhere at home, most start in the kitchen or the bedroom.

Fires usually are caused by carelessness, and most can be prevented. Follow fire and burn prevention safety rules.

Watch for flammable items that could catch fire on the stove. *Flammable* items catch fire easily or burn quickly.

- Never leave the kitchen when food or grease is heating on the burners—not even for a moment.
- Keep potholders and dish towels away from burners.
- Remember that electrical burners may be hot enough to ignite a fire for several minutes after they are turned off.
- Don't let grease build up on the stove or the exhaust hood where it can catch fire.

## Protect Yourself from Burns in the Kitchen

- Turn handles away from the front of the stove, but not directly over another burner, so pots and pans don't get knocked over.
- Use well-padded, dry potholders to remove hot pans from the oven.
- Keep your hands away from hot oil.
- Turn off appliances and the stove when you're finished cooking. Check the controls to make sure that they are all the way to the "off" position.
- Tilt lids on pots away from your face when you remove them to protect yourself from steam.
- Use wooden spoons when stirring hot foods because they don't conduct heat.

- Keep lightweight, flammable items, such as paper towels, away from the stove; they can be blown or knocked onto burners.
- Don't hang anything that could ignite, such as curtains or a paper towel rack, near the stove.
- Don't wear long, dangling sleeves when you're cooking.

Handle appliances and electrical cords properly. Don't overload outlets by plugging in too many appliances at once. Don't use electrical cords near the stove. Replace frayed or cracked cords on appliances.

Have household heating equipment checked regularly for safety. Keep chimneys and flues clean and in good condition. Be alert for leaks around gas appliances. Check space heaters to make sure they are in good working condition. Use a screen in front of fireplaces.

Be careful with candles, matches, and lighters. Never leave a room where candles are burning. Keep matches and lighters out of the reach of children and away from flammable products.

Handle flammable chemicals carefully. Never store cleaning fluids, paint and turpentine, or aerosol sprays near heat. Ventilate a room when using these products because they can give off dangerous vapors. Never use gasoline, charcoal, or fire starter inside the house.

Don't allow anyone in your family to smoke in bed!

### FIRE SAFETY PLAN

Inexpensive smoke detectors save lives because a buzzer goes off when smoke starts filling a room. This alerts the people to the danger and they have time to get out of the house. Every home should have at least one.

Experts recommend one detector for each floor of a house. Since smoke rises, attach them to the ceiling, at least six inches away from the walls. Most smoke detectors are battery-powered. Check them monthly to be sure the battery is working.

Having a smoke detector is only part of a fire safety plan. You and your family also must know what to do if the alarm goes off! As part of your plan do the following:

- Establish an escape plan for every room in the house, especially the bedrooms. Tell overnight guests how to leave their bedroom safely in an emergency.
- Have a rope or chain ladder by the window of any upper-floor bedrooms.
- Have a fire drill with your family every so often—even at night.
- Decide who will rescue small children.
- Don't risk your life to rescue pets.
- Choose a place outside, away from the house, where your family will meet if you have to escape quickly.

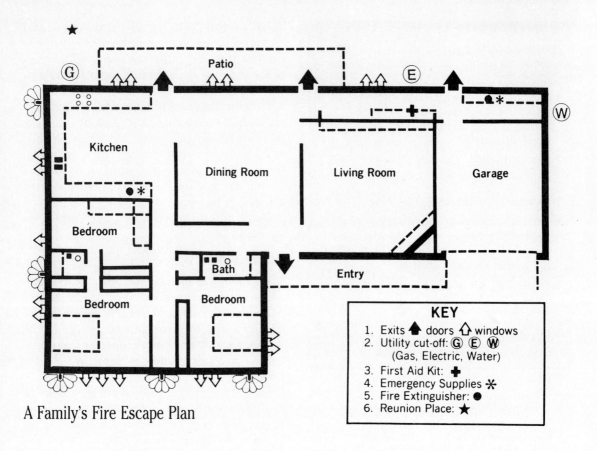

A Family's Fire Escape Plan

**KEY**
1. Exits ⬆ doors ⇧ windows
2. Utility cut-off: Ⓖ Ⓔ Ⓦ
   (Gas, Electric, Water)
3. First Aid Kit: ✚
4. Emergency Supplies: ✳
5. Fire Extinguisher: ●
6. Reunion Place: ★

• Keep fire extinguishers where you can easily get to them. You should have one in the kitchen and perhaps near a fireplace or in a basement workroom, a utility room, and a garage.

### IN CASE OF FIRE

Eighty percent of deaths in home fires are caused by smoke inhalation. *Smoke inhalation* is when smoke fills the lungs, and the victim cannot get enough oxygen to breathe. He or she suffocates. Most people who die in home fires are sleeping when fires break out, and they never wake up. That's why smoke detectors are so important!

What would you do if a fire started in your house? React in a smart, safe way, and don't panic. If the fire is small, you may be able to control it. If you can't put it out or don't know what to do, leave the house immediately. Call the fire department from a neighbor's home.

Never try to extinguish a grease fire with water because it will splatter. Pour baking soda, if it's handy, over the fire. Or use a fire extinguisher made for grease fires. You often can smother a small grease fire in a frypan by completely covering it with a lid.

If you have to escape from a burning building, crawl on your hands and knees.

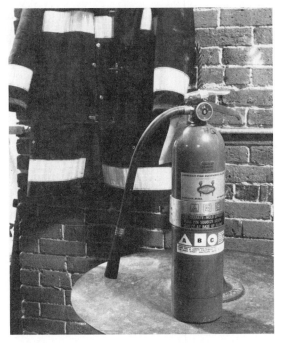

*Fire extinguishers have three classifications: type A for trash, wood, and paper; type B for liquids and grease; and type C for electrical fires. A multipurpose fire extinguisher uses a dry chemical that is effective on all types of fires.*

Smoke rises so there's more oxygen near the floor. Before opening a door, feel the air coming through underneath. If it's hot, don't open it; instead, find another way out. Never go back into a burning building once you've escaped.

If your hair or clothes catch fire, follow these three steps:

- STOP immediately.
- DROP to the ground.
- ROLL to smother the flames.

## Falls

Falls injure millions of people every year. Some sustain minor injuries; others are se-riously hurt. Deaths from falls are the second leading cause of accidental deaths. You can take many precautions to prevent falls around your home.

### PREVENTING FALLS INSIDE

Prevent falls inside your home. Wipe spills, and avoid walking on wet floors. Keep floors and steps well lighted and clutter free. Secure the corners of loose throw rugs to prevent tripping. Put hand rails along stairs and near the tub for safety, especially for young children and older adults. Put non-skid strips in the tub. Keep drawers and cupboard doors closed so no one bumps into them and trips. If you need to reach something above your head, use a step stool, not a chair.

### PREVENTING FALLS OUTSIDE

There are many opportunities for falling outdoors. You can trip over toys and tools left in the yard. A garden hose stretched across the lawn can trip someone. In the winter, ice or snow on steps and sidewalks is hazardous.

If you are using a ladder, inspect it for safety. Is it in good condition? If not, don't use it. Place the ladder at a safe angle. Set the base one foot away from the wall for every four feet you're climbing. Make sure the base is on firm footing and won't slip and slide. Wear clean, dry shoes when you climb so you won't slip. It's best to climb only to the third-highest rung on the ladder so you don't get top-heavy and tip.

## Cuts

Cuts are caused by careless handling of sharp items, such as yard tools and kitchen utensils. Cuts can cause severe bleeding, pain, scars, and infections, if they aren't treated properly.

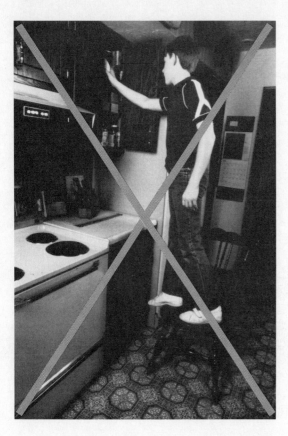

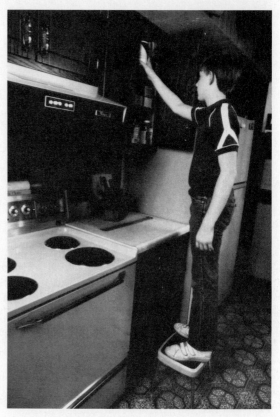

*Use only a ladder or stepstool to reach high shelves. Chairs or boxes may look sturdy enough to stand on, but they are not balanced properly to hold a person safely.*

Careful handling of sharp items can prevent cuts:

- Keep knives and scissors in a rack or use blade covers. Don't leave them loose in a utensil drawer.
- Work with kitchen knives on a cutting board. Cut down and away from you.
- After using sharp items, clean and store them immediately.
- Pick up and hold sharp items by the handles, never the blades.
- If a sharp item falls, don't try to catch it. Back away instead.
- Never run with anything sharp in your hands. You might fall.

- Pick up broken glass with a paper towel or by wearing garden gloves.
- Keep hands away from moving blades on yard and kitchen appliances.

## POISONS

Accidental poisoning can happen to young children, the mentally handicapped, and older adults who don't know or can't see the dangers of household chemicals. *Poisons* are

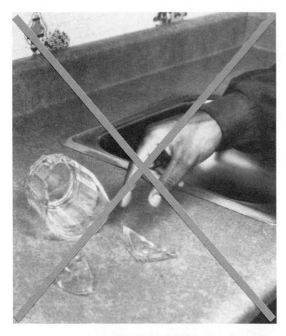

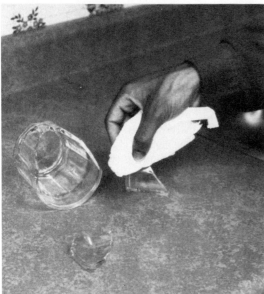

*Do not pick up broken glass with your bare hands. Use a paper towel or sweep it up.*

substances that cause injury or death when they're taken into the body by swallowing or breathing in. The most common poisons are household products, medicines, and plants.

Household chemicals should be stored carefully so that they aren't swallowed accidently:

- Store cleaning products away from food and dishes in the kitchen.
- Keep toothpaste, mouthwash, and other items you put in your mouth on different bathroom shelves from shampoo and other personal hygiene products.
- Keep household chemicals far out of reach and sight of children. Lock chemicals up, if necessary, or keep them on high shelves.
- Keep medicines and other products in their original containers. Make sure you can read the labels and warnings.
- Replace caps securely on medicines, cleaning products, and other chemicals. If children are around, use products with child-resistant caps.

Household cleaners, chemicals, and other poisons should also be used and disposed of safely:

- Read the directions for chemicals before using them.
- Don't mix two or more different chemicals together. They might form *toxic*, or poisonous, fumes.
- Cover or remove food and dishes where you're cleaning with household chemicals or spraying for insects.
- Use sprays, such as insecticides or paint, only in well-ventilated places. Wear a mask if the vapors are strong. Protect your eyes from sprays that can cause injury.
- Supervise children when they use potentially harmful products, such as glue.

- Be responsible for dangerous products you're using. If you leave the room even for a moment, take the product with you.
- Wash your hands thoroughly after using chemicals. Remove and wash your clothes if the chemical has come in contact with them.

Carbon monoxide fumes from a car's engine are deadly even though they're invisible and odorless. Never start the car's engine in a closed garage. For the same reason, don't cook on a charcoal grill in the garage or the house. Kerosene space heaters do not emit toxic fumes; however, they must be handled carefully so that they don't start fires.

Medicines can become poisons when they're not handled responsibly. As stated earlier, always keep medicines in their original containers. Read the label carefully to make sure that you have the right medicine and that you are following all directions properly. Never take or give a medicine at night without turning on a light. Only give prescription medicines to the person the doctor prescribed it for. Flush outdated medicines or those no longer used down the toilet; then rinse the containers and throw them away. Never call medicine "candy" when talking to children.

Since some plants are poisonous, train children early not to chew on plants of any kind. Don't keep poisonous plants around small children.

## Food Poisoning

Like chemicals, contaminated food or water is toxic. In improperly handled food and water, tiny but harmful organisms called bacteria grow rapidly, making them unsafe to eat and drink. Some bacteria simply cause a mild stomachache and perhaps a low fever that pass in time. Without medical treatment, other food-related illnesses

°F

| 250 | |
| 240 | Canning temperatures in pressure canner. |
| | Canning temperatures for fruits, tomatoes, |
| 212 | and pickles in waterbath canner. |
| | Cooking temperatures destroy most bacteria. |
| | Time required to kill bacteria decreases as |
| 165 | temperature is increased. |
| | Warming temperatures prevent growth but |
| 140 | allow survival of some bacteria. |
| 125 | Some bacterial growth. Many bacteria survive. |
| | DANGER ZONE |
| | Foods held more than 2 hours in this zone are |
| | subject to rapid growth of bacteria and the |
| 60 | production of toxins by some bacteria. |
| 40 | Some growth of food poisoning bacteria may occur. |
| 32 | Slow growth of some bacteria that cause spoilage. |
| | Freezing temperatures stop growth of bacteria, |
| | but may allow bacteria to survive. Do not store food |
| 0 | above 10° F for more than a few weeks. |

FOR FOOD SAFETY
KEEP HOT FOODS HOT
COLD FOODS COLD

can be fatal if symptoms are severe or if the victim is very old, very young, or in poor health.

Prevent food poisoning in these ways:
- Keep foods which spoil easily, such as dairy products, cooked eggs, meat, poultry, and fish, cold. Bacteria grow fastest between 60° F and 125° F—a range that includes normal room temperature. In the summer heat, don't take these foods on picnics unless they can be kept cold.
- Don't eat foods with signs of spoilage. Often the appearance or smell are clues, but not always. When in doubt, throw them out—don't taste them first.
- Thaw frozen foods in the refrigerator, not at room temperature where bacteria can grow quickly.
- Put leftovers in the refrigerator or freezer immediately. Don't let them cool on the counter.

## How to Purify Water

Use one of these four methods:

- Boil water for 5–10 minutes.

- Add 10 drops of a household bleach solution per gallon of water. Mix it well, and let it stand for 30 minutes. A slight smell or taste of chlorine indicates that the water is safe to drink.

- Add household tincture of iodine in the same manner as the bleach described above.

- Use commercial purification tablets, such as Halazone or Globaline. Follow the package's instructions.

- Throw away bulging canned foods.
- Always wash your hands before preparing food.
- Wash knives and cutting boards after handling raw meat so other foods don't get contaminated.

Water supplies get contaminated from time to time during floods and other natural disasters. Streams that campers or hikers might choose to drink from usually are unsafe. In these instances, drink safe, bottled beverages or purify your water supply. The chart on this page tells how to purify water so it's safe to drink. If you're not sure about the safety of your home water, ask the local public health service.

## Lawn Mower Accidents

Power lawn mowers can cause serious cuts, fires, and inhalation of gasoline fumes when people aren't careful. Get thorough instructions on handling a mower so that you avoid injury. Before you start mowing, follow these rules for mower safety:

- Fill the mower's gas tank outside the garage so fumes are well vented.

- Don't let anyone smoke near the gas tank while it's being filled because the fumes may ignite.
- Clear the yard of rocks, sticks, or anything the mower could hurl in the air.
- Mow only when the grass is dry so you don't slip on wet grass after a rain or heavy dew.
- Wear heavy-duty shoes with rough nonskid soles to protect your feet, and wear long pants to protect your legs.
- Plan to finish while there is still sufficient light to see what you're doing.

While you mow, follow these mower safety practices:

- Never leave the mower unattended with the motor on.
- Look out for children or pets who could run into your path.
- If the chute clogs, turn off the motor and clear the chute with a stick or tool; never use your hand around a sharp blade.
- Turn off the motor to repair the mower, adjust the mower height, or empty the grass bag.
- On a hill, mow across the lawn with a walk-behind mower to avoid slipping under it; on a riding mower, mow up and down the hill to avoid tipping.

## Back Injuries

Eight out of ten people injure their backs at home, school, or work, or during recreational activities. The average medical cost for a back injury is $800 to $1000! Back strains, sprains, and slipped discs happen because people aren't careful.

Most back injuries can be prevented. Help prevent back injuries by using good posture when you sit, stand, walk, and carry things.

Back injuries from lifting aren't caused by the weight of the load, but instead by lifting and carrying objects improperly. You can injure yourself while picking up a pencil if you

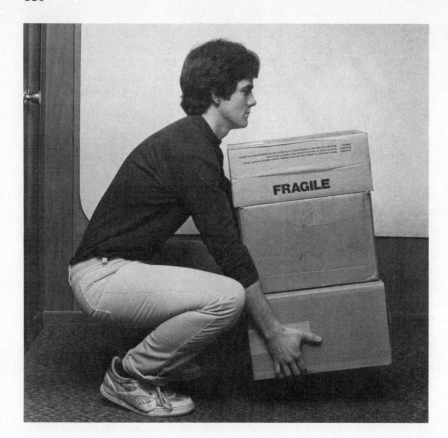

*Bend your knees to lift a heavy object. Don't bend at your waist. You'll protect your back from injury if you lift objects properly.*

do it incorrectly. There is, however, a safe way to lift and carry loads. First, wear non-skid shoes. Be sure the floor is clean and dry. Then follow this technique:

1. Stand close to the object with your feet a hip's width apart, possibly with one foot slightly ahead of the other.
2. Bend your knees and hips into a squatting position. Keep your back straight, with a slight arch.
3. Grasp the object on opposite ends. Make sure the load is balanced and close to your body.
4. Tighten your stomach muscles.
5. Stand up smoothly, using your leg muscles. Keep your back straight with a slight arch.

6. Lift the load to your waist or chest level, no higher.

Don't hold your breath when lifting and carrying. If you feel you have to hold your breath to muster the strength to lift, the load is too heavy to lift alone.

To move a heavy object, slide the object along the floor by pushing or pulling, or ask another person to help. The two of you need to lift together, in the way just described. If the load is very heavy, use a dolly or wheelbarrow.

## Choking on Food

People choke when the air passage to their lungs gets blocked. If they can't breathe again quickly, they don't get the oxygen needed to stay alive. Usually, the body can dislodge something that gets caught in the throat by coughing. If not, the Heimlich maneuver or abdominal thrusts described in Chapter 6 can save a life.

People can choke on anything they put in their mouths, but they choke on food more than anything else. Choking is the nation's sixth leading cause of accidental death! Young children, who put everything in their mouths, have the most choking accidents. Pieces of hot dog, candy, nuts, and grapes account for 40 percent of all children's deaths due to choking.

Among young children, most choking accidents can be avoided by following these suggestions:

- Only give children food they can chew completely and swallow easily.
- Avoid giving children nuts and hard candies.
- Cut children's food into small bites.
- Create a calm atmosphere when children are eating. Excited and distracted children are more likely to choke.
- Remove bones and seeds from food which children could choke on.
- Don't give children toys with small pieces they could swallow.

Teenagers and adults can reduce the chance of choking on food, too, by following these guidelines:

- Don't talk and eat at the same time.
- Eat slowly.
- Take reasonably-sized bites of food.
- Avoid eating when you're drowsy.
- Try not to laugh while you're eating.
- Remember that people who are under the influence of alcohol are more likely to choke on food.

## Safety on Wheels

More teenagers die every year in the United States from motor vehicle accidents than any other type of accident. Last year alone, 18,000 people under the age of 24 died. Motor vehicle accidents usually are caused by the carelessness of drivers or their passengers. Fifty percent of all fatal car accidents are related to alcohol consumption.

Rain also contributes to unsafe driving conditions. When the pavement first gets wet, rain mixes with grime on the roads making the surface very slick. In time, rain washes grime away, but even wet streets are slick. On slick streets, vehicles have a harder time stopping and controlling sharp turns. If you're driving in the rain, allow plenty of time to get where you're going, and leave extra room between vehicles.

Federal and state laws have been enacted to protect motor vehicle occupants. For example, federal law limits the speed to 55 m.p.h. on the nation's roads and has ordered that cars manufactured from 1986 on have back window brake lights. States have enacted laws requiring car occupants to wear seat belts and requiring child restraint devices for babies and young children under four years of age. But the real solution to safety on wheels is individual responsibility.

## Automobiles

Personal safety in a car depends on the use of seat belts and the skill, attitudes, and habits of the driver.

The simplest and most effective way to protect yourself from injury in a car accident is to wear a seat belt. Seat belts reduce injuries and deaths in car accidents by 50 to 60 percent. Some people complain that seat belts are uncomfortable, but after a while most people feel more secure with them on. Properly adjusted belts help you maintain a riding posture that keeps you more alert. Wear your seat belt, and encourage everyone in the car with you to do the same.

Young children need to be buckled into restraint devices. Chapter 9 provides more information about car seats for youngsters.

## Seat Belts Make a Difference

**MYTH:** Wearing seat belts doesn't significantly affect the number of deaths in a vehicular accident.
**FACT:** Approximately 50 percent of deaths in vehicular accidents could be prevented if seat belts were worn.

**MYTH:** Children should wear seat belts, but it's not really that important for adults to wear them.
**FACT:** A common cause of death and injury to children in automobiles is being crushed by adults who aren't wearing seat belts.

**MYTH:** I'm a good driver—I don't need to wear seat belts.
**FACT:** Drivers wearing seat belts have more control over their cars in an emergency and are therefore more likely to avoid an accident. Being a good driver doesn't necessarily protect you from bad drivers on the road.

**MYTH:** If I get in an accident, it's safer for me to be thrown out of the car.
**FACT:** The chances of death or serious injury in an accident are 25 times greater if victims are thrown out of the vehicle.

**MYTH:** I might drown or be burned to death if I wear seat belts.
**FACT:** Fewer than one half of one percent of all injury-producing accidents involve submersion or fire. Even if victims were unrestrained in these instances, they would probably be unconscious or unable to get out of the vehicle.

In the sun, the metal buckles on belts get burning hot. When you get into a car that's been sitting in the sun, check the buckles before securing them around yourself or a child.

Each driver has a personal responsibility for preventing vehicular accidents. This includes not only driving skill, but also safe attitudes and habits behind the wheel. As a safe driver, you should:

- Keep the car in good working condition. Have the brakes, lights, windshield wipers, and tires checked regularly. Many states require safety inspections yearly.
- Drive defensively and always be prepared for other drivers to make mistakes that can cause accidents.
- Obey driving laws. Heed the speed limit and passing, stop, yield, and warning signs.
- Avoid tailgating, or driving too close to the car in front of you. Allow one car length's space for every 10 m.p.h. the car is traveling.

*Driving too close to the car in front of you can cause a serious accident if the other driver stops suddenly.*

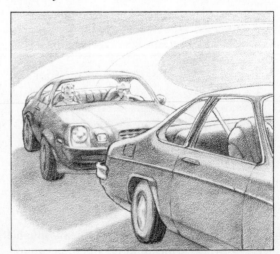

- If possible, avoid driving when weather conditions are dangerous, such as in snow, ice, or fog.
- Avoid driving when you're sleepy. On long trips, take breaks, and walk outside to refresh yourself.

What would you do if you were a passenger in a car with an unsafe driver? Ask the person to drive safely. For your own well-being, don't ride with anyone who won't listen. Never ride with a driver who has been consuming alcohol.

Even with diligent safety practices, minor accidents and injuries occur, so keep a first aid kit in the car.

## Cycles

Although there are fewer bike and motorcycle accidents than car accidents, injury and death rates are higher. That's because a cyclist has less protection. For this reason, cyclists need to be especially cautious about driving safely.

Many states have laws to protect cyclists. They may be required to wear helmets and may not be allowed on interstate highways.

A motorcylist can decrease the risk of accidents by following these safety rules:

- Obey all traffic laws with no trick riding or weaving between cars in traffic or on the road's shoulder.
- Yield to all trucks and cars; they can't stop or maneuver as easily as a motorcycle.
- Turn on the headlight, even in the daylight, to make the cycle more easily seen.
- Wear safety equipment such as a helmet, goggles, heavy shoes, and heavy gloves.

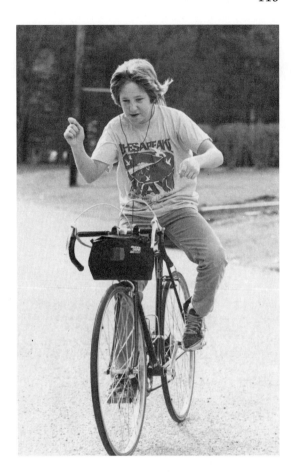

- Protect against weather exposure, especially on long trips.

Bicycling is a popular form of recreation, but it can be dangerous in traffic. Bikers must obey the same traffic laws as motorists. This includes obeying all traffic signs and signals, riding on the right side of the road, and signaling for turns. As a bicyclist, you can also reduce accidents by following safety reminders:

- Wear a hard-shell helmet for protection in case of a fall.
- Don't give anyone a ride because the extra, unbalanced load can make you lose control of the bike.

- Secure books and personal items to your bike in a way that allows you to keep both hands on the handlebars.
- Wear bright-colored clothes, and put reflectors on your bike.
- At dusk, wear a reflector vest and have lights front and back.
- Confine stunt and trick riding to tracks for that purpose.
- Use a band or clip to keep pant legs from catching in the chain or spokes.
- Avoid riding on wet pavement or on gravel where you can skid.
- When riding with others, form a single file near the curb.

As a driver, you have a responsibility to cyclists. Move away from them on the road, and slow down when you pass them. Don't frighten them unnecessarily by honking.

## Buses

Many teenagers get to school on a bus. After hours, you may use the bus to get around town. Although a bus is a fairly safe way to travel, there are some precautions you can take as a rider.

- Remain seated while the bus is moving.
- Avoid behavior or loud yelling that might distract the driver.
- Buckle up if the bus has seat belts.
- Don't throw anything from the bus, even at slow speeds; tossed items can inflict injury to a passerby.

## Outdoor Safety

Your body can withstand moderate temperatures. But when the thermometer dips below 60° F or rises above 90° F take precautions.

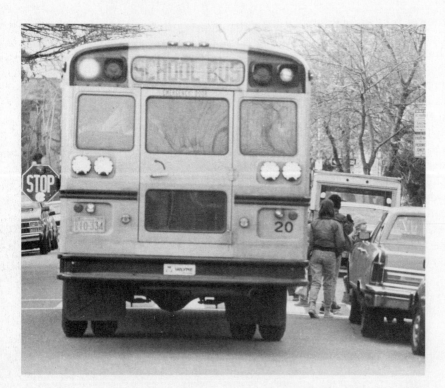

*In all states, drivers going in either direction on an undivided road must stop while children get on and off a school bus. As a driver, you are responsible for these children's safety.*

# Protection from Sun

Sun can be your worst summertime enemy. Prolonged exposure to sun can cause severe sunburn, more rapidly age your skin, and potentially cause skin cancer. Fair-skinned blonds tend to be more vulnerable to the sun's rays than people with olive skin that never burns but tans well. The skin of black people also can be sun damaged.

Sun is most intense and damaging midday—between 11 a.m. and 3 p.m. (Daylight Savings Time). But early morning or late afternoon sun can cause a bad burn. Even on cloudy days, 75 percent of the sun's rays may get through. The sun's rays even penetrate summer clothing.

Protect yourself from the sun's damaging rays. Cover up by wearing a hat or visor, sunglasses, and lightweight clothes. Avoid direct sun exposure, particularly midday. Use a sunblock, which deflects the sun's harmful ultraviolet rays, to protect your nose and lips because they burn easily. Sunscreens are lotions that can protect your skin from the sun; they slow burning or tanning but do not prevent it. Sunscreens are given a *sun protection factor* rating that indicates the degree of protection provided. Apply a sunscreen with a sun protection factor appropriate for your skin type, and reapply it every two hours and after you swim, wash, or perspire heavily. See the chart on the upper right for the sun protection factor recommended for your skin type.

Skin damage from the sun won't show for many years, but its effect accumulates over time and is irreversible. No moisturizers, cosmetics, or medicine can remove wrinkles or fully heal damaged skin.

Prolonged, intense sun exposure can also damage your eyes temporarily or permanently. It is best to protect your eyes with sunglasses that don't transmit much light. The lenses should be dark enough so you

## Sunscreens Protect Your Skin

Buy a sunscreen with an SPF (sun protection factor) that's right for your skin!

| Skin Type | | SPF Range |
|---|---|---|
| I | Very fair. Always burns. Never tans. | 10–15 |
| II | Fair. Usually burns. Sometimes tans faintly. | 6–12 |
| III | Sometimes burns. Usually tans. | 4–6 |
| IV | Almost never burns. Always tans. | 2–4 |

can't see your eyes in a mirror when you wear sunglasses.

# Protection from Heat

High temperatures, especially combined with high humidity, can be dangerous to health. Even healthy people can die from too much heat and sun exposure.

Perspiration is part of your body's natural air conditioning system. But hot air temperature and high humidity make it harder for your body to cool itself down. Heat and humidity combine to make up a *heat index* which indicates the impact of heat on the body. See how the heat index is calculated on the chart on page **122**.

To protect yourself from heat hazards, stay out of the sun, preferably in a cool, air-conditioned place. Avoid sunburn since it impairs the body's ability to cool itself. Wear light colored, loose-fitting clothes that don't retain body heat. Minimize your physical activity so your body doesn't get overheated. Drink plenty of liquids to replace fluids lost through perspiration, but avoid alcohol. If

## Heat Index

Match the temperature with the humidity to find out what the temperature feels like.

### Relative Humidity

| | 22% | 26% | 30% | 34% | 38% | 42% | 46% | 50% | 54% | 58% | 62% | 66% | 70% | 74% |
|---|---|---|---|---|---|---|---|---|---|---|---|---|---|---|
| 80° | 77 | 78 | 79 | 79 | 80 | 80 | 81 | 81 | 82 | 83 | 84 | 85 | 85 | 86 |
| 82° | 79 | 80 | 80 | 81 | 82 | 83 | 84 | 85 | 85 | 86 | 87 | 88 | 89 | 90 |
| 84° | 81 | 82 | 82 | 83 | 84 | 85 | 86 | 86 | 87 | 88 | 90 | 91 | 92 | 93 |
| 86° | 83 | 84 | 85 | 86 | 87 | 87 | 88 | 90 | 90 | 92 | 93 | 94 | 95 | 97 |
| 88° | 86 | 87 | 87 | 88 | 90 | 90 | 91 | 92 | 94 | 95 | 97 | 99 | 100 | 102 |
| 90° | 87 | 88 | 90 | 91 | 92 | 93 | 95 | 96 | 98 | 100 | 101 | 104 | 105 | 107 |
| 92° | 90 | 91 | 92 | 93 | 95 | 97 | 98 | 100 | 103 | 105 | 106 | 110 | 112 | 114 |
| 94° | 93 | 94 | 95 | 96 | 98 | 100 | 102 | 104 | 107 | 110 | 113 | 115 | 118 | 121 |
| 96° | 95 | 97 | 98 | 99 | 101 | 104 | 106 | 109 | 111 | 115 | 119 | 120 | 125 | 129 |
| 98° | 97 | 99 | 101 | 104 | 105 | 108 | 111 | 114 | 118 | 121 | 125 | 130 | | |
| 100° | 100 | 102 | 104 | 108 | 110 | 113 | 115 | 120 | 124 | 126 | 130 | | | |

*Temperature*

☐ Alert:          Possible harm with prolonged exposure

◻ Caution:      Harmful effects possible

◼ Hazard:       Heat-related harm likely

*Source: NOAA/National Weather Service, U.S. Department of Commerce*

you feel weak or dizzy from the heat, get help immediately.

## Protection from Cold

Exposure to cold causes loss of body heat which in turn causes illness and injury. Babies, young children, and older adults are especially affected by cold temperatures. Hypothermia and frostbite, which you'll learn more about in Chapter 6, are serious injuries that result from too much exposure to the cold.

Wind makes cold temperatures more severe because it carries body heat away. Just how cold you feel depends on the combined effects of temperature and wind, called the *windchill factor*. See the chart on page **123** to see why it's so important to protect yourself properly, even on a day that doesn't seem too cold.

## Windchill Factor

| Estimated wind speed (in mph) | Actual thermometer reading | | | | | | | |
|---|---|---|---|---|---|---|---|---|
| | 50° F | 40° F | 30° F | 20° F | 10° F | 0° F | −10° F | −20° F |
| | Equivalent Temperature | | | | | | | |
| Calm | 50 | 40 | 30 | 20 | 10 | 0 | −10 | −20 |
| 5 | 48 | 37 | 27 | 16 | 6 | −5 | −15 | −26 |
| 10 | 40 | 28 | 16 | 4 | −9 | −24 | −33 | −46 |
| 15 | 36 | 22 | 9 | −5 | −18 | −32 | −45 | −58 |
| 20 | 32 | 18 | 4 | −10 | −25 | −39 | −53 | −67 |
| 25 | 30 | 16 | 0 | −15 | −29 | −44 | −59 | −74 |
| 30 | 28 | 13 | −2 | −18 | −33 | −48 | −63 | −79 |
| 35 | 27 | 11 | −4 | −20 | −35 | −51 | −67 | −82 |
| 40 | 26 | 10 | −6 | −21 | −37 | −53 | −69 | −85 |

(Wind speeds greater than 40 m.p.h. have little additional effect.)

☐ LITTLE DANGER (for properly clothed person) Maximum danger of false sense of security.

▨ INCREASING DANGER
Danger from freezing of exposed flesh.

▩ GREAT DANGER

You can preserve body heat and remain comfortable and warm in cold temperatures. Dress warmly, using several layers of loose-fitting clothes; each layer traps in air as an insulator. Wear mittens instead of gloves so your fingers stay warmer. Wear a hat, perhaps a scarf over your mouth; your body loses over half of its heat through your head. Keep dry; wetness increases loss of body heat. Keep moving to generate body heat, but don't overexert yourself. Don't drink alcoholic beverages. They increase loss of body heat and impair your judgments about the situation.

## Protection from Lightning

Lightning, another outdoor hazard, can severely injure, even kill. It usually strikes the highest object on a landscape, then searches for the fastest path to the ground. Standing on the ground or being in the water is dangerous when lightning strikes nearby.

Protect yourself from lightning. In a storm, come indoors and stay there until the storm passes. Or, if necessary, stay in a car, but don't lean on anything metal since metal is a good electrical conductor. Avoid using the telephone because current can travel

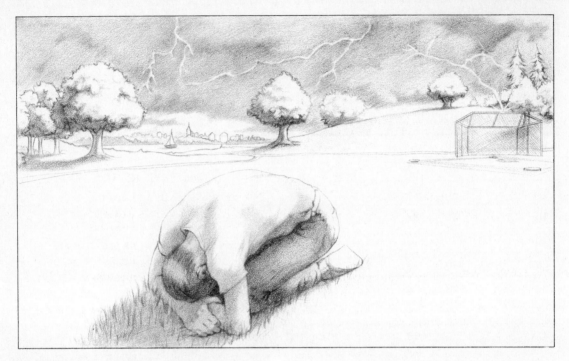

*Tuck yourself in a protective position if you're caught outside in a lightning storm.*

through the lines when lightning strikes them.

If you can't get inside, stay away from tall objects, especially trees since lightning usually strikes them first. If you're in an open field, bend down on your knees and tuck your head down so you're a small target; don't flatten yourself on the ground. If you feel your hair stand on end, drop to your knees. Don't stand on or near anything that conducts electricity, such as water or metal.

## Protection from Insects

Insects are both annoying and potentially dangerous. The stings of ants, bees, wasps, and yellow jackets are painful and, to some victims, can cause death. Bites of fleas, mosquitoes, and chiggers itch but rarely cause a serious reaction. Some biting insects transmit diseases, such as malaria and sleeping sickness.

Protect yourself from insects. Dress wisely. Wear long sleeves and pants to cover your arms and legs. Stinging insects are attracted to dark colors, and biting insects, to bright floral prints. Use insect repellents, but know that they only repel biting insects. Keep yourself clean, and don't wear perfumes, aftershave lotion or scented hair sprays because insects are drawn to strong body odors, good or bad. Don't provoke stinging insects by swatting them; instead, stay calm and walk away slowly. On picnics, keep sweets covered and stay far from garbage cans, which insects love. If possible, stay within a well-screened area.

# Safety and Recreation

Leisure time is an opportunity for relaxation and pleasure. But any time people actively participate in outdoor activities there is potential for accidents, weather exposure, or insect bites.

Alcohol doesn't mix with recreation. Drinking alcohol affects a person's balance, reaction time, and judgment. When people are drowsy or clumsy from alcohol, they can't swim or cycle safely, respond to sudden hazards, or tolerate extreme weather. They may be a danger to others around them.

## Water Safety

Drownings happen where there's water— a pool, lake, river, even a well, bathtub, or bucket. About 100 million people take part in some recreational water activity every year, and about 2,500 of them drown. Approximately 4,000 people drown every year in non-recreational water accidents.

Good swimming skills and knowledge of water hazards are part of water safety. Many times a person who can't swim is the victim of drowning. The American Red Cross recommends the following guidelines for recreational water safety:

- Learn to swim well enough to survive in an emergency.
- Never swim alone. Swim with a buddy who has the ability to help when needed.
- Swim only in supervised areas.
- Follow the rules set up for the particular place where you are swimming.
- Don't overestimate your swimming ability.
- Stay out of water when you are overheated, overtired, or chilled.
- Dive only into known waters of sufficient depth.
- Don't substitute inflated tubes, air mattresses, or artificial supports for swimming ability.
- Always swim a safe distance away from diving boards and platforms.
- Be especially careful in areas of strong currents, slippery rocks, or white water where you might lose control.
- Call for help only when you need it.
- If you're boating, have enough life preservers for everyone. Don't overload the boat.

## Safety for Jogging and Walking

Jogging and walking are popular ways to keep fit, but they have their hazards.

Warming up before exercise and cooling down after exercise helps prevent muscle injuries. You learned about safe exercise patterns in Chapter 1. You may exercise hard, but don't overexert.

Dress appropriately to avoid injury when you jog or walk. Wear running shoes with well-cushioned soles and wide, built-up heels to avoid foot injury. In warm weather, wear lightweight clothes that breathe. In cold weather, wear layers of clothes, a hat, and mittens to keep you warm. If you're out after dark, wear reflective strips on your clothes so motorists will see you.

Jog or walk in safe places, if possible, where there's little or no traffic. On the streets, stay on the left side so you face oncoming traffic. Avoid running or walking where exhaust from motor vehicles is heavy; the pollution damages your heart and lungs.

## Safety at Work

Many accidents occur at the workplace. Many of these are caused by workers who don't know or don't follow safe practices. In other cases, unsafe equipment and employee fatigue are causes.

Government agencies are responsible for the protection of employees and consumers from hazardous conditions. The Occupational Safety and Health Administration

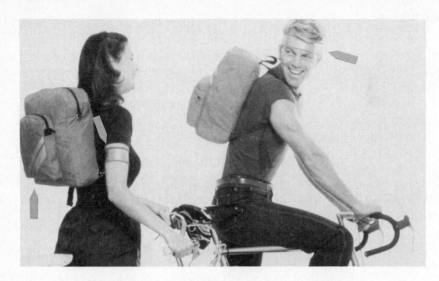

*Reflective material on headbands, jackets, gloves, jogging suits, backpacks, and helmets makes people more visible to drivers in the dark. When light bounces off this material, drivers know to proceed with caution.*

(OSHA) sets safety standards in the workplace and inspectors check regularly. This is especially important around industrial machinery. For example, some jobs require workers to wear hard hats or safety goggles.

Public health agencies have regulations for safety and sanitation in restaurants and other places where food is handled. For example, workers must wash their hands after using the toilets. Refrigerators and steam tables must be kept at certain temperatures. And workers must be checked regularly in their use of slicing machines.

## Safety from Assault

Anyone, regardless of sex or age, can be the victim of *assault*, or a physical attack. Assault results in both physical harm and emotional trauma, with possible long-term effects. Safety includes protecting yourself from physical attack—at home, outdoors, and in the car.

Prevent dangerous situations at home. Keep outside areas well lighted. Don't hide extra keys around the outside of your home; instead keep them with neighbors you trust.

Don't let people know you're home alone, including those who phone you. Keep your ground floor windows and doors locked at all times and your curtains or shades drawn at night. Don't open the door to strangers; use a peephole to see who's at the door. If you are coming home and it appears that someone has broken into your home, don't go in; call the police from a neighbor's phone.

More parents work outside their homes, so more children are left unsupervised after school and on weekends. Children who let themselves in and out with a key because their parents aren't home are called latchkey children. These youngsters need to protect themselves from danger when they're home alone. They also need to know how to call for help or reassurance if they need it.

Unfortunately, dangers lurk on the streets and in parks. So be alert to your surroundings when you're outside—day or night. Watch for suspicious people. At night, stay in well-lighted, busy places. Avoid alleys, doorways, and other dark places where people can lurk. Walk in the middle of the sidewalk, not too close to the street or buildings.

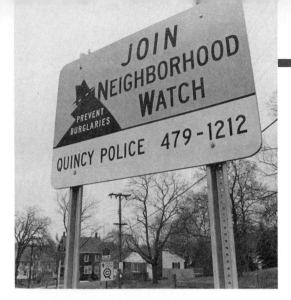

# NEIGHBORS HELPING NEIGHBORS

Everybody needs help sometime. Preventing crime, loneliness, and fear in your neighborhood is a way to help and show you care. Either informally or as part of an organized group, you can help make your neighborhood a better place to live.

## Neighborhood Watch

Neighborhood Watch is a program of citizen involvement that discourages residential crime and may help prevent assault. In addition, it encourages neighbors to look out for the well being of one another. Through periodic meetings, people learn how to burglar-proof their own homes. They learn to look for suspicious activities, vehicles, and strangers. They also have a system to report quickly and accurately to the police. In this way, crime may be averted, help can be obtained fast, and the neighborhood is a safer place to live.

## Latchkey Care

Organizations, such as the YMCA, sponsor child-care programs for children during the hours before and after school. This way, the children aren't home alone when parents are at work. This helps protect them from accidents and crimes in their own neighborhood.

## Helping Hand

In some neighborhoods, "safe" homes are designated with a special sign in the window. This sign lets children know where they can go for help if they're in trouble. The Helping Hand program is often organized through the schools where parents who are home during the day look out for neighborhood children.

## What Can You Do?

Your own neighborhood may have these or similar programs. You can be a program volunteer, or possibly you might help organize a program in your area.

If your neighborhood doesn't have organized groups for community safety, it becomes each citizen's individual responsibility to look after and help neighbors. The elderly, the impaired, and young children especially can benefit from your help.

- Offer to babysit for unattended children.
- Watch for and report strange people or vehicles in your neighborhood.
- Be alert for suspicious activities.
- Offer to run errands for people who are homebound.
- Check on your neighbors periodically, especially if you don't see them for several days.

Make the choice to work together to help one another. You and your neighbors will enjoy a safer and more secure place to live.

When possible, walk with friends; there's safety in numbers. Don't hitchhike. If someone follows you while you're walking, go quickly to the nearest home or business. Always let your family know where you are going to be.

Sometimes people get boastful or careless about their money. Don't make yourself the target of assault. Handle money discreetly. When you carry a schoolbag or a purse, hold it close. Usually, it's safer to carry a small billfold that you can tuck out of sight. If your bag is grabbed, let it go. It's better to lose your bag than to get hurt.

When you're out driving, protect yourself from assault. Keep your gas tank full so you aren't stranded. Drive on well-lighted, well-traveled roads. Never pick up a hitchhiker, no matter how safe or needy the person looks; go to a nearby phone to call if the person needs help. Drive into a police, fire, or gas station if you suspect you're being followed. Carry a "SEND HELP" sign to use if you have car trouble, and only accept help from the police. In public places, always park in a busy, well-lighted place; roll up the windows and lock all doors before leaving. When returning to a parked car, have your keys ready. Check the inside of the car before getting in. Keep your windows closed and doors locked while driving.

## Safety and Preparedness

The more you know about protecting yourself and your family from the hazards around you, the better prepared you can be! The more you practice what you know, the safer you are.

In your home, keep lists of emergency numbers by all phones. At night, keep a phone by the bed in case someone in the family must make an emergency call.

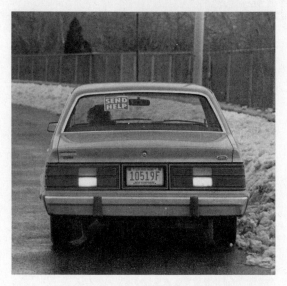

*Keep a "Send Help" sign in your car. In case you're stranded, put it in your window for other drivers to see. Stay in your locked car until the police come to help.*

Information about safety is easily available. Magazines and television carry safety information. Organizations and public services in many communities sponsor safety programs.

- Police departments sponsor crime-watch groups.
- Fire departments give programs on fire prevention.
- The Safety Council sponsors safety seminars and information pamphlets.
- The American Heart Association and American Red Cross offer courses, such as cardiopulmonary resuscitation, first aid, and water safety.
- Pools offer swimming lessons.
- The Highway Patrol sponsors car safety programs.

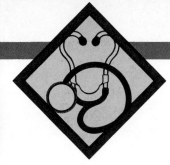

# CHAPTER CHECKUP

## Reviewing the Information

1. Name five ways to prevent kitchen fires.
2. Why should your family have a fire safety plan?
3. How can people protect themselves from smoke inhalation in a fire?
4. What is the safe way to use a ladder?
5. What are five ways a person could avoid serious cuts?
6. Why do people become victims of accidental poisoning?
7. What would you do if you weren't sure if food was spoiled?
8. What is the safe way to lift an object?
9. How can you prevent a child from choking on food?
10. Why can driving fast on wet pavement be dangerous?
11. What are five rules for riding a bicycle safely?
12. Name five tips for handling a lawn mower safely.
13. Why is overexposure to sun and heat so dangerous?
14. How could you protect yourself from cold temperatures?
15. How could you protect yourself from drowning while you were swimming?
16. Why can insect bites be dangerous?
17. What could you do to protect yourself from personal assault while you walk in the dark?

## Thinking It Over

1. How would you protect a young child at your home from accidental poisoning?
2. What would you do if your friend was driving recklessly?
3. What would you say to a friend who refused to wear a seat belt?
4. What is your correct SPF factor?
5. Why can the temperature feel like 22° F below zero even though the outside temperature is 20° F above zero?
6. Tell what conditions are unsafe for swimming.
7. What should you do if you're caught outside in a thunderstorm?

## Taking Action

 1. Write a fire safety plan for your home. Have your family practice it. Discuss the results.

 2. Write a newspaper article about your school's fire drill plan. Suggest improvements.

 3. Calculate today's windchill factor or heat index.

 4. Read about one case of personal assault in the newspaper. How might the victim have prevented the crime?

5. Pick up a heavy object in a way that protects your back.
6. Examine your kitchen and bathroom to make sure you store household chemicals and medicines safely.
7. Call two local organizations to learn what safety training is available.

# 6 Emergency Response and First Aid

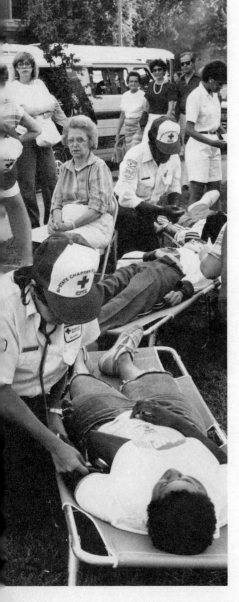

After reading this chapter, you should be able to:

- describe the contents of a basic first aid kit.

- identify several emergency services.

- tell how to report an emergency.

- describe first aid for emergencies.

## Terms to Understand

| | |
|---|---|
| antidote | hemorrhaging |
| asphyxiation | hypothermia |
| cardiopulmonary resuscitation (CPR) | infection |
| | life support equipment |
| first aid | rescue squad |
| fracture | shock |
| heatstroke | wound |
| Heimlich maneuver | |

$A$ccidents are part of everyday life. No matter how careful you are, collisions, fires, and other accidents happen which can have serious consequences. Statistics show that accidents are the leading cause of death among people from 1 to 38 years of age. These facts tell how important it is to prepare for emergencies. With skills, knowledge, and supplies, you can quickly and efficiently respond to medical emergencies. You might save a life!

If you're like most people, you've never saved a life or responded to an emergency. Have you ever thought how you would react if an emergency arose? Many people think they would panic or freeze. Most people, however, perform the tasks necessary to help the victim if they know what to do.

## Preparing for Emergencies

Being prepared is the first step in offering first aid. *First aid* is immediate and temporary care for anyone who is injured or ill. Even if you never use your first aid skills, knowing what to do is good insurance.

Two steps in being prepared are to have a first aid kit ready and to learn how to respond to emergencies. This is called emergency preparedness.

### First Aid Kit

A first aid kit has supplies needed for immediate medical care. Every home, office, school, and public building should have a first aid kit in a convenient, visible location. People should know where it is and how to use its supplies. The picture below shows the contents of a basic first aid kit.

*Supplies for a basic first aid kit include:*
- *24 adhesive strip bandages in many shapes and sizes*
- *12 sterile gauze pads in 2-, 3-, and 4-inch squares*
- *6 gauze rolls in 1-, 2-, and 3-inch widths*
- *2 triangle slings*
- *roll of 1-inch adhesive tape*
- *bandage scissors*
- *ice bag*
- *pair of tweezers*
- *12 cotton swabs*
- *thermometer*
- *safety pins*
- *soap*
- *first aid manual*
- *phone numbers of local emergency services*

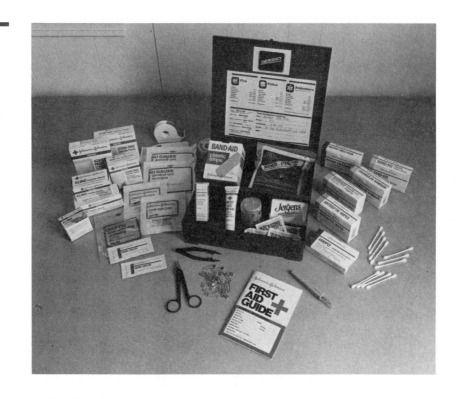

Medicine and other supplies don't last forever. Replace the contents of the first aid kit by the expiration date. You can use old bandages and gauze for practicing first aid.

Bring a first aid kit when you travel, camp, or participate in sports and recreational activities. Small, portable first aid kits fit in backpacks, under car seats, or on the back of a bicycle.

First aid kits are available at most drugstores and department stores, or you can make your own kit and stock supplies for your special use. For example, if you live in a very cold climate, you should include a lightweight, thermal blanket. Or if you're allergic to certain insect bites, include allergy medicine.

Store first aid supplies in a waterproof container, and label the container clearly as first aid supplies. Store the kit out of the reach of children, and inform family and friends of its location.

## Emergency Preparedness Training

You prepare for emergencies through training. Training will teach you what to do and, as importantly, what not to do. Some courses you might want to take to prepare for emergencies are:

- Water Safety, where you'll learn to swim and, in advanced classes, how to rescue someone who's drowning.
- First Aid, to learn how to give immediate treatment for injuries and sudden illnesses.
- Cardiopulmonary Resuscitation (CPR), to learn to revive someone whose heart or breathing stops.

Training provides you with new skills or reinforces what you already know. At the time of an emergency, you want to be prepared and feel confident that you can handle the situation safely.

## Identifying the Emergency

A call for help from a struggling swimmer or billowing smoke from a building are obvious signs of an emergency. They require urgent attention. You would respond immediately because you know that someone's life might depend on it. Other times, someone may be injured or take ill in less noticeable, less dramatic ways.

Knowing just what to do depends on how you size up the situation. Ask yourself these questions when you arrive at the scene of an accident or see someone in medical trouble:

- What is the emergency? Perhaps it's a fire, a car crash, or a person having an apparent heart attack.
- Is someone injured? Could someone die?
- Can I help?
- Am I alone?
- How and where can I get help?

Gathering information about the emergency is also important. The subtle details are as valuable as the obvious information. Suppose a young boy has fallen from his speeding bicycle. The obvious clues to what has happened would be his cries, a bleeding wound, or his foot caught in a pedal.

Less noticeable clues also provide valuable information. In the same example, torn clothes might mean a cut or scrape underneath. The place where he fell or slid might suggest dirt in his wounds. The position of his body might indicate a twisted ankle or broken bone.

How thoroughly you gather information determines how accurately you can report an emergency. When professionals or other persons arrive, be prepared to answer these questions:

- What is the emergency?
- When did it happen?
- How did it happen?
- Who is hurt or sick?

*In some states, medical information is provided on the back of a driver's license.*

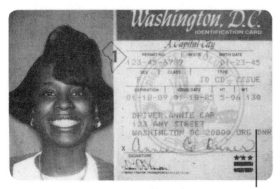

People can state their intention to donate their body organs if they die an accidental death.

Certain health conditions, such as vision problems or paralysis, require driving restrictions, but not all restrictions relate to health.

**RESTRICTION CODE**

1. With proper glasses or contact lenses.
2. Valid only in the District of Columbia.
3. May operate only pleasure vehicles without compensation prior to age 18.
4. Armed Forces vehicles only.
5. Left outside rear view mirror properly placed.
6. To operate Motorcycles only.
7. May also operate Motorcycles.
8. Diabetic.
9. Holder is required to display Official Document stating special conditions, upon demand.

Some driver's licenses tell others about health conditions they should know about before giving emergency first aid.

- How badly are they injured? Or how sick do they seem to be?
- What aid have you given?

If a victim is unconscious, look for a Medic Alert tag on a bracelet or a necklace. It tells about health problems the person has, and it may help you learn what's wrong. Medic Alert tags indicate the person may have a disease, such as diabetes, takes special medicine, is allergic to drugs or other substances, wears a special device, such as a pacemaker for the heart, or has seizures.

## Communicating the Emergency

What do you do once you've identified an emergency? You tell others, if possible, so you can get help. Communicating the emergency is important for several reasons. The emergency may require special equipment.

*The Medic Alert emblem can help prevent tragic—even fatal—mistakes in emergency medical treatment. The emblem, worn on a necklace or bracelet, alerts emergency medical workers to health conditions that can't be easily seen—such as heart conditions, diabetes, severe allergies, and epilepsy.*

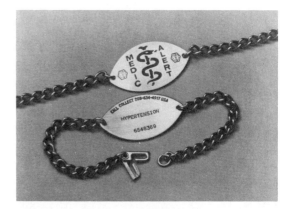

You may not be able to provide all the necessary aid by yourself; skills of specially-trained professionals may be needed. The victim may need to be transported to a hospital.

If there are bystanders, enlist their aid. Ask them to go for help. Meanwhile, remain at the scene to give first aid and try to calm the victim.

## A Call for Help

In most parts of the country, you can dial 911 to connect with help from the police, the fire department, or an ambulance. In places that don't have the 911 emergency system, dial the telephone operator who will connect you with the right emergency service. Be prepared by learning the emergency numbers where you live and posting them next to the phone.

To get fast, appropriate help by phone or face to face, you need to convey certain information about the emergency:

• type of emergency
• condition of the victim
• exact location of the victim
• your name
• what help the victim is getting

When you call for help, never be the first to hang up. There may be additional questions. Let the person you call end the call.

Emergencies often happen in isolated places with no one within shouting distance to help. Suppose you and a friend are hiking in the countryside. Suddenly your friend falls and breaks an ankle. You remember

*Good Samaritan laws in many states protect citizens from liability if they stop at the scene of an accident to give first aid.*

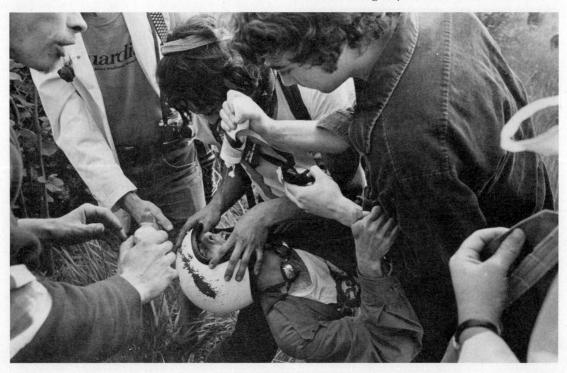

that the nearest phone is a half mile back. What do you do?

Since every emergency is unique, you must rely on your training and judgment. In this situation you have these choices:

- Stay with your friend and wait for a passerby. With a broken bone that's fine, if you expect someone to pass by. But some emergencies can't wait.
- Leave your friend to go for help fast.
- Transport your friend in a makeshift manner to get aid. You would only want to do this if you were sure the injury was minor and only if you could protect the ankle while you transported your friend.

What you do depends on many things. Most importantly, you must consider the condition of your friend.

## Emergency Services

Who should you call for help? Every community has access to a police department, fire department, and an ambulance service. Many towns and cities also have an emergency room, a rescue squad, and poison control center. To save time, contact the most useful emergency service first—know what each one does.

### POLICE DEPARTMENT

When you're not sure which emergency service you need, call the police. Since they cruise or walk their local beat, they are often close by. They can be on the scene of an emergency quickly. They'll know what, if any, additional emergency services should be called.

Police are trained to provide basic first aid. Upon arrival, they will take over the responsibility for handling an emergency.

### FIRE DEPARTMENT

Firefighters respond mainly to fires. But sometimes they handle bomb threats, people trapped in cars and buildings, chemical spills, and building collapses. If you need to rescue someone from a dangerous place, call the fire department.

### AMBULANCE SERVICE

Ambulance services are for the emergency transportation of victims. Some ambulances have life support equipment, and others have none. *Life support equipment* is highly technical equipment which can sustain or revive someone in a near-death condition. When you call for an ambulance, the type of ambulance dispatched will be determined by your description of the victim's condition.

### EMERGENCY ROOM

Emergency rooms (ERs) in hospitals provide emergency medical services. Health professionals there are specially trained to handle emergencies. Very ill and severely-injured persons should come to a hospital ER. These are some emergencies which are best handled there: heart attacks, heavily bleeding cuts, unconscious accident victims, badly broken bones, and drowning victims. Many ambulance services contact emergency rooms by radio so the hospital ER is ready for the crisis when the victim arrives.

Free-standing emergency facilities, or those not part of a hospital, are a new health care trend. They provide walk-in services for people who are mildly ill or have minor injuries, such as sprains.

### RESCUE SQUAD

Many local communities have rescue squads as part of their police or fire departments. *Rescue squads* are staffed with highly-trained medical technicians who can give emergency care at the scene of the emergency. The rescue squad vehicles are equipped with rescue equipment, such as

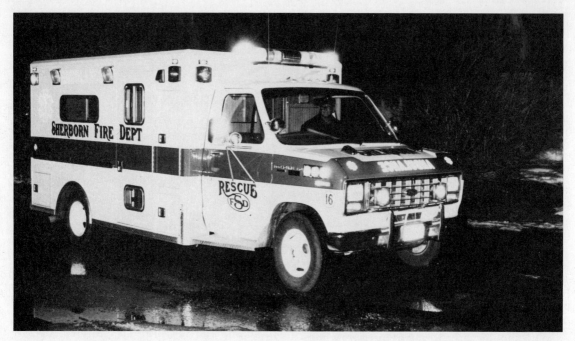

*If you're driving, pull to the side of the road to allow emergency vehicles to pass.*

stretchers, splints, neck braces, oxygen tanks and masks, medical supplies and equipment, and "jaws of life." Jaws of life are a special tool used to remove accident victims from their crushed vehicle.

Most rescue squads also transport and care for the victim on the way to the hospital. When the rescue squad brings the victim to the emergency room, the hospital takes over the victim's care.

### POISON CONTROL CENTER

Poison control centers are staffed with health professionals, too. They have information on most chemical products used in households and businesses. This enables them to provide instructions for emergency first aid for swallowing most substances.

If you call a poison control center, be prepared to tell:
- the name of the poison.
- the ingredients in the poison. Find the ingredient list on the label.
- the manufacturer of the poison.
- how much of the poison was swallowed.
- how the victim reacted to the poison.
- what first aid was given, if any.
- the victim's age and health.

The poison control center will explain what you should do. Sometimes they tell what antidote the victim should take. An *antidote* is a substance that counteracts a poison. They may recommend that the victim go to the nearest emergency facility.

There are many poison control centers across the United States. Look in the Yellow

Pages of the phone book under "Poison Control."

## Providing First Aid

As stated earlier, first aid is immediate and temporary care given for anyone who is injured or ill. It is given according to a set of basic rules of emergency care, and it requires common sense.

The first aid information in this book is not meant to take the place of a first aid course. Instead, it's a brief explanation of important first aid rules to refer to. All people, teens and adults, should take certified first aid training regularly. When you use the skills learned in a first aid course, you can give good, safe emergency care.

In an emergency, give first aid quickly and efficiently. Then get medical help as soon as you can. Injuries and illnesses requiring first aid include wounds, shock, broken bones, heart attacks, choking, poisoning, burns, and many others.

## Wounds

Wounds require first aid. A *wound* is any break in the skin that might bleed. It may be as simple as a mild scrape, or it may be as severe as a deep, tearing cut. There are five types of wounds:

- abrasion, or a skin scrape, such as scraping your knees when you fall off a bicycle
- incision, or a cut from a sharp object, such as a knife or glass
- laceration, or a jagged cut from an irregular object, such as a fishhook or barbed wire
- puncture, or a piercing cut down into the skin, such as from stepping on a nail
- avulsion, or skin or a body part torn from the body, such as when a finger is cut off by a saw

# Types of Wounds

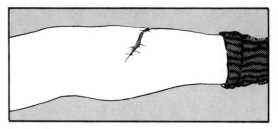

Laceration

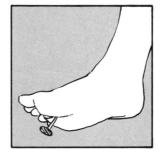

Puncture

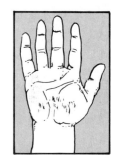

Abrasion

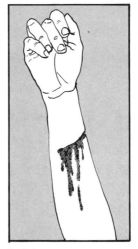

Incision

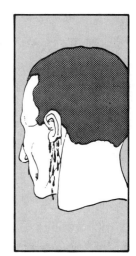

Avulsion

Bleeding and infection are dangers of any wound. First aid protects against both. An *infection* occurs when germs get into the wound. Signs of an infected wound are redness, swelling, and possibly the appearance of a thick, yellowish liquid called pus.

The first and most important rule in first aid for a wound is to control the bleeding. For minor wounds, applying firm, direct pressure over the wound usually stops the bleeding. Use a clean compress over the wound, placing the palm of your hand over the compress and pressing firmly. A clean handkerchief, a wad of tissue, or even a newspaper can serve as a compress. In an emergency, use your bare hand or fingers until someone can get a compress for you. Firm, constant pressure usually controls bleeding. If blood soaks through the first compress, add another, press more firmly, but don't remove the first compress.

Raising the wounded part of the body above the level of the victim's heart helps slow bleeding, too. (Don't move the injured part if it's broken, however.) Keep pressure over the wound even while it's raised.

Sometimes bleeding is so severe that direct pressure on the wound won't control it. Very heavy or uncontrollable bleeding is *hemorrhaging*. If this happens, put pressure on the artery which leads to the wound. This is called the pressure point. Arteries are the blood vessels carrying blood under high pressure, from the heart to all parts of the body. Compressing the artery against the underlying bone stops blood flow into the affected body part and stops bleeding from the wound. Continue to apply pressure to the wound and keep the wounded body part raised while using the pressure point technique. Don't use the pressure point technique for any longer than it takes to control bleeding because it cuts off blood flow to the entire area.

Sometimes a tourniquet is used to control prolonged bleeding. A tourniquet is a band of cloth or a belt placed on the pressure point above a wound and twisted tightly to cut off blood flow. Only trained professionals should use tourniquets which can cause serious damage if used improperly.

*Severe bleeding can be controlled by elevating the arm or leg and applying direct pressure on the wound and pressure points.*

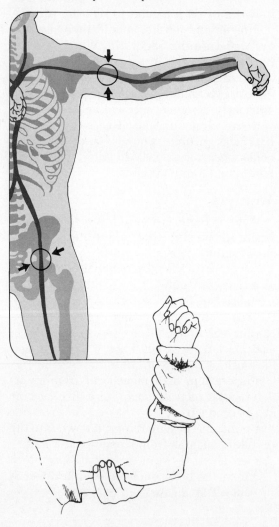

There are several pressure points in the body. The pressure point for the arm is half-way between the elbow and the armpit on the inside of the arm. The pressure point for the leg is in the leg crease of the groin area.

Open wounds can become infected. Once bleeding stops, preventing infection becomes the top priority. These steps will clean and protect the wound:

1. Wash your hands thoroughly.
2. Wash in and around the victim's wound with soap and water.
3. Rinse with clean water.
4. Dry the wound by gently patting with a clean cloth.
5. Apply a clean dry bandage. In many cases, you can use prepackaged adhesive bandages which come in many shapes and sizes. Avoid using ointment or first aid cream. Unless it's washed off and changed frequently, it does more harm than good.
6. If signs of infection appear, see a doctor.

## Shock

*Shock* is the disruption of blood flow in the body. Often it's caused by a large blood loss. It occurs with many major injuries, such as a car accident, severe bleeding, or serious burns.

When you see a victim bleeding, always look for signs of shock: pale, cool, and moist skin; weakness; rapid heart beat (over 100 beats per minute); restlessness; and shallow breathing.

Shock is a medical emergency. If you suspect shock, give first aid quickly. Acting quickly can make the difference between life and death. These are the rules when giving first aid for shock:

- Keep the victim lying down.
- Raise the victim's legs.
- Cover the victim with a light cover for warmth.

- Don't give the victim anything to drink.
- Get medical help as fast as possible.

## Asphyxiation

*Asphyxiation* means not breathing. When someone stops breathing, it's important to get breathing started again immediately. In most adults, brain damage begins after four minutes of not breathing. The first rule of first aid is to remove the cause of asphyxiation quickly.

- If someone is choking on something, remove it. The next section of this chapter discusses choking more fully.
- If an electrical shock causes asphyxiation, move the victim with a dry wooden pole, wooden chair, or broom, or turn off the source of the electric current. Current cannot travel through wood. Be careful to avoid the electrical current yourself. It could kill you.
- If poison gases cause asphyxiation, move the victim to fresh air.
- If you suspect a drug overdose, keep the air passage to the lungs open by lifting up on the chin and pushing down on the forehead.
- If the victim has a crushed chest, remove the crushing force, if possible.
- If the victim is drowning, remove the victim from the water, if possible.

After you remove the cause, help the victim start breathing again with mouth-to-mouth breathing. Begin mouth-to-mouth breathing as fast as possible:

1. Tip the victim's head so that the chin points up.
2. Pinch the victim's nose shut.
3. Take a deep breath, seal your mouth around the victim's mouth, and blow into the victim's mouth with two quick, full breaths.
4. Watch the victim's chest. It should fall as air leaves.

## Artificial Respiration

IF A VICTIM APPEARS TO BE UNCONSCIOUS — TAP VICTIM ON THE SHOULDER AND SHOUT, "ARE YOU OKAY?"

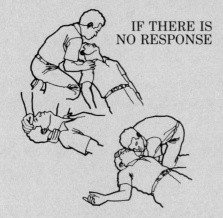

IF THERE IS NO RESPONSE — TILT THE VICTIM'S HEAD, CHIN POINTING UP. Place one hand under the victim's neck and gently lift. At the same time, push with the other hand on the victim's forehead. This will move the tongue away from the back of the throat to open the airway.

IMMEDIATELY LOOK, LISTEN, AND FEEL FOR AIR.
While maintaining the backward head tilt position, place your cheek and ear close to the victim's mouth and nose. Look for the chest to rise and fall while you listen and feel for the return of air. Check for about 5 seconds.

IF THE VICTIM IS NOT BREATHING — GIVE FOUR QUICK BREATHS.
Maintain the backward head tilt, pinch the victim's nose with the hand that is on the victim's forehead to prevent leakage of air, open your mouth wide, take a deep breath, seal your mouth around the victim's mouth, and blow into the victim's mouth with four quick but full breaths just as fast as you can. When blowing, use only enough time between breaths to lift your head slightly for better inhalation. For an infant, give gentle puffs and blow through the mouth and nose and do not tilt the head back as far as for an adult.

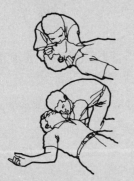

If you do not get an air exchange when you blow, it may help to reposition the head and try again.

AGAIN, LOOK, LISTEN, AND FEEL FOR AIR EXCHANGE.

IF THERE IS STILL NO BREATHING — CHANGE RATE TO ONE BREATH EVERY 5 SECONDS **FOR AN ADULT.**

**FOR AN INFANT,** GIVE ONE GENTLE PUFF EVERY 3 SECONDS.

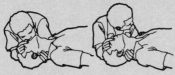

*This is not intended to replace a first aid or CPR course. Everyone should learn how to perform basic first aid and CPR skills. Call your local chapter of the American Red Cross for more information about these and other lifesaving courses.*

5. Begin a cycle of one breath every five seconds for a teen or adult.

Continue mouth-to-mouth breathing until the victim begins to breathe or until medical help arrives.

## Choking

It's easy for objects to get caught in the air passage to the lungs and cause choking, especially in children. When people choke, they aren't breathing enough air to survive. You need to respond quickly, or asphyxiation will result.

How will you know if someone is choking? Look for violent coughing, squealing breathing sounds, the victim grabbing his or her throat with both hands and unable to speak, bluish color of the face and neck, and possibly unconsciousness.

The purpose of first aid for choking is to get the victim breathing again. To do this, have the person sit down and try to cough up the object. If this doesn't work, begin the *Heimlich maneuver,* or abdominal thrusts, recommended by the American Heart Association and the American Red Cross:

1. Wrap your arms around the middle of the victim's body between the belly button and the ribs.
2. Make a fist with one hand. Place the thumb side of the fist against the victim's abdomen slightly above the navel. Grasp the fist with the other hand.
3. Apply the Heimlich maneuver by pressing the fist into the victim's abdomen with a quick upward thrust. Each new thrust should be a separate and distinct movement.
4. Look in the mouth for the expelled object. If it is not expelled, repeat the Heimlich maneuver.
5. When the object is expelled, if the victim is not breathing, give mouth-to-mouth breathing.

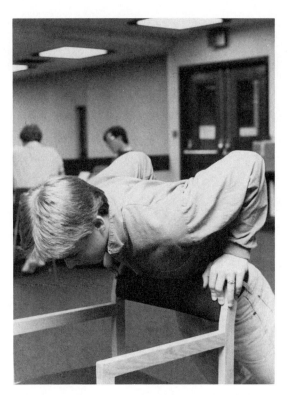

*If you're alone and start choking on food, lean over the back of a chair. Press your abdomen against the chair so that the air is forced out of your lungs. This should force the food loose from your throat.*

## Drowning

Most drownings occur within reach of safety. They occur close enough to shore or in shallow water, so the victim can be reached and rescued. Sometimes you may be able to rescue someone in the water without swimming yourself.

Only people trained in advanced lifesaving should attempt a swimming rescue. Even if you know how to swim, you may not be able to get and bring to safety a frantic drowning victim. You're more likely to be drowned yourself.

# First Aid for Choking

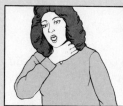

- **ASK: Are you choking?**
- If victim cannot breathe, cough, or speak . . .

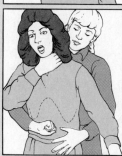

- **Give the Heimlich Maneuver.**
- Stand behind the victim.
- Wrap your arms around the victim's waist.
- Make a fist with one hand. PLACE your FIST (thumbside) against the victim's stomach in the midline just ABOVE THE NAVEL AND WELL BELOW THE RIB MARGIN.
- Grasp your fist with your other hand.
- PRESS INTO STOMACH WITH A QUICK UPWARD THRUST.

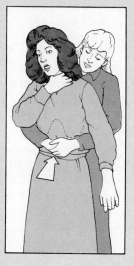

- **Repeat thrust if necessary.**

- **If a victim has become unconscious:**

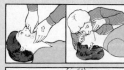

- Sweep the mouth.

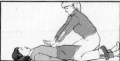

- Attempt rescue breathing.

- Give 6–10 abdominal thrusts.
- Repeat Steps 4, 5, and 6 as necessary.

**LOCAL EMERGENCY TELEPHONE NUMBER:** _____

Everyone should learn how to perform the steps above for choking and how to give rescue breathing and CPR. Call your local American Red Cross chapter for information on these and other first aid techniques. Caution: The Heimlich Maneuver (abdominal thrust) may cause injury. Do not *practice* on people.

**American Red Cross**

If a swimmer is in trouble near a dock, bridge, or pool edge, lie down and extend your hand, or look for a towel or branch to extend so you can pull the victim to safety. If you can't reach the victim, toss something that floats such as a buoy, an inner tube, or a board. The person can cling to this while you go for assistance. If a boat is nearby, row out. The victim can grab the boat or your oar.

If the victim is unconscious, get someone trained in advanced lifesaving. Mouth-to-mouth breathing should be begun as soon as possible, even while the victim is still in the water. This procedure should continue until the victim can breathe unaided.

## Poisoning

Almost all chemical substances are potential poisons. They are all around you at home, at school, and in public places. Think how often you see these potential poisons: cleaning products, such as bleach and ammonia; cosmetics and beauty aids; some house plants; medicines; paints and thinners; and spoiled food.

How do you know if someone has swallowed poison? If the victim can talk, ask. Suspect poisoning if you see any of these signs: burns on the mouth and lips, strange breath odor, stomach pain, vomiting, or an open container near the victim.

Poisoning is a life-or-death situation. You must respond quickly.

First aid for poisoning depends on whether the victim is conscious or not. If the victim is conscious, follow these procedures:

1. Dilute the poison by having the victim drink a glass of water or milk. But stop if the victim starts vomiting.
2. Call the poison control center.
3. Follow the poison control center's instructions. Give the antidote they recommend.

4. Take the victim to an emergency facility immediately. Take the container of poison along, if possible.

If the victim isn't conscious, follow these procedures:

1. Keep the airway open by tilting the chin up and pushing the forehead down.
2. Call 911 to get the victim to an emergency facility as quickly as possible.
3. Start doing mouth-to-mouth breathing, if necessary.
4. Don't give the victim anything to drink.
5. If possible, save a sample of the victim's vomit for the poison control center.
6. Give the container of poison to the personnel at the emergency facility.

## Burns

Burns most often are caused by steam, hot liquids, the sun, or by touching hot surfaces such as stove-tops. Burns also happen when people handle matches, fireplaces, and outdoor grills.

Burns are categorized by how severe they are:

- First-degree burns. The outer layers of skin redden.
- Second-degree burns. Skin blisters.
- Third-degree burns. All skin layers are damaged. Burns such as these are very serious.

Burns are painful, even first-degree burns. A burn is also a place where infections can start. Treat burns quickly for the victim's comfort, and cover quickly to prevent infection. First aid treatment depends on the degree of the burn.

Most first-degree burns heal rapidly and usually don't require professional medical treatment unless the burns cover a large part of the body. For first-degree burns, give the following first aid treatment:

1. Soothe the burn in cold water, but never put ice on a burn.

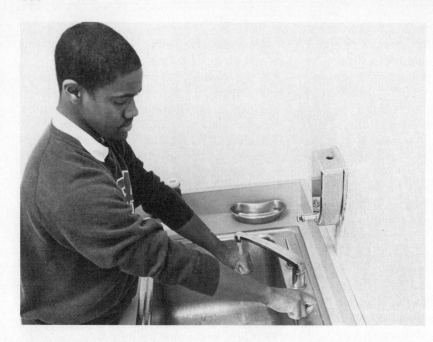

*Soothe minor burns with cold water to minimize blistering.*

2. Cover the burn with a dry piece of gauze or a bandage, if necessary.

Second-degree burns are more serious than first-degree burns. For second-degree burns, give the following first aid treatment:

1. Soothe the burned skin with cold water to relieve pain. Again, don't use ice.
2. Dry the burned area by gently patting the skin with a dry cloth.
3. Cover the burned area with a dry piece of gauze or bandage.
4. Don't apply ointments or salves. They aren't necessary for healing and may lead to infection.
5. Don't pop blisters or peel the skin. This increases the chance for infection.
6. Get medical attention for facial or large burns or if signs of infection occur.

For third-degree burns, get medical help immediately. However, if this isn't possible, give the following first aid treatment until medical help comes:

1. If clothing is causing continued burning, such as clothing absorbed with hot oil, remove it. Never, however, remove clothing which sticks to burned skin.
2. Cover the burn with clean, moist cloths. Don't apply salves or ointment.
3. Elevate burned arms or legs.
4. Watch for signs of shock, and treat accordingly.

## Heat Exposure

In warm temperatures, your body is exposed to heat, and perspiration cools you down. Too much heat, however, can be hard on the body.

### HEAT CRAMPS

Heat cramps are one effect of heat exposure. Heat cramps are muscle spasms that occur in the abdomen, arms, and legs.

Give first aid by replacing salt and water lost through sweating. Offer sips of salt water (one teaspoon of salt in one cup of water). Give a half cup every 15 minutes. Be careful that the person doesn't take in too much salt at one time. Allow the victim to rest in a cool place. Gently rubbing the muscles helps relieve cramps, too.

### HEAT EXHAUSTION

Heat exhaustion happens when the body no longer can cope with heat. It's brought on by the body losing a lot of salt and water through perspiration. When the heat is severe, a victim of heat exhaustion may have these symptoms: pale and clammy skin, profuse sweating, listlessness, an upset stomach, dizziness, and close to normal body temperature.

Give first aid for heat exhaustion at the first signs by following these steps:
1. Take the victim to a cool place.
2. Lie the victim down with the feet up a few inches to increase blood circulation back to the heart.
3. Give the victim salt water as you would for heat cramps.
4. Pat the victim's face and neck with a cool, damp cloth.
5. Get medical help.

### HEATSTROKE

*Heatstroke* is a severe physical response to heat. The victim has an extremely high body temperature and loses the ability to sweat. Because people with heatstroke can't sweat, they have no way to cool their bodies.

Heatstroke is a medical emergency, requiring immediate treatment. If you don't treat it fast and in the right way, the victim will die. You can recognize heatstroke by these symptoms: very high body temperature, higher than 105° F; hot, red, dry skin; fast heartbeat; and non-alert behavior, possibly unconsciousness.

The goal of first aid for a heatstroke victim is to cool the body as fast as possible. When you recognize heatstroke, be sure to act quickly:
1. Sponge the body with cool water or rubbing alcohol.

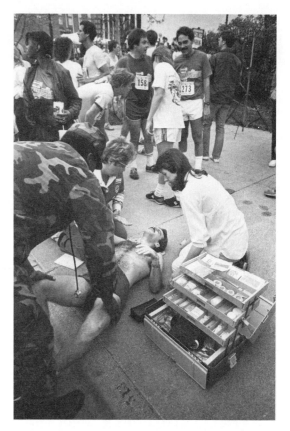

*Treat a victim of heat exhaustion immediately. These paramedics will cool the runner's body by applying damp cloths to his face and neck.*

2. If available, apply cold packs, such as an ice bag to the head, neck, armpits, and groin.
3. If possible, put the victim in a tub of cold water, but don't use ice.
4. Use drafts of cool air from fans or air conditioners to cool the victim.
5. Check the temperature often. When the body temperature drops below 102° F, stop these drastic measures, and treat the victim as you would for a fever. But if the victim's temperature starts to rise again, resume first aid for heatstroke.
6. Call a doctor immediately.

# Cold Exposure

Exposure to cold can't always be avoided. If you live or visit in cold climates, you are exposed to its dangers. Cold temperatures can harm the body in different ways.

### FROSTBITE

Have you ever been outside in cold weather without gloves? Or have you gone snow skiing without a face mask? After 30 minutes, how did your fingers or your face feel? How did they look?

Frostbite is when your skin and underlying body tissues freeze. It affects the parts of the body that are exposed to cold for too long. It occurs most often to the ears, face, fingers, and toes.

These are the signs of frostbite: pink skin that turns gray, pale, and glossy; pain, then numbness in the frostbitten part of the body; blisters on the skin; and possible mental confusion. When these signs appear, the skin is already frozen and may be dead.

Frostbite is dangerous, and it requires emergency first aid. Immerse the frozen part of the body in warm, not hot, water immediately. If you have no warm water, wrap the frostbitten area gently in warm blankets. See a doctor right away.

These are some things you must not do because they damage frostbitten skin:

- Don't apply anything hot, such as a hot water bottle or a heating pad.
- Don't break blisters. Remember that this can cause an infection.
- Don't rub the frostbitten area.
- Don't put on bandages except between the toes and fingers to keep them from touching each other.
- Don't allow the victim to walk on frostbitten toes.

### HYPOTHERMIA

Exposure to cold can cause *hypothermia*. This is a gradual cooling of the body's inner core. It causes all of the body systems to slow down, and unless heat loss is reversed, death results.

It doesn't take freezing temperatures to cause hypothermia. People can lose dangerous amounts of heat when the outside temperature is 40° to 50° F especially if it's windy or raining or if their clothing is wet. You can recognize hypothermia by these symptoms: body temperature below 94° F, uncontrollable shivering, slurred speech, increasing clumsiness, drowsiness, mental confusion, and in the later stages, unconsciousness.

When you give first aid for hypothermia, act quickly, especially if the victim is already unconscious. It can be a matter of life or death. First aid for hypothermia includes these procedures:

1. If the victim isn't breathing, use mouth-to-mouth breathing.
2. Bring the victim to a warm, sheltered place.
3. Remove any wet clothes.
4. Redress the victim in dry warm clothes and wrap him or her in warm blankets.
5. If the victim is conscious, give warm liquids, such as soup, coffee, or tea.
6. Get medical help.

# Sprains and Fractures

Falls are the most common accidents. When you fall, you hit the ground—hard! The force of impact from falls and other accidents can cause sprains and fractures. *Fractures* are broken bones. A sprain is an overstretched or torn part of a muscle, ligament, or joint.

Fractures and sprains often happen from falls and car accidents. They also happen during recreational and sports activities. If you play contact sports such as football, hockey, or soccer, you've probably been knocked down. That's when injuries often happen.

*Give hot fluids, such as tea and soup, to victims of cold exposure. Contrary to popular belief, don't give alcohol because it causes the body to lose its warmth more quickly.*

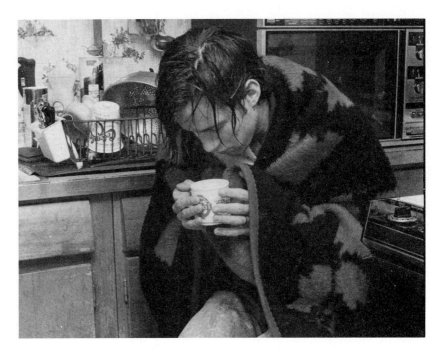

The ankle is the most common site of a sprain. How do you recognize a sprain? Look for swelling, pain when you move or touch the injured joint, redness, and bruising. What is first aid for a sprain?

1. Loosen tight clothing around the sprain.
2. Raise the injured part of the body above the level of the victim's heart to prevent swelling.
3. Apply a cold pack, such as an ice bag, for the first 24 hours after injury.
4. After 24 hours, apply warmth with a hot water bottle or a heating pad.
5. Go to the doctor.
6. Don't use the injured part of the body—rest.

A sprain may not seem serious. You give first aid and think that's enough. But even a minor sprain should be examined by a doctor. Maybe it's worse than you think. There may be bleeding in the joint or a chipped bone. The only way to be sure is to get an X-ray.

Sometimes the victim knows a bone is broken by hearing or feeling the bone break. Perhaps the victim feels the bone pieces grating together. Or maybe the victim can't control the way the injured part of the body moves. Of course, there may be a great deal of pain, too.

The person giving first aid needs to look for any of these signs of a fracture: swelling, redness and bruising, pain when the injured area is touched, inability to move or put weight on the injured part, an injured part that looks bent, a broken bone that can be seen through torn skin.

Some signs of a fracture and a sprain are the same. A doctor can tell the difference by looking at an X-ray. When in doubt, give first aid for a fracture until the victim gets to an emergency facility.

A splint is used when giving first aid for a broken bone. This keeps the victim from moving the injured part of the body. It's important to keep the injured part still to prevent further injury. It also helps relieve pain.

A splint can be made from different materials. You may have to be resourceful and use whatever rigid material you can find, such as a straight stick or branch, a rolled magazine or newspaper, a piece of stiff cardboard, or a rolled blanket or towel. A splint can be tied in place with different materials, too. You can use scarves, belts, neckties, or strips of cloth. This is how you apply a splint:

1. Put a pad between the splint and the skin. Include the joints above and below the fracture in the splint.
2. Tie the splint on snugly, but not too tight, in two places, one above and one below the fracture. Watch the injured part. If it turns blue, the ties are too tight; loosen slightly.
3. If the injured part is bent out of line, splint it in that position. Do not try to straighten it out.

## Animal, Snake, and Insect Bites

Many types of animals, snakes, and insects bite humans. They cause wounds, such as punctures, lacerations, and even avulsions, which you learned about earlier in this chapter.

You need to treat animal bites quickly to control bleeding, prevent infection, and guard against rabies. Rabies is a disease of mostly wild animals that's spread by their saliva. Once rabies is in its final stage, there is no cure. So anyone bitten by an animal should be given first aid and then quickly taken for medical treatment.

Bites from pets, such as dogs and cats, are the most common animal bites, but bites from wild animals, such as snakes, squirrels, and raccoons happen, too. First aid for animal bites is to do the following:

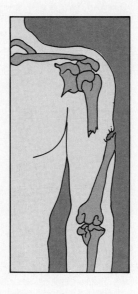

*With an open fracture, you need to give first aid for both the wound and the broken bone.*

1. Control bleeding as you would for any wound.
2. Wash the wound with soap and water.
3. Flush the wound several times with water.
4. Cover the wound with a clean bandage.
5. Limit the victim's movement until he or she can be seen by a doctor.

If possible, catch the animal and turn it over to the authorities. The animal, even if it's a pet, must be observed for signs of rabies. If the animal has rabies, the victim needs to be treated with a vaccine.

Snakebites can be very dangerous if the snake is poisonous. Such bites need to be treated with special first aid. In the United States, only a few snakes are poisonous.

To recognize a snakebite, look for: puncture wounds, swelling, a red or bluish color around the wound, and complaints of pain from the victim. With snakebites from a poisonous snake, there also may be signs of general sickness from the poison, or venom. Look for weakness, nausea, breathing difficulty, and blurred vision.

The purpose of first aid for a poisonous snakebite is to prevent the venom from getting into the victim's bloodstream. Act quickly to do the following:
1. Keep the victim lying down and very still.
2. Keep the bitten area below the level of the heart.
3. Get the victim to a doctor.

Someone with advanced first aid training might apply a snug band above the bite or possibly cut the bite and suck out the venom. This should not be attempted by anyone who has not been trained!

People are bitten by insects all the time. Insect bites are usually no more than an annoyance. Bites from mosquitoes, fleas, ants, and chiggers cause itching or a little pain, but these symptoms usually are gone in a day or two. First aid is for comfort, and it includes the following:
1. Wash the bitten area of the body with soap and water.
2. Apply an ice pack or a cool cloth.
3. Apply calamine lotion or rubbing alcohol to the skin to stop itching.
4. Discourage the victim from scratching the bitten area because it could cause infection.

Bites from other insects, such as wasps and black widow spiders may be dangerous and need additional treatment if the person has an allergic or severe reaction. Act quickly to:
1. Apply ice to the area to reduce the swelling.
2. Keep the bitten or stung part below the level of the heart and don't let the victim move it.
3. Get the victim to a doctor immediately.

As with a snakebite, a trained person may apply a snug band to prevent any insect venom from going into the victim's circulation. But this takes special training!

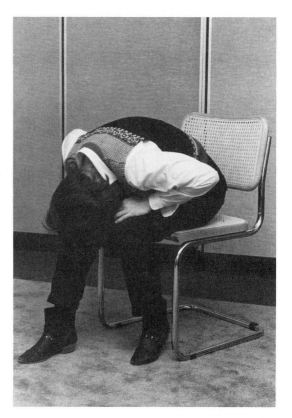

*If you feel like fainting, bend over or squat down with your head on your knees. This may prevent you from fainting. Or at least you won't fall and hit your head.*

## Fainting

Sometimes a person collapses without warning. It can happen for many reasons, such as emotional shock or overly strenuous exercise. It's caused by too little circulation of blood to the brain. Usually the victim recovers within two or three minutes after falling or lying down.

Often you can tell when someone is about to faint. The person may be pale, sweaty or clammy, dizzy, or nauseous. Or perhaps the victim's vision is blurred.

You can help someone prevent fainting. Have the person lie down if possible. Or have the person bend over and, with head placed on the knees, squat or sit down.

If the person still faints, follow these steps:

1. Keep the victim lying down.
2. Loosen the victim's clothes.
3. Keep the airway open so the victim can breathe.
4. Pat the victim's head and neck with a cool cloth.
5. Don't give the victim anything to drink.
6. Check for injuries if the victim has fallen.
7. Take the victim to an emergency facility.

## Heart Attacks

Not all emergencies requiring first aid are caused by injury. Some, such as heart attacks and seizures, are caused by illness.

Heart attacks can happen to people of all ages, but they usually occur to older adults. They happen during strenuous activity, but they also happen to people at rest. A heart attack is a life-or-death emergency. Treat it quickly and seriously.

Would you be able to recognize a heart attack victim? These are the signs: chest pain, especially if it moves into the neck, shoulders, or arms; gasping for breath; pale or blue skin; upset stomach; weakness.

React immediately to these signs. The victim's life may depend upon it. First aid for a heart attack is to:

1. Lie the victim down.
2. Raise the head if the victim can't breath.
3. Call 911, your local rescue squad, or the phone operator if neither of the first two is available to you.
4. Be prepared to give CPR.

*By taking classes in CPR, people become trained and certified to help victims of heart attacks.*

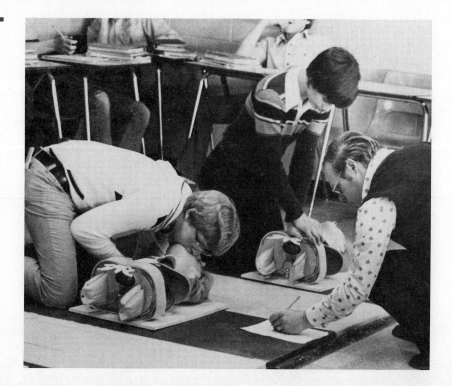

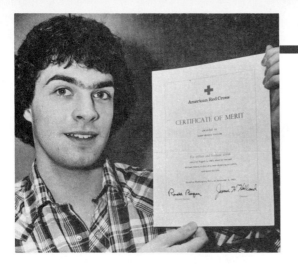

# TEENS SAVE LIVES

$S$adly, accidents and sudden illnesses claim many lives. But that's what first aid, CPR, and water safety training are all about. Anyone, no matter what age, with the ability to study and master these skills can save a life. And that's just what John and Molly did.

In 1983, 17-year-old John Taylor was at summer camp. While hiking near the Montreal Falls, he and a group of friends decided to go for a swim. One person in the group wanted to dive into the water at the foot of a dangerous waterfall. While out on the rock by the falls, he slipped in and was quickly pulled under the water by the churning current. He surfaced briefly and then went under again, this time loosing his life jacket to the force of the water. Screams of the group alerted John to the emergency. He saw his friend pulled out of reach.

No one else in the group felt capable of attempting a rescue, but John had just taken the Red Cross Advanced Lifesaving and Water Safety Instructor training earlier in the summer.

John swam to his friend, dived under water to grab him, and brought him to the surface. John then replaced his friend's life jacket, which was floating nearby, and carried him over 125 feet through the water until he reached shore. Without John's heroic rescue, his friend surely would have drowned.

In the summer of 1986, 14-year-old Molly Nordstrom often babysat for eight-month-old Tamra. Babysitting usually involved the routine tasks of feeding, diapering, and playing with Tamra. But on June 26, Molly faced a much bigger challenge.

While looking in on Tamra as she slept, Molly noticed that the baby was perfectly still and blue colored. Scared about what she should do, she hesitated for just a moment and began to cry. But then she remembered the CPR she'd learned in school. "I grabbed Tamra out of the crib and laid her on the sofa. I started mouth-to-mouth breathing and then CPR." When Tamra started to breathe, Molly called 911 and Tamra's mom.

The paramedics took Tamra to the hospital where she made a full recovery from what doctors think was sudden infant death syndrome, or crib death, which you'll read about in Chapter 9. Thanks to Molly's lifesaving skills, a child who would otherwise have died now enjoys a healthy, happy life.

*Cardiopulmonary resuscitation* (CPR) is the emergency treatment for someone whose heart stops beating. It includes mouth-to-mouth breathing and pressing on the chest in a special way. To perform this lifesaving skill, you need to take a special training course in CPR. You learn this skill by practicing on a manikin, or life-size doll. Both the American Red Cross and the American Heart Association offer CPR courses. Cardiopulmonary resuscitation follows three steps. They are as simple as A-B-C.

A = airway opened
B = breathing returned
C = circulation of blood returned

To keep the airway open, tilt the head and lift the chin up so the airway is not blocked. By giving mouth-to-mouth breaths, breathing returns. You can bring back circulation by pressing on the lower half of the victim's breastbone in a rhythmic motion with your palms. By doing these things, you breathe for the victim and squeeze the heart. This forces blood to circulate. You keep the victim alive until emergency services arrive.

## Seizures

A seizure is a symptom of several conditions. A person with epilepsy, a high fever, brain damage, or an emotional upset might have a seizure. Nearly four million people in the United States have a condition which causes seizures. Most of these people take medicine as prevention.

During a major seizure, often called a grand mal seizure, a person loses consciousness and has jerky movements of all parts of the body. A seizure usually lasts for about 45 seconds.

First aid for seizures helps protect the person from harm and ensures that breathing starts again after the seizure is over. If you see someone having a seizure, go to their aid immediately. Do the following:
1. Move objects away from the victim.
2. If possible, put something soft under the victim's head.

After the seizure, provide this first aid treatment:
1. Loosen the clothing around the neck.
2. Make sure the air passage to the lungs is open by lifting up on the chin and pushing back on the forehead.
3. Check for breathing. Give mouth-to-mouth breathing if necessary.
4. Keep the victim lying down.
5. Get medical help.

The following practices are not safe:
- Never put anything between the victim's teeth.
- Don't throw water on the victim during or after a seizure.
- Don't restrain the victim in any way.
- Don't try to give the victim medicine or anything to drink during the seizure.

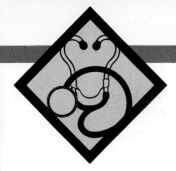

# CHAPTER CHECKUP

## Reviewing the Information

1. Where should a first aid kit be kept?
2. Name three safety courses that prepare you for an emergency.
3. What is the Good Samaritan Law?
4. List four questions to ask yourself when you arrive at the scene of an accident.
5. What is the three-digit phone number to call in an emergency?
6. What information should you convey about an emergency when you call for help?
7. What does a Medic Alert tag tell you?
8. Name four emergency services you can call for help.
9. Describe the five types of wounds.
10. What is the first and most important rule in giving first aid for wounds?
11. What are the causes of asphyxiation?
12. How would you treat someone in shock?
13. How do you give mouth-to-mouth breathing?
14. What is the Heimlich maneuver?
15. What is basic first aid for poisoning?
16. What injuries occur from exposure to cold? Heat?
17. How do you treat a victim of heat stroke?
18. To splint a fractured leg without a first aid kit, what materials could you use?
19. What is CPR?

## Thinking It Over

1. To what public recreational events should you bring a first aid kit?
2. What emergency services should be called to a fire in a senior citizens' apartment building?
3. Name five substances in your house that are potential poisons and what you would do if someone swallowed them.
4. What is the difference between treating a first-degree burn and a third-degree burn?
5. Why could someone suffer from hypothermia in 45° F temperatures?
6. What would you do if your friend fainted, and no one was nearby?

## Taking Action

 1. List the supplies in a homemade first aid kit. Calculate the total cost of the kit.

 2. Read and then report on an article in your local newspaper that involves an emergency situation or rescue.

3. Prepare lists of phone numbers for local emergency services. Post them beside all phones in your home.
4. Using a map of your community, star the locations of emergency services.
5. Find the pressure points on your own body. You'll feel the artery pulsing.
6. Obtain and read emergency preparedness brochures from your local American Red Cross chapter.

# 7 Disease Control

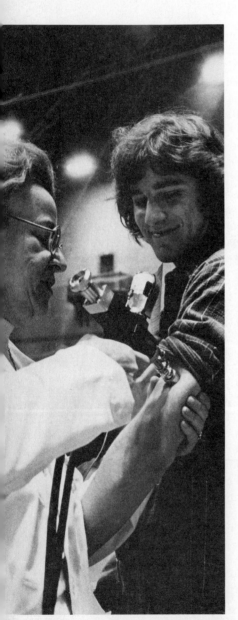

After reading this chapter, you should be able to:

- list practices that prevent communicable diseases from spreading.

- explain the causes of several chronic diseases.

- describe mental illness.

## Terms to Understand

| | |
|---|---|
| antibiotics | immunity |
| carcinogen | immunization |
| carrier | incubation period |
| chemotherapy | pathogens |
| chronic | psychotherapy |
| communicable disease | risk factors |
| contagious | vaccine |

Nobody likes to be sick. Being ill is inconvenient, it takes up time, and it's no fun. Most people do get sick now and then, and they usually get well soon—if they take good care of themselves.

Lifestyle affects health, the chances of becoming sick, and the speed of recovery. Maintaining good health requires a nutritious diet, good personal hygiene, regular exercise, routine medical checkups, and adequate rest. Avoiding cigarettes, alcohol, and illegal drugs promotes health, too. You can prevent many illnesses. The choice is yours.

## Disease—What Is It?

Disease is the term for most sicknesses. There are many different types of diseases that vary in many ways.

First, diseases can be spread in different ways—by people, animals, objects, or through the air.

Some diseases are contagious; others aren't. *Contagious* diseases are those which can be spread from one person to another, such as by coughing, sneezing, or using the same eating utensils. Chickenpox is contagious, and heart disease isn't.

Some diseases affect almost the whole body; others affect only one part. For example, the flu affects the chest, throat, stomach, joints, and other body parts. Athlete's foot only affects feet.

Some diseases are common while others are rare. Practically everybody gets colds, but there are many diseases that only a handful of people ever get.

The cause of a disease may or may not be known. We understand the causes of polio, for example, but not of cancer. Some diseases have physical causes, while others have emotional causes.

The outcome of a disease, or its prognosis, can be good or bad. For a disease such as flu the prognosis is usually good—usually complete recovery. However, for many diseases, such as colon cancer, the prognosis may be poor. Victims may have to live the rest of

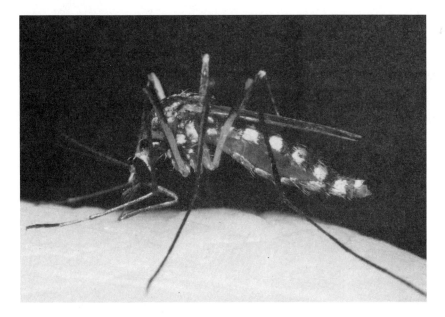

*The bite of a mosquito can carry many different diseases, such as malaria, yellow fever, and skin diseases.*

their lives with the effects. Some diseases are incurable and eventually result in death. Even people with many incurable diseases can live a relatively good life, if they carefully follow the physicians' guidelines.

Some diseases are hardly noticed, while others are severe. The difference is in the way they affect life or the family's ability to continue usual routines. For example, how often have you gone to school with a mild cold or athlete's foot? These diseases aren't serious because they have little or no effect on your life.

Some diseases, such as a serious case of pneumonia, heart disease, or most types of cancer, seriously disrupt life. These diseases cause emotional stress as everyone worries about the threat to the person's health and life. Doctor visits and possibly hospitalization are inconvenient. Medical expenses may be a financial burden. A sick child may not be able to attend school, and a sick adult may not be able to work.

## Infectious Diseases

Infectious diseases occur when pathogens get into the body and then start growing and multiplying. *Pathogens* are tiny disease-carrying organisms. Most pathogens are called germs and can only be seen through a microscope. Pathogens include a wide variety of bacteria and viruses. Bacteria are one-celled organisms; the streptococcus bacteria, for example, cause strep throat. Viruses cause diseases, such as chickenpox, flu, and colds.

Other pathogens are not classified as germs because they are not microorganisms—you do not necessarily need a micro-

scope to see them. These pathogens include tapeworms, roundworms, and flatworms. This chapter deals only with pathogens most commonly referred to as germs.

When a pathogen first attacks your body, you don't even know you're ill. The infection stays and grows in your body for hours or days without any signs of disease. This is the *incubation period* of the infection—before the first symptoms appear. When signs eventually appear, you realize that you're sick.

Every day your body is exposed to pathogens from many sources. People are the most common source. If someone outwardly shows

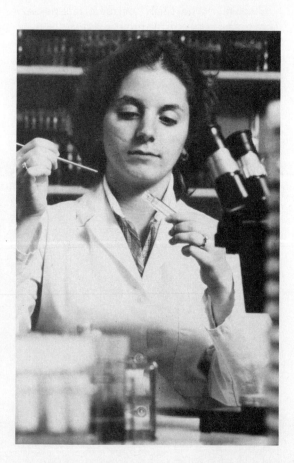

*A health professional examines pathogens under a microscope as part of diagnosing a disease.*

signs of illness, you know to stay away from him or her. But some people have the pathogen in their bodies and don't show any signs of disease. Perhaps they've recovered from the disease already, or they have a very mild case. These people can still infect you with the disease even though they don't appear sick. They are disease *carriers*.

Infections are spread from one person to another by touching or through tiny droplets of mucus or saliva passed in a sneeze or a kiss. Pathogens are also spread by objects, such as dishes or bathroom towels, handled by an infected person.

Not all infectious diseases are spread by people. Some diseases, such as encephalitis, are spread by insects which bite an infected person then spread the disease by biting an uninfected person. Animals with a disease such as rabies spread that disease when they bite another animal or a person. Still other infections can be caught by eating spoiled or contaminated food or by drinking contaminated water.

The healthier you are, the better your resistance to disease. Resistance is your body's ability to fight off infections when you're exposed to germs. When your resistance is low, germs invade your body and may cause infectious disease. When your resistance is high, your body fights off the germs, and you don't get sick.

Bacterial infections can be treated with *antibiotics*. These medicines help keep germs from multiplying and destroy those already in your body. Penicillin and tetracycline are commonly used antibiotics. Viral infections cannot be treated with antibiotics.

## Communicable Diseases

Infectious diseases are caught from pathogens. When an infectious disease is spread from one person to another, it is called a *communicable disease*. When you have a communicable disease you are contagious to people around you.

Colds, flu, mononucleosis, hepatitis, and sexually-transmitted diseases are the most common communicable diseases in the United States today. Many childhood diseases are communicable, too. You'll learn more about these in Chapter 10.

Not too many years ago, people died by the thousands of communicable diseases, such as smallpox, typhoid fever, and tuberculosis, that couldn't be controlled easily. Today very few people in the United States ever get these diseases because we know how to control them. If found early enough, most communicable diseases can be cured.

## Common Cold

A cold is never fatal. It rarely leads to serious illness. However, more people in the United States miss work and school because of colds than from any other disease.

Colds are caused by several different viruses. These viruses often change so frequently it's not possible to have medicine for every one. Because cold viruses are so contagious, they're easy to pass along. Smokers and people under stress tend to have more colds, but no one knows exactly why.

Signs of a cold are familiar: a stuffy, runny nose, sneezing, and sometimes a sore throat, headache, and fatigue. Usually with a cold, there's no fever unless you develop an accompanying infection.

| Look for These Common Symptoms of Illness | |
|---|---|
| • Cough | • Itch |
| • Fatigue | • Pain |
| • Fever | • Sore throat |

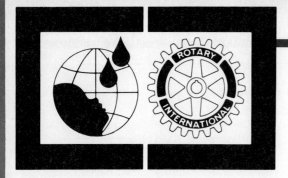

# POLIOPLUS

Imagine a disease-free world. If an organization called the Rotary Foundation of Rotary International has its way, the world will at least be free of polio! Since 1979, Rotary International has been involved in the fight against this dreaded disease. In 1985, it launched "PolioPlus."

Polio is a word that strikes fear in the hearts of parents. Over the years, this infectious disease of the nervous system has killed and crippled hundreds of thousands, many of them children and teens. When the oral vaccine came into widespread use in the 1960's, there was hope that the disease would be completely eliminated. In fact, today in the United States, less than 20 cases are reported a year.

The hope to eliminate polio in other parts of the world, however, hasn't been realized. In underdeveloped countries, especially in Africa and Asia, millions of children don't even get the vaccine. The World Health Organization estimates every year polio strikes up to 275,000 people. At least one in every 200 children born in the developing world will suffer the crippling effects of polio.

"PolioPlus" is the Rotary's answer. This program plans to provide regular polio immunizations to all children worldwide by the year 2005. Through "PolioPlus," the

Rotary Foundation will supply the following to countries:

- Vaccine for up to five years
- Teams of health professionals to plan and provide the immunization program by request only
- Support to the countries' existing health resources
- Assistance in educating people about the need for immunizations

Already, massive immunization has taken place in Paraguay, Turkey, Mexico, and the Sudan. There are 42 other countries currently on the list targeted for "PolioPlus." The foundation is also working with many other governments and world-wide health agencies. The Rotary Foundation has a worthy, yet ambitious, goal!

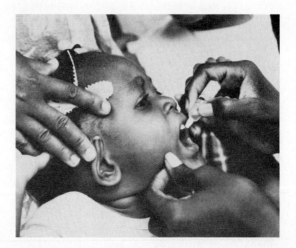

Name of Product

Net Volume

*Over-the-counter drugs are labeled according to federal law for your protection. Read them carefully, and follow the directions and warnings for safety.*

Dosage

Active Ingredients

Warning

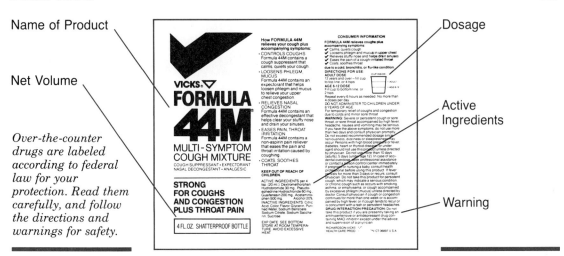

Medicines are available at the drugstore to relieve cold symptoms, but there are no cures. Aspirin or acetaminophen help relieve achiness. Nasal decongestants and antihistamines are medicines that can help dry up stuffy noses and relieve itchy eyes. Antiseptic or salt water gargles sometimes provide relief from a sore throat. Always be sure to check with your doctor before taking any medicine.

The most reliable way to recover from a cold is to rest and to drink plenty of liquids. Stay home from school, work, and social activities for a few days, preferably in bed, or at least rest quietly. Drink liquids, such as fruit juices, water, and broth. A cool-air humidifier may help you breathe more comfortably. If a cold lasts longer than a few days or gets worse, call your doctor.

To dispel a common myth, large doses of vitamin C do not prevent or cure a cold. In fact, taking too much (over 100 or 200 milligrams daily) may be hard on the kidneys. You get enough vitamin C in a daily serving of citrus juice.

Colds spread easily to others. So stay home while you're sick. And cover your mouth and nose when you cough or sneeze to keep germs from spreading.

The best way to avoid catching a cold is to get plenty of rest, eat nutritious foods, avoid becoming chilled, and stay away from people with colds since they're contagious. During the winter months, when colds are common, avoid crowds.

## Influenza

Influenza, or the flu, is caused by viruses. But there are so many different types of flu-causing viruses that your body can never build up resistance to all of them. Some people have several bouts with flu every year. Each bout may be caused by a different virus.

Influenza is very contagious. Over time, it has killed millions. In World War I, 24,000 soldiers died of influenza!

The flu is an infection of the respiratory system, similar to a cold. The respiratory system includes the nose, sinuses, throat, bronchial tubes, and lungs. Unlike a cold, the flu is a systemic infection, or one which infects the entire body. It causes fever, chills, muscle aches, and overall weakness. The biggest danger is that it often leads to pneumonia, a serious respiratory disease. This is especially true for elderly people and people who aren't healthy to begin with. These people should do everything they can to avoid the flu, including being immunized.

Treatment for influenza is similar to treatment for a cold—treat the symptoms. Stay home in bed, rest, drink lots of liquids, and eat nutritious foods. Take medicines on the advice of the doctor.

## Mononucleosis

Mononucleosis, usually called mono, is a viral infection characterized by a severe sore throat, a feeling of tiredness, and sometimes swelling of two body organs—the lymph nodes and spleen. Lymph nodes and the spleen help fight infection.

Mono is a common disease among teenagers. It's been nicknamed the "kissing disease" because it was once thought that the virus was spread through saliva when kissing. Kissing is one means of spreading the disease, but it's also thought to be spread in other ways.

A typical case of mono might follow this course:

1. Three or four days of fatigue
2. Five to 10 days of sore throat, 101° F fever, swollen lymph nodes in the neck, upset stomach, and possibly a swollen spleen
3. One to three weeks of gradually diminishing fatigue

Mononucleosis that lasts for three to six months is rare. Teenagers with mono usually return to school within a few weeks. Some people with mononucleosis have no symptoms. These people are still carriers, however.

Early symptoms of mononucleosis are similar to those of a cold or the flu. If you have cold or flu symptoms that don't go away in a few days, see your doctor. A simple blood test can confirm the disease. If the disease shows you have mono, stay home and rest until you recover.

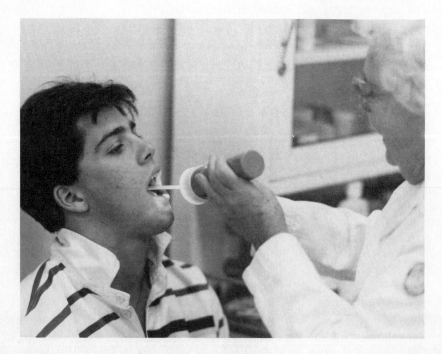

*One of the first signs of mononucleosis is swollen lymph glands of the neck. Have a nurse check them if you feel very tired.*

# Hepatitis

Hepatitis is a viral infection of the liver. The liver is the largest body organ and is essential to life. Hepatitis has been around for hundreds of years but has become more common in this century.

There are two different viruses that cause hepatitis, virus A and virus B. The viruses usually are passed on, or transmitted, to people in different ways, and strike people of different age groups.

The type A virus in infectious hepatitis can be found in both the bloodstream and the intestines. The virus may be passed along when someone eats or drinks something that contains the virus. Anything that comes in contact with any of the body secretions—blood, mucus, saliva, urine, or feces—of a person infected with hepatitis A becomes contaminated with that virus. Children, teens, and young adults are the most susceptible to hepatitis A.

Type B virus, called serum hepatitis, is found only in the bloodstream. Drug users can get it from sharing dirty needles. Very few people get it through blood transfusions. Serum hepatitis more likely occurs in people over age 30.

The symptoms are the same for both types of hepatitis. With hepatitis B, the symptoms are more severe, and they usually last longer. The most noticeable symptom of both types is jaundice, which is yellowing of the skin and the whites of the eyes. Other symptoms include some or all of the following: upset stomach, loss of appetite, dark urine, very light-colored bowel movements, weakness, fever, and a swollen and sore liver.

People with hepatitis should be under a doctor's care. Rest, a nutritious diet, and lots to drink are important in treating the disease and for protecting the body from permanent damage. Cleanliness is important because the body can reinfect itself.

The incubation period for hepatitis can be up to six months. By the time symptoms appear, it's hard to trace the source of the disease.

Since hepatitis is so contagious, be very careful around someone who has it. Follow guidelines for protecting against communicable disease.

# Sexually-Transmitted Diseases

Sexually-transmitted diseases (STDs), previously called venereal diseases (VDs), are spread through direct contact during sexual activity. Their spread is a serious health problem. Every year more than 10 million Americans contract a sexually-transmitted disease. These diseases are second only to colds and flu as the most common communicable diseases in the United States.

*In many doctors' offices you will find an assortment of brochures that will help you better understand diseases and their control.*

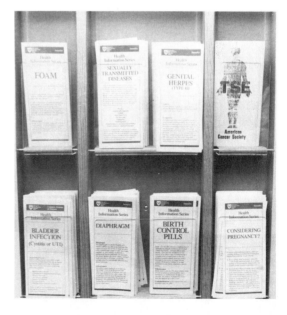

The only way to guarantee prevention of STDs is avoid sexual intercourse. To reduce the spread of STDs infected persons must be identified quickly so their sexual contacts can be identified and treated. STDs won't go away on their own, and there are no home remedies. Professional medical treatment is always necessary.

## GONORRHEA

Gonorrhea is a common STD. Two million cases are reported each year. It's caused by certain bacteria. Gonorrhea has a short incubation period, three to 14 days, so symptoms show up quickly after someone is infected. This makes it easier to identify and treat others who have been infected by that person.

A man with gonorrhea has a yellowish pus-like discharge from his penis. He also has burning when he urinates. If it's not treated, the disease goes through the whole body. Then the man has a fever, swelling in the groin, and can't urinate. Untreated, gonorrhea can lead to sterility, or inability to reproduce.

Women with gonorrhea may have a yellowish discharge from the vagina, pain when they urinate, and itching. But many have no symptoms at all. Without treatment, women develop infections in their female organs which can cause sterility.

In both men and women, the outward symptoms may go away temporarily, leading them to think the disease cured itself. But the disease continues to grow inside their bodies, and they can also infect other people. Babies of infected pregnant women can get gonorrhea when they pass through an infected birth canal.

There is a simple test that confirms the presence of gonorrhea. Once it's detected, the disease can usually be treated successfully with the antibiotic, penicillin. Follow-up treatment is wise to be sure that the gonorrhea bacterium has been completely destroyed.

## SYPHILIS

Syphilis is a destructive STD. Untreated, it infects all systems of the body. It kills over 50,000 people in the United States every year and infects five times that many.

Syphilis is caused by another bacterium. It is almost always transmitted by sexual intercourse. Then, through the bloodstream, it goes to other parts of the body. There are three stages of syphilis.

In the first stage, a painless sore, called a chancre, may appear on the penis or in the vagina. This occurs one to 10 weeks after sexual contact and goes away on its own even without treatment. However, the disease continues to develop and spread throughout the body.

About six weeks into the disease, the second stage begins with a rash on the hands, feet, or face. Also some hair falls out, sores develop in the mouth, and the victim may develop a sore throat and a general feeling of sickness. These symptoms may disappear without treatment. The disease is still there. During the first two stages, the person is very contagious.

In the final stage of syphilis, all the symptoms disappear. They may not show again for one to 30 years. All this time, the pathogens grow and invade organs of the body such as the heart, lungs, and brain. When symptoms reappear, the person may have a heart attack, blindness, nervous condition, or brain damage.

Untreated, syphilis in pregnant women can cause a miscarriage, or termination of pregnancy before the baby can survive on its own. Or the baby can be born with a form of the disease.

Obviously, with such dangerous conse-

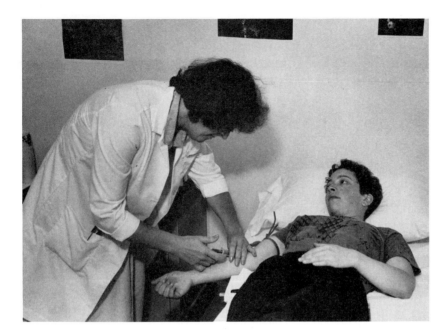

*In many states, a blood test for syphilis is required before a marriage license can be issued.*

quences, early detection and treatment of the syphilis are extremely important. A simple blood test can detect it. Especially in its early stages, syphilis can be successfully treated with penicillin. In the final stage, little can be done, and the person eventually dies.

### CHLAMYDIA

Chlamydia is the most widespread STD, striking 3 million Americans a year. It attacks the urinary and reproductive systems. If untreated, chlamydia can cause permanent damage, leading to sterility.

Symptoms of the disease may appear two to four weeks after exposure to someone who has the infection. These symptoms include: burning and itching around the external reproductive organs, a discharge, a burning sensation when urinating, and for females, pain in the abdomen.

Most men and some women have no noticeable symptoms. Responsible partners may tell them that they've been exposed. A simple test confirms the presence of the disease. Then they can be treated with an antibiotic for a complete cure.

### TYPE II HERPES

Herpes infections of the sex organs almost always come from the herpes simplex virus type II. (The type I herpes virus causes fever blisters and cold sores of the lips and mouth.) Type II herpes infections are spread by sexual contact. The major symptom is blisters in the area around the sex organs. These blisters break and form raw sores. Other symptoms include fever, painful urination, and a general feeling of sickness.

About one third of the people exposed to herpes get the disease. The herpes virus stays in their bodies, causing periodic outbreaks of blisters. The outbreaks can be triggered by other illnesses, emotional stress, and physical irritation such as tight clothing.

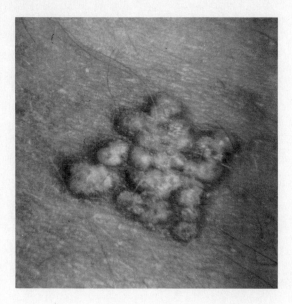

*Sometimes sores from type II herpes break out on the upper thighs.*

Even several days before a herpes outbreak, the victim is very contagious. Itching, tingling skin is a signal. The sores that follow contain the active virus. Sexual activity when blisters or sores are present can easily infect the partner, so contact at that time should be avoided to prevent spreading the disease.

Pregnant women need to be careful about passing the disease to their babies at birth. Also women with herpes have a five times greater chance of developing cancer of the uterus. Therefore, frequent checkups are important.

There's no cure for herpes, so it can reoccur, and even the newest medicines don't always help. Warm-water soaking and heat-lamp treatments relieve some pain from the sores.

## ACQUIRED IMMUNE DEFICIENCY SYNDROME (AIDS)

*AIDS* is the abbreviation for a deadly disease called Acquired Immune Deficiency Syndrome. It affects the body's ability to

*Sometimes sores from type II herpes break out on the upper thighs.*

fight infection and disease. This lowered resistance leaves the body vulnerable to pathogens. The body can't fight them off. It is these infections, not AIDS itself, that are so deadly.

The AIDS virus is not passed from person to person by casual contact. It is passed through intimate contact, such as sexual intercourse. You can't get AIDS from being in the same room with someone who has it or even from touching that person. You can safely live, work, and attend school with someone who has AIDS. Studies of families with an AIDS victim at home show this to be true.

The disease is also passed in breast milk and by pregnant women to their unborn children. In the past, a few people contracted AIDS through blood transfusions. However, stricter screening of blood donors virtually eliminated this problem.

Once the AIDS virus gets into the bloodstream, it does not always cause the person to get the disease. Some develop only a few symptoms. Many stay completely healthy. However, anyone with AIDS virus is considered a carrier and can pass the virus along to others. Remember, a carrier does not necessarily have any symptoms of the disease.

The symptoms of AIDS actually are symptoms of other diseases and conditions acquired because AIDS lowers the body's resistance. AIDS victims often develop a rare form of pneumonia and a rare form of skin cancer.

About three fourths of AIDS victims—those with the active disease—die within two years after they're diagnosed.

Exposure to the AIDS virus can be identified in the body with a blood test. But the

*Because the incidence of AIDS is rapidly increasing, the public should learn more about this disease. Free information is available from the public health department.*

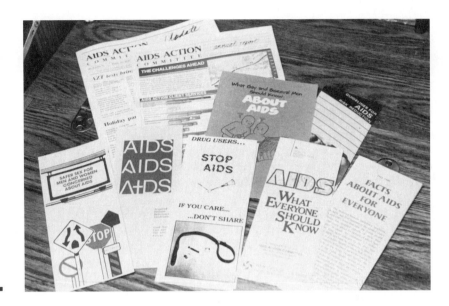

blood test doesn't distinguish between a carrier of the virus and the person who actually has the disease.

AIDS strikes all groups of people. It has spread more quickly among homosexuals and drug users who use needles.

Currently no treatment can cure AIDS. The AIDS virus destroys immunity. AIDS *Immunity* is the body's own ability to fight off infection. So to stay well for as long as possible, AIDS victims need to protect themselves from as many infectious diseases as possible.

People with AIDS and those whose blood test shows they have been exposed to AIDS have another responsibility. They must protect others from contracting their disease. By learning about AIDS and how it's spread, they can take appropriate precautions.

Having AIDS causes emotional strain. Its victims, their families, and their friends face the consequences of a deadly illness. And there's a social stigma associated with being contagious or possibly being homosexual. There are support groups for AIDS victims

in large cities. Several toll-free hotline phone numbers are available to comfort and inform AIDS victims, their families, and friends.

## Controlling Communicable Diseases

Germs are everywhere. They're in the air you breathe, the water you drink, and even on your own skin. You know that germs are spread in many ways. They can enter your body through any opening—mouth, eyes, nose, wounds, and others—causing infections and disease. You and your family can control the spread of these diseases.

When a communicable disease attacks many people in one area, it is called an *epidemic*. When an epidemic occurs, the community takes steps to control its spread. In Chapter 15 you'll learn how.

### Personal Habits

Your own personal hygiene and habits can protect you from getting sick and from passing your germs along to others.

Be careful when you're with family or friends who have colds, flu, mono, hepatitis, and other communicable diseases. Stay away if you don't need to be together. You might catch their illness or infect them with your own illness if their resistance is low.

Even when your hands look clean, they can carry germs. So keep your hands away from your nose and mouth. Wash your hands with soap frequently to destroy germs, especially when you have open cuts or sores. Always wash your hands:

- before putting anything in your mouth.
- before and after blowing your nose or sneezing.
- after touching someone who is ill.
- after using the toilet.
- before handling or eating food.
- after touching pets.
- after handling things that other people have handled, such as money, store items, or school equipment.
- after taking out the trash.
- after handling soiled clothing, like dirty diapers.

You can also prevent your own illness and avoid passing a disease on to others by being immunized against certain preventable diseases. An *immunization* with a vaccine produces an immunity in a person. A *vaccine* consists of small amounts of dead or weakened bacteria or viruses that stimulate a person's body to build up resistance to a disease. Vaccines are given by mouth or injection. The chart in Chapter 10 gives more information on immunizations.

## Family Habits

When someone in your family has a cold, it may be a matter of time before everyone catches it. Family members can avoid spreading disease to each other.

If someone in your house has a contagious disease, keep him or her in a separate room if possible. It'll just be for a few days. Insist that the contagious person cover both nose and mouth with tissues when coughing or sneezing.

Even when no one in the family is sick, you should all practice healthy habits. All

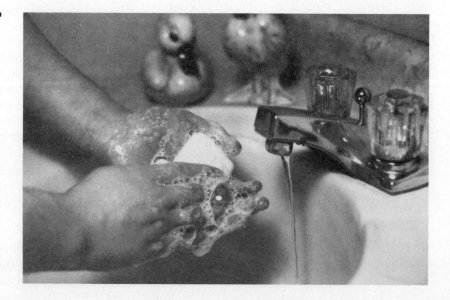

*Soap is important when you wash your hands because it destroys bacteria that cause disease.*

family members should have their own drinking glasses, bathroom towels, and soap; avoid sharing—that's how germs get passed. Wash dishes in hot, soapy water to help destroy germs.

Keep your home clean and fresh. Exposure to sunlight and air kills many germs. Weather permitting, open the windows. Dust and clean the home regularly. Use household disinfectants such as cleaning aids. Removing dirt and crumbs keeps away bugs which can carry and spread disease. Regular fumigation, especially in warm climates is important to kill insects and other household pests that carry germs.

Handle food in a safe manner. Germs multiply on food, so store food that can spoil in the refrigerator or freezer. Cover food so that bacteria from the air doesn't contaminate it. Don't let a sick family member prepare food for the family.

## Chronic Diseases

Not all diseases come on quickly like infections do. Some diseases develop slowly, often silently, and last for a lifetime. These diseases are *chronic*; they are never cured. The sick person may get better for a while, then the disease flares up. Chronic diseases may always require medicine or treatments to keep them under control. Chronic diseases aren't caused by pathogens.

Chronic diseases strike older people more than any other age group, but most chronic diseases are not limited to a particular age group. Alzheimer's Disease, arthritis, cancer, cardiovascular disease, diabetes, and osteoporosis are common chronic diseases.

Like communicable diseases, many chronic diseases can be prevented, or at least their progress can be slowed with lifestyles that promote health. Refer to Chapters 1 and 2, which focus on healthy living and decision making for you and your family.

## Alzheimer's disease

Until a few years ago, few people had heard of Alzheimer's disease, but this disease has been around for a long time. Many people just thought it was the forgetfulness that often seems to come with getting old. Alzheimer's disease is much more than forgetfulness, and people don't need to be old to get it. There are middle-aged people who have been diagnosed with Alzheimer's disease. This disease is now thought to be the fourth leading cause of death in the United States.

Physical changes within the brain cause people with Alzheimer's disease to gradually deteriorate mentally, physically, emotionally, and socially. A person with this disease has a gradual, steady loss of memory until the time comes when he or she may no longer recognize close family members. Forgetfulness is only one of many symptoms which include: increasing loss of judgment, inability to make even the simplest decisions, rambling and confused speech, aimless wandering, personality changes, emotional outbursts, and a decreasing ability to use and control muscles.

No one knows what causes this disease or how to treat it. Drugs may help control some symptoms, but no medicine or treatment can keep the disease from progressing.

As the disease gets worse, Alzheimer's victims can do less and less for themselves. They may get lost around their own homes. They may not be able to feed, bathe, or dress themselves. Eventually everything must be done for them, and they need constant attention.

## Arthritis

Arthritis is actually about 100 different diseases. They all cause aches, pains, and damage to the joints. Arthritis can be a crippling, lifelong disease.

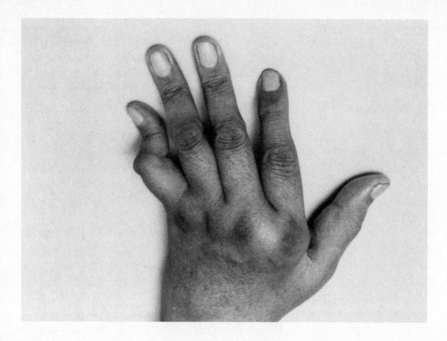

*Arthritis, a crippling disease, causes joints to swell and stiffen.*

Over 36 million Americans have some form of arthritis. Arthritis usually strikes older people; most people over the age of 60 have it to some degree. However, 250,000 infants, children, and teens have the disease, too.

The symptoms of arthritis come and go. They tend to be more severe early in the morning and in cold weather. People with arthritis have some or all of the following symptoms: swollen joints; painful joints, especially when the affected area is used a lot; joints which are difficult or nearly impossible to move; and popping and grating sounds coming from the joints.

Like other chronic diseases, arthritis can't be cured, but its victims can keep the symptoms of their disease under control by following a doctor's advice. This advice probably would include some combination of exercise, heat or cold applications, aspirin, and possibly splints or braces. For very deformed joints, surgery may help.

## Cancer

Cancer affects one of every three Americans. No disease strikes fear into people like a diagnosis of this dreaded disease, not even heart disease which actually causes more deaths. This is because a diagnosis of cancer once was considered a death sentence—no hope for a cure. Today, however, there have been great strides in cancer treatment, and people can be more optimistic about their chances of survival. The American Cancer Society predicts that of the people who get cancer today, 40 percent will be alive five years from now. Every day researchers learn more about the causes of cancer.

What is cancer? Cancer is not completely understood, even by the scientists. Cancer seems to come from repeated or long-term contact with one or more cancer-causing agents, called *carcinogens*. Alcohol, sunlight, and cigarette smoke are carcinogens.

With cancer, normal cells become abnormal and start to grow out of control. The

## Cancer's Warning Signals

Early detection is the key to controlling cancer. Look out for these warning signals. Check with your doctor if you notice these symptoms. And remember, none of these signals necessarily means cancer:

- Change in bowel or bladder habits
- A sore that doesn't heal
- Unusual bleeding or discharge
- Thickening or lump in the breast or elsewhere
- Indigestion or difficulty swallowing
- Obvious change in a wart or mole
- Nagging cough or hoarseness

new cells don't look or act like other body cells. Often these new cells become a tumor which can hurt the body in several ways: by pushing against other body organs, upsetting their work; by pressing on blood vessels, cutting off blood supply to parts of the body; by robbing the rest of the body of its nutrients; and by causing pain.

In time, cancer cells spread to other parts of the body. It is easier to treat and cure cancer before it spreads, so it is important to find cancer in its early stage. Regular exams are a good idea. About half of all cancers start in parts of the body that a doctor checks routinely during a visit.

Usually before the disease spreads, symptoms appear that you can detect. See the American Cancer Society's warning signs at the top of this page.

You can reduce your chances of getting cancer by the choices you make in your daily life, namely by reducing your exposure to carcinogens. These personal guidelines help protect against cancer:

- Don't smoke. Request nonsmoking sections in public places. Breathing in smoke increases the risk of lung cancer.
- Eat a high-fiber, low-fat diet, that is low in calories. High-fiber foods protect against colon and rectal cancers because food passes through the intestine faster and so the absorption of carcinogens into the body is decreased.
- Protect skin from direct sunlight. Cover up and use a sunscreen. Exposure to sun increases the risk of skin cancer.
- Avoid alcohol. The physical irritation of alcohol might affect the gastrointestinal tract, which in turn seems to increase the risk of cancer of the mouth, throat, esophagus, and liver.
- Avoid unnecessary X-rays, and wear an X-ray shield to protect other parts of your body. Overexposure to X-rays over time increases the risk of cancer.
- Follow worksite health and safety rules at your job. Wear protective clothing, and use safety equipment provided for you.

*A leaded shield protects your body from radiation when you get dental X-rays.*

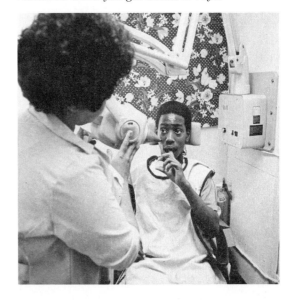

Cancer is really many diseases. There are several types of cancer for every organ of the body. See the chart at the bottom of the page which shows common cancer sites in men and women. Certain cancers tend to strike particular groups of people. The most common cancer among teens is leukemia, or blood cancer.

Cancer is treated in several ways. Removing tumors with surgery is common. Cancer can also be treated with medicines, usually injected into the bloodstream. This is called *chemotherapy*. Some types of cancer are treated with radiation delivered by a special machine. Radiation is a form of energy. All of these treatments can successfully cure many cancers if they're found early. And new and better cancer treatments are discovered every day.

You can get more information about cancer and the early detection of this disease by contacting the Cancer Information Service: 1-800-4-CANCER.

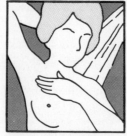

**1  IN THE SHOWER:** Examine the entire area of each breast in the bath or shower, since fingers glide more easily over wet skin. Check for any lump or thickening.

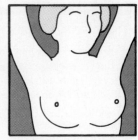

**2  BEFORE A MIRROR:** Inspect your breasts first with arms overhead, and then by placing hands on hips and flexing your chest muscles. Look for any changes, i.e., dimpling or swelling.

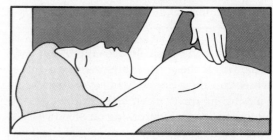

**3  LYING DOWN:** To examine your right breast, place a pillow or folded towel underneath your right shoulder and place your right hand behind your head. With fingers flat, press the breast in small, circular motions around an imaginary clock face. Repeat for the left breast. Then squeeze each nipple. Any discharge should be promptly reported to your physician.

*Each month, after a menstrual period, women should check their breasts for a lump or thickening. If one is discovered, the woman should see a doctor immediately. Usually the lump or thickening is harmless, but it can also be a sign of breast cancer.*

## Cancer Deaths in Men and Women

| Men | | Women | |
|---|---|---|---|
| SKIN | 2% | SKIN | 1% |
| ORAL | 3% | ORAL | 1% |
| LUNG | 35% | BREAST | 18% |
| COLON & RECTUM | 11% | LUNG | 19% |
| PANCREAS | 5% | COLON & RECTUM | 14% |
| PROSTATE | 10% | PANCREAS | 5% |
| URINARY | 5% | OVARY | 5% |
| LEUKEMIA & LYMPHOMAS | 9% | UTERUS | 4% |
| ALL OTHER | 20% | URINARY | 3% |
| | | LEUKEMIA & LYMPHOMAS | 9% |
| | | ALL OTHER | 21% |

*Source: American Cancer Society*

## Cardiovascular Disease

Cardiovascular disease includes any medical condition that affects how well the heart and blood vessels in your circulatory system work. When they're not working right, you can have serious health problems. Artery diseases, high blood pressure, heart attacks, and strokes are cardiovascular diseases.

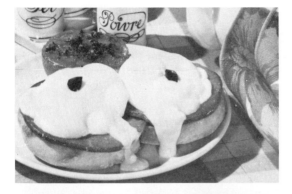

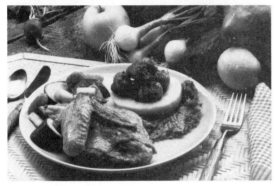

*If you were placed on a low-cholesterol diet, which of these meals would be better for you? Why?*

Some lifestyle habits and personal characteristics increase the chances of developing one or more of these cardiovascular diseases. These are called *risk factors*. You can control some of them:

- Smoking. Smoking causes blood vessels to constrict, or draw together and narrow, and the heartbeat to speed up as the heart works harder to pump blood.
- Obesity. Excess weight puts an added strain on the heart and blood vessels. It's healthier to drop extra pounds, and then maintain desirable weight.
- Sedentary lifestyles, or inactivity. The heart is a muscle which needs exercise. Exercise allows it to pump more blood

per heartbeat, then it doesn't have to work as hard. Exercise your heart with 20 minutes of aerobic activity, three times a week.

- Diet. For some people, diets high in saturated fats, cholesterol, and even excess calories can lead to cardiovascular disease. Diets high in sodium are harmful to people with high blood pressure. People can protect themselves by avoiding too much fat, cholesterol, and sodium in their foods.
- Stress. Anger and tension can affect blood pressure. It's good to find healthy ways, such as exercise, to release these emotions, and to learn to relax.
- Inadequate medical care. Cardiovascular disease often goes undetected because the symptoms aren't easily felt or noticed. Through regular medical checkups, which include blood pressure checks, it can be diagnosed and treated early.

The following risk factors for cardiovascular disease can't be controlled:

- Age. The older you get, the higher your risk.
- Heredity. Cardiovascular disease tends to occur in families. If your blood relatives had these diseases, there's a greater chance that you will, too.
- Sex. More men than women have cardiovascular disease. But women are catching up fast, possibly because of changes in their lifestyles. Work-related stress and increased smoking may be among the causes.
- Race. Black Americans are more likely to get cardiovascular disease.

## ARTERY DISEASES

Arteries are the vessels that carry blood from the heart to the rest of the body. In some people fatty deposits build up on the inner lining of the arteries. Over time these

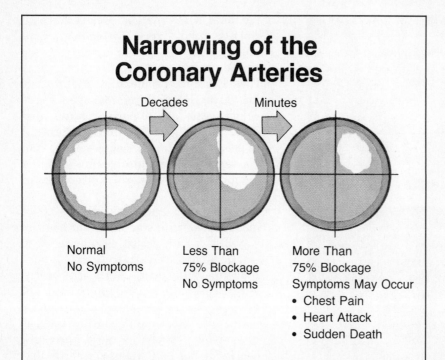

# Narrowing of the Coronary Arteries

Decades →　　　Minutes →

Normal
No Symptoms

Less Than
75% Blockage
No Symptoms

More Than
75% Blockage
Symptoms May Occur
• Chest Pain
• Heart Attack
• Sudden Death

*The arteries that surround the heart can gradually become blocked with fatty deposits. This happens over the years without apparent symptoms. Within a matter of minutes, a severe blockage can cause a heart attack and even death.*

deposits narrow the passageway and interfere with the blood flow. This condition is called atherosclerosis.

Atherosclerosis can also contribute to hardening of the arteries. When arteries harden, they lose their elasticity and narrow so they cannot regulate blood flow properly. Arteries harden as part of the natural aging process, but fatty deposits make the arteries even narrower and less able to expand with blood flow.

## HIGH BLOOD PRESSURE

Blood pressure is the force of your blood as it goes through the blood vessels to all parts of the body. Blood pressure can be measured with special equipment by those with proper training. The normal measurement is 120 over 80 (120/80). The top number is the systolic pressure, which is the greatest

pressure produced by the heart's contraction to pump out blood. The bottom number is the diastolic pressure, which is pressure when your heart has relaxed to permit the inflow of blood. Your blood pressure is different from your pulse which just measures the number of heartbeats per minute.

In some people, the force of the blood is greater than it should be. This is called high blood pressure, or hypertension. Over 50 million adults and 2.5 million young people under the age of 17 have hypertension.

High blood pressure is bad for the heart. It makes the heart work harder to circulate blood. The constant high force causes damage to the arteries. It can even damage the kidneys or cause a stroke.

People can have high blood pressure without knowing it. A few people get dizzy or have a headache, but many have no symptoms at all. The only way to find out if you have high blood pressure is to have your blood pressure checked by your doctor or at a clinic or public health service.

Once it's detected, high blood pressure can usually be controlled. Following the guidelines on page **171** for reducing risk factors is helpful. Also the doctor may prescribe a specific low-sodium diet and medicine. The medicine must be continued even though it doesn't make a difference in the way a person feels.

### HEART ATTACK

Every year 1.5 million Americans have heart attacks. One-half million of them die. This is the country's leading cause of death. Heart attacks often happen to older people. More and more people are stricken in their middle years. It's rare for young people to have heart attacks. That only happens if there's already a heart condition or if drugs, such as amphetamines or cocaine, are involved.

What causes a heart attack? When the blood supply to the heart is blocked, the heart can't get all the oxygen and nutrients it needs. Part of the heart dies. Then the heart can't function as it should to pump blood through the body. This can cause death. The blockage can be caused by atherosclerosis or a blood clot.

The keys to surviving a heart attack are recognizing it and getting medical treatment fast. People having a heart attack often have these symptoms: pain, starting in the chest and sometimes going to the neck or arm; sweating; upset stomach; dizziness; and shortness of breath.

These symptoms require immediate medical treatment. This is a medical emergency. When someone shows signs of a heart attack, call an ambulance at once. In the minutes before the ambulance arrives, you may be able to save his or her life if you know CPR. See Chapter 5 for first aid instructions for a heart attack.

### STROKE

Just like the heart, the brain requires blood to survive. A stroke occurs when the blood flow to the brain is interrupted. When the blood flow to the brain stops, part of the brain dies. Whatever activity that part of the brain controlled is lost—speech, memory, emotions. The body can't heal brain cells or make new ones, so the damage is permanent.

The effects of strokes can be mild or severe. The face, arm, or leg feels numb or weak suddenly. This may end up in paralysis, which is the loss of feeling in and inability to move the affected part of the body. Perhaps the victim can't speak or understand another's speech, or the victim may have trouble seeing, particularly in one eye.

Recovering from a stroke can be long and hard. If there's paralysis, victims try to relearn how to use the affected part of the body. Many people recover from strokes.

Fifty million Americans have strokes every year, but strokes can be prevented. High blood pressure is the leading cause, so finding and treating it early is good prevention. You also can reduce your risk by making choices in your daily life that reduce cardiovascular disease later.

## Diabetes

Diabetes is a disease in which the pancreas, a body organ, doesn't make enough insulin. Insulin is an important hormone which helps move blood sugar from the bloodstream into body cells where it can be used. Without an adequate insulin supply, high levels of sugar circulate in the blood. This is called hyperglycemia. With hyperglycemia, the body's cells aren't properly

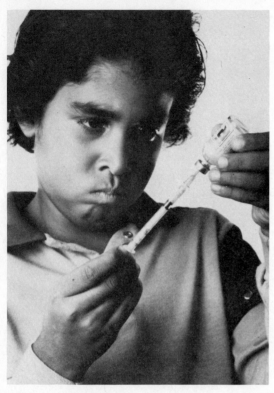

*With proper instruction, diabetics can give their own insulin injections.*

nourished, and the body can become permanently damaged.

About 11 million people in the United States have diabetes, and 3 million of them are children and teenagers. People who are overweight, middle-aged, or have relatives with diabetes have a higher chance of getting the disease.

People with diabetes have some or all of these symptoms: frequent urination, excessive thirst, tremendous appetite, inability to gain weight even after eating more, and fatigue.

Simple blood and urine tests are able to diagnose diabetes. While there is no cure for diabetes, diabetes can be controlled with a low-carbohydrate, low-fat diet, regular exercise, and, in some cases, daily injections of insulin. But there are still dangers—insulin shock or hyperglycemia. See the chart below.

Medical researchers continue to search for new diabetes treatments. Transplanting part of the pancreas from a healthy person into someone with diabetes has had some success. This may lead to a cure in the future.

## Dangers of Diabetes

Diabetes can result in insulin shock and hyperglycemia.

|  | Insulin Shock | Hyperglycemia |
|---|---|---|
| Cause | Too much insulin taken<br>Not enough sugar eaten | Not enough insulin taken<br>Too much sugar eaten |
| How to Recognize | Shakiness<br>Headache<br>Fast, shallow breathing<br>Cool, wet skin<br>Loss of consciousness | Fruity breath odor<br>Extreme thirst<br>Increased appetite<br>Loss of consciousness |
| What to Do | Quickly eat a high-sugar food. Call the doctor. | Quickly take insulin. Call the doctor. |

# Osteoporosis

How many times have you heard, "Drink your milk"? There are plenty of reasons for that. Milk is a food rich in calcium. Lack of sufficient calcium in the diet, among other factors, is related to a chronic disease called osteoporosis.

Bone loss is a normal part of aging. Osteoporosis, often called "brittle bone disease," is actually excessive bone loss. When bones lose much of their mass they may become too weak to support a person's weight so fractures, such as a broken hip, happen when the person does everyday activities. The pictures on the right show a healthy bone and an osteoporotic bone in the spine.

Osteoporosis causes other problems, too. The stress of body weight on weak bones may cause pain. And as the backbone collapses, the person may get shorter and even develop a hunchback. Osteoporosis can also keep fractures from healing properly. Bone loss from the jawbone also causes loss of teeth.

Certain people are more prone to osteoporosis: people with small body frames, people with calcium-deficient diets, women, the elderly, smokers, inactive people, and those under extreme stress.

Bone loss among women and men starts in middle age and progresses slowly, over many years. After menopause, women lose bone faster than they did as young adults. Menopause is when the menstrual cycle stops during middle age. Usually osteoporosis develops for years before people know they have it. By the time symptoms show,

*A healthy bone (bottom) is much more dense than an osteoporotic bone (top). For that reason, a healthy bone is less likely to break.*

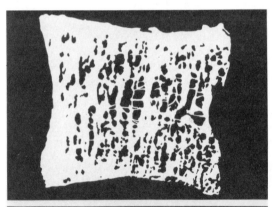

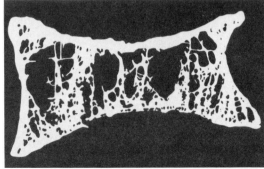

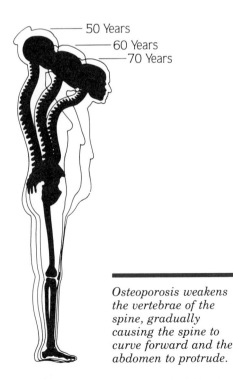

50 Years
60 Years
70 Years

*Osteoporosis weakens the vertebrae of the spine, gradually causing the spine to curve forward and the abdomen to protrude.*

## Enjoy These Calcium-Rich Foods

| | |
|---|---|
| 1½ cups flavored milkshake | 376 milligrams |
| 1 cup whole milk | 304 milligrams |
| 1 cup flavored yogurt | 290 milligrams |
| 1 ounce cheddar cheese | 202 milligrams |
| ⅖ cup canned salmon, with bones | 196 milligrams |
| 3½ ounces tofu | 128 milligrams |
| ½ cup cottage cheese | 106 milligrams |
| ½ cup greens | 104 milligrams |

it's too late. You can't cure osteoporosis if you get it, but you may help prevent it.

Start preventing osteoporosis while you're still young. Bones grow stronger and more dense into early adulthood. Help make your bones strong now so that you enter middle age with an advantage. Eat plenty of calcium-rich foods, such as those listed in the chart above. Teens need at least 1,200 milligrams of calcium daily. Exercise regularly. Weight-bearing activities, such as jogging, help your bones grow stronger. Avoid smoking and stress.

Calcium pills aren't the best source of calcium. Most don't provide enough calcium. And they don't have other nutrients which allow calcium to be absorbed into the body. Remember that pills can never provide all the nutrients found in a balanced diet.

## Mental Illness

Physical illness strikes most everyone, but 10 percent of Americans also suffer from mental illness, or diseases of the mind. A fever or pain may be symptoms of physical illness. Abnormal behavior is the symptom of mental illness. Mental illness keeps people from living normal, healthy lives.

There are many causes of mental illness. Some have a definite physical cause, resulting from a head injury, atherosclerosis, infection, or alcohol or drug use. Others have an emotional cause, such as severe stress or severe inner conflicts.

Mental illness resulting from emotional problems has a high recovery rate when patients receive prompt competent care. Psychotherapy is often effective treatment, but it can be a long, slow process. *Psychotherapy* involves the patient talking through emotional problems with a professionally trained therapist.

## Neuroses

Neuroses are mild mental disorders in which people overreact to emotional stress. They suffer from excessive fears, anxiety, or both, but they seldom lose touch with reality. People who suffer from a neurosis are called neurotics. Neurotics usually live fairly normally but with more effort and less personal satisfaction than healthy people. Severe anxiety, phobias, and hypochondria are examples of neuroses. Anorexia, which was discussed in Chapter 3, is considered by many to be a neurosis, too.

### SEVERE ANXIETY

Most people have experienced and coped with mild anxiety. Severe anxiety, however, can keep people from coping well with normal life. Their bodies may react physically to extreme tension. Overly anxious people may take tranquilizers, or drugs which calm them down and mask their problems. The best treatment, however, is psychotherapy.

### HYPOCHONDRIA

People with hypochondria are abnormally concerned about their health. They exaggerate trivial symptoms and often are convinced they're suffering from a serious ailment. In fact, no physical cause exists for their complaints.

Hypochondriacs may go from one doctor to another looking for one who will confirm an illness. Doctors, family, and friends repeatedly hear their worrisome complaints. In addition to psychotherapy, hypochondriacs need to be listened to and reassured by those around them.

### PHOBIAS

Phobias are severe, irrational fears, of something that poses little or no real threat. Victims react uncontrollably and unreasonably to the object or situation they fear. The reaction includes heart palpitations, sweaty palms, shaky voice, and weak knees. The phobic person usually avoids or runs from the source of fear.

There are many types of phobias. Nosophobia, fear of being sick, is one type. Other phobias are acrophobia (fear of heights), agoraphobia (fear of open spaces), ariaphobia (fear of flying), claustrophobia (fear of closed spaces), hydrophobia (fear of water), and zoophobia (fear of animals).

Phobias can be overcome, often with professional help. Medication, psychotherapy, and hypnosis often are used. A new treatment called desensitization has been effective. With the help of a psychotherapist, the phobic person can gradually confront and overcome their fear in controlled surroundings.

## Psychoses

Psychoses are severe mental disorders in which the affected person can't cope with life and may withdraw from the real world. Often these people can't distinguish between what is real and what is fantasy. They may hallucinate, or see and hear things that aren't there. A person who suffers from a psychosis is called a psychotic. Some psy-

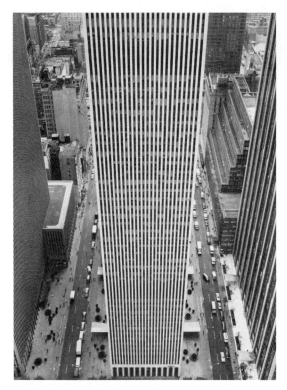

*Fear of heights, or acrophobia, is one of the more common phobias.*

chotics harm themselves and others. They may require hospitalization.

### SCHIZOPHRENIA

Schizophrenia, characterized by disturbed and disorganized thinking, moods, and behavior, is the most common psychosis. Often schizophrenics live in the private world of their own minds.

The onset of schizophrenia usually occurs between the adolescent and middle-age years. The cause is yet unknown but may be a combination of environmental and physical factors. Schizophrenia may be treated successfully with medication, hospital care, and psychotherapy.

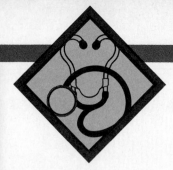

# CHAPTER CHECKUP

## Reviewing the Information

1. Name four requirements for maintaining good health.
2. Name five ways that diseases differ from each other.
3. What causes an infection?
4. Define communicable disease.
5. What are the causes and symptoms of a cold?
6. What is the appropriate treatment for influenza?
7. What are two ways that mononucleosis is spread?
8. What are the symptoms of hepatitis?
9. What can be done to reduce the spread of sexually-transmitted diseases?
10. Describe the three stages of syphilis.
11. How is the AIDS virus passed from one person to another?
12. Describe five conditions under which people should always wash their hands.
13. How can a family control the spread of a contagious disease at home?
14. What is Alzheimer's disease?
15. List the seven warning signs of cancer.
16. What are the risk factors for heart disease?
17. What is athlerosclerosis?
18. What is diabetes?
19. What factors contribute to the incidence of osteoporosis?
20. What's the difference between a neuroses and a psychosis?
21. What causes mental illness?

## Thinking It Over

1. Think about your lifestyle. List your habits that are healthy and those that are unhealthy. Which is longer?
2. How could you avoid spreading disease to your classmates at school?
3. What might you do now to protect yourself from getting cardiovascular disease later in life?
4. What might you do to protect yourself from getting cancer?
5. What does a blood pressure reading of 160/90 suggest?
6. What steps can you take now to help prevent osteoporosis later?
7. What is the difference between a fear and a phobia?

## Taking Action

 1. Write an article for the school paper on ways to prevent spreading disease at school.

 2. Notice the headlines in grocery store tabloids for arthritis and cancer cures. How truthful do you think they are? Explain.

 3. Contact the American Cancer Society for information on how teenagers can cope with cancer. Write a report.

4. Contact the local public health service for current statistics on a particular disease.
5. Volunteer in a local hospital or nursing home where there are people with chronic diseases.

# Prenatal Care and Birth

## 8

After reading this chapter, you will be able to:

- describe the changes in a fetus and mother-to-be during pregnancy.

- explain good health practices during pregnancy.

- explain the mother's and father's roles during childbirth and the postnatal period.

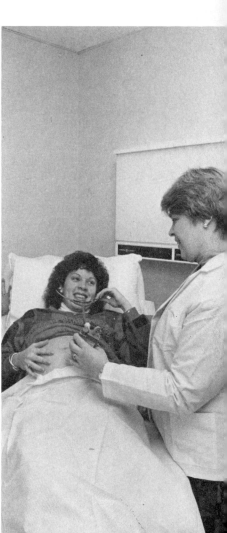

## Terms to Understand

| | |
|---|---|
| bonding | neonate |
| caesarean section | obstetrician |
| fetal alcohol syndrome | placenta |
| fetus | trimester |
| miscarriage | umbilical cord |

Pregnancy is a very special, exciting time. The months of pregnancy are filled with wonder and anticipation for a living being— a baby. Pregnancy brings great joy. It also means responsibility in order to have a safe and healthy pregnancy.

Prenatal care is the special way a woman cares for herself during pregnancy. *Prenatal* means before birth. Prenatal care includes healthy habits, medical care, and emotional support.

Prenatal care officially begins the moment a woman learns she is pregnant. But actually, a woman can prepare for pregnancy almost her entire life by practicing good health habits. The healthier a woman is before and during her pregnancy, the better the chances her baby will be healthy, too.

Pregnancy is divided into three sections of three months each, called *trimesters*. Only three percent of pregnancies last exactly 280 days. Almost all pregnancies deliver a little early or late.

To prepare for the baby's birth, parents do many things. There are tasks to be completed such as arranging time away from work, buying baby clothes, and finding a pediatrician, or doctor who specializes in child care. Preparing to be a parent also involves anticipating the child's nurturing needs such as attention, love, and guidance.

As a pregnancy progresses, the mother feels very close to the developing baby, called a *fetus*. The more involved the father is in the activities surrounding pregnancy, the closer he feels to the baby, too.

To have a safe pregnancy, parents need to learn as much as they can. There are important guidelines to know about prenatal care, delivery of the baby, and care afterward. Parents-to-be also can do many things that help reduce the risks of problems in a pregnancy.

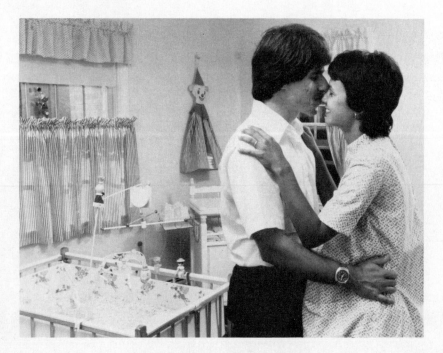

*Pregnancy can be a time of emotional closeness between a couple.*

# Signs of Pregnancy

As pregnancy progresses, there are many changes in a woman's body. At first, she is probably unaware of most changes, but they eventually become noticeable.

Usually the first clue to pregnancy is a missed menstrual period. This is caused by changes in the woman's body hormones. Hormones are glandular secretions that stimulate many body functions. An interruption in the menstrual cycle can have many causes. If pregnancy is suspected, a simple lab test one to two weeks after a missed period will indicate if the woman is pregnant. Any vaginal bleeding during pregnancy should be reported to a doctor immediately.

The majority of pregnant women experience morning sickness. This is a feeling of nausea, sometimes with vomiting, that tends to occur in the early months of pregnancy. A definite cause isn't known, but it's probably due to hormonal changes. Even though it's called morning sickness, the queasy feelings can occur at any time of the day or even last all day. Some women find relief by eating dry toast or saltines in the morning before getting out of bed. For severe cases, the doctor may prescribe medicine. Morning sickness is frustrating and uncomfortable, but usually it subsides after the first trimester.

Other signs of pregnancy are breast changes. The breasts enlarge and become tender. These changes are in preparation for breast feeding. The milk ducts and glands inside the breasts swell and fill with fluid, as early as the fourth month.

As the fetus grows, so does the uterus. As you learned in Chapter 1, the *uterus* is the female organ that holds the fetus during pregnancy. As it grows, the fetus puts pressure on the urinary bladder. This causes a feeling of having to urinate, sometimes as often as every hour or two. Frequent urination occurs early in pregnancy and is one sign of pregnancy. Often frequent urination occurs again in the last months.

Feeling tired is also typical early in pregnancy. Carrying a growing fetus is demanding. It is a physical stress that the body needs to adjust to. Eating healthful foods and avoiding additional stress is helpful. Adequate rest is essential.

A doctor looks for scientific signs of pregnancy, such as hearing the fetus' heartbeat and conducting blood and urine tests to detect pregnancy. Women can also test their own urine with pregnancy testing kits from the drugstore, but these tests sometimes are inaccurate.

# Changes in the Mother and Baby

As pregnancy progresses, the mother and fetus grow and change in many ways. Although every woman's pregnancy is different, most changes occur in the same order during each trimester.

## First Trimester

Pregnancy begins with conception. In the fallopian tube, the male sperm and female egg unite; the fertilized ovum then implants in the uterus during the week. During the first trimester, the fetus grows from that two-cell joining to many millions of cells. It becomes about three inches long and weighs one ounce by the end of the first trimester. The beginnings of human features develop, such as arms, legs, ears, eyes, and internal organs during this time, too.

Most women don't look pregnant in the first trimester, but critical fetal growth and development are taking place. Early growth is delicate, for all of the new baby's organs are forming during the first two months. It can be disturbed by drugs, alcohol, disease,

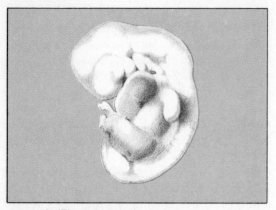

1 month (First trimester)

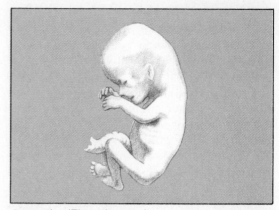

3 months (First trimester)

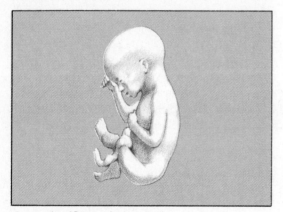

6 months (Second trimester)

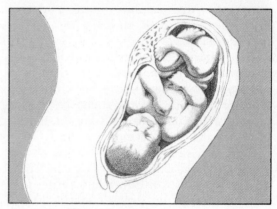

9 months (Third trimester)

and poor nutrition. These conditions can cause birth defects. It's important for a woman to maintain healthful habits as soon as she suspects she is pregnant, even while she is trying to become pregnant.

During the first trimester, many expectant couples experience feelings of joy about the idea of pregnancy. But they may also have some doubts about their ability to be parents and how the baby will affect their lives. These conflicting and uncertain feelings are normal.

## Second Trimester

In the second trimester, the fetus grows to about 12 inches in length and weighs 2½

pounds. The skin is wrinkled and covered with downy hair and a thick creamy covering for protection. Fine features such as eyelids and lashes, toothbuds, fingernails, fingerprints, and facial features develop. A fetus born toward the end of the second trimester can survive with today's medical technology.

For the mother, the second trimester is the most enjoyable time of pregnancy. She's not grown too large yet, and there are usually few discomforts. She displays what is called the "glow of pregnancy." It's also during the second trimester that she feels quickening, which is the fetus' movement inside her. This is a wonderful event that helps her view the fetus as a separate being from herself. By placing his hand on the woman's stomach, the father can feel the fetal movements, too.

In the second trimester, the mother's uterus enlarges to the level of her navel. By the sixth month, she has gained about one half of her total pregnancy weight.

## Third Trimester

The fetus grows rapidly in size during the third trimester—to about 20 inches in length and 7½ pounds in weight. It's not unusual for a baby to weigh eight or nine pounds at birth, however. As the fetus accumulates fat, the wrinkled skin disappears. Other features and organs fully develop in final preparation for birth:

- The bones harden.
- The brain develops.
- The fetus moves around, "exercising" its muscles and joints.
- Scalp hair grows.
- All body systems mature.

- Some antibodies to fight disease are acquired, but it takes several months for the baby's immune system to work well.

A pregnant woman gains weight rapidly during her last trimester, but less of the weight gain goes to her own body fat. Instead, it becomes a reserve of body fat for the fetus and also includes fluid accumulation. The uterus enlarges up to the level of the ribs. The effects of the weight gain plus the enlarged abdomen make a woman feel uncomfortable. This is the time she experiences the discomforts of pregnancy that will be discussed later. She may have some shortness of breath as the uterus presses up into her lung space. Her breasts will grow and fill in preparation for breast feeding.

During the third trimester parents-to-be become impatient for the birth. They also begin thinking about the realities of having a baby at home. The mother may have fears about the delivery and may even dream about it. These concerns are normal. But it's a good idea to talk to the doctor about them.

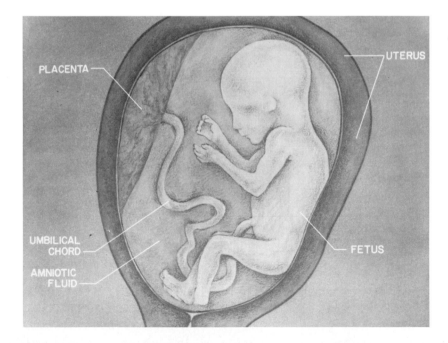

*The uterine environment protects and nourishes the developing fetus.*

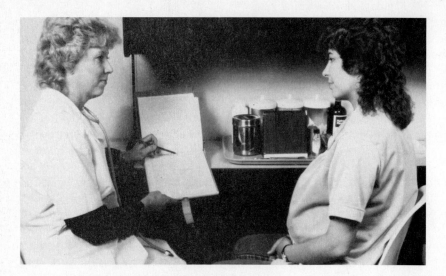

*Regular visits to the doctor or nurse practitioner are an important part of prenatal care.*

# Good Health Practices During Pregnancy

Throughout pregnancy, the fetus receives all of its oxygen and nourishment from the mother. All of this passes in the blood from the placenta through a lifeline, called an *umbilical cord*, to the fetus. The *placenta* is a blood-rich organ on the wall of the uterus that provides nourishment to the fetus.

Almost everything that the mother eats, breathes, and does affects the fetus. So the most important thing a pregnant woman can do for her developing fetus is to practice good health habits. This is an appropriate time for the father to adopt good health practices with the mother.

## Routine Care

Routine care for a pregnant woman includes doctor visits, nutrition, rest, activity, and avoiding potential dangers. She also needs emotional support. These are good habits to continue after pregnancy.

### DOCTOR VISITS

As soon as a woman suspects she is pregnant, she should see an appropriate health professional. This would probably be an obstetrician or a nurse practitioner. A doctor who specializes in pregnancy is called an *obstetrician*. Registered nurses who care for pregnant women are usually called certified nurse midwives or nurse practitioners. Nurse midwives work under the guidance of an obstetrician.

Regular medical care is important throughout pregnancy. For the first two trimesters, visits are usually scheduled every three or four weeks. In the last trimester, it's best to go more often, every one to two weeks.

During these periodic visits, the doctor discusses diet, exercise, rest, and possible medical treatment. A history of past illness and operations will also be recorded. Questions and concerns of the mother and father are discussed, too.

A typical prenatal examination includes: weighing in, a blood pressure check, a blood test to check for iron, a urine test to check for sugar and protein, and an examination of the pelvic area and the uterus.

During visits in the last trimester, the doctor may perform a pelvic exam. This is an exam of the internal reproductive organs, done through the vagina. A pelvic exam provides information about how close a woman is to delivery and how capable her body is of handling childbirth.

There are some special tests to check a pregnant woman and the fetus for certain conditions:

- A blood test for the Rh factor measures how compatible the fetus' and mother's blood are. If they're not compatible, there can be problems with any pregnancies the mother has after the first one. The doctor can deal with this.
- A blood test detects antibodies to rubella, or German measles. If the mother gets the disease during pregnancy, it can seriously harm a growing fetus.
- Blood tests detect some infectious diseases, such as sexually-transmitted diseases (STDs), which can harm the baby as it passes through the birth canal.

### NUTRITION

Good nutrition is essential for the health of the fetus and the mother. An adequate supply of nutrients helps the baby develop normally, protects the mother from damaging her own health, and improves the mother's ability to breast feed later if she chooses. The mother and baby need to share the nutrients she consumes, so an adequate supply is essential.

Nutritional guidelines for pregnancy follow the same general principles you learned about in Chapter 1. However, during pregnancy, women need slightly higher amounts of some nutrients and more calories. For example:

- extra calcium is needed for the fetus' teeth and bone formation. When pregnant women don't consume enough of this mineral, calcium for the fetus may be taken from the mother's bones and teeth.

- more iron is needed for blood formation. Anemia may develop if a woman doesn't consume enough iron. Often the doctor recommends an iron supplement.
- because new body cells are forming at a rapid rate, women need more protein.

Food choices should supply adequate amounts of essential nutrients for the mother and fetus. The Daily Food Guide has specific recommendations for pregnant and breast-feeding women. The chart below shows these guidelines.

There's an old wive's tale that a pregnant woman needs a lot more food because she's eating for two. That just isn't so. Eating too much, especially in the first two trimesters, puts extra pounds of body fat on the mother. This can make pregnancy more difficult. Pregnancy requires only about 300 additional calories per day. Increasing the quality of foods, rather than eating a lot more quantity, makes good nutrition sense.

Desirable weight gain during pregnancy is between 20 and 30 pounds. Slow, steady gain is a sign of a healthy pregnancy. If a

### Daily Food Guide for Pregnancy and Breast Feeding

| | Recommended Servings | |
|---|---|---|
| Food Group | Pregnancy | Breast Feeding |
| Milk and Cheese | | |
| Adults | 4 | 4 |
| Teenagers | 6 | 6 |
| Meat, Poultry, Fish, and Beans | 3 | 2 |
| Vegetables and Fruit | 4 | 4 |
| Bread and Cereal | 4 | 4 |

baby weighs only seven to nine pounds, what does the other weight go to? Weight gained during pregnancy is distributed approximately as follows:

- fetus                                           7.5 pounds
- placenta                                    1.5 pounds
- amniotic fluid (The am-          2.0 pounds
  niotic fluid surrounds
  and protects the fetus.)
- increased weight of              2.0 pounds
  uterus
- increased weight of              1.0 pound
  breast tissue
- excess fluids                          5.0 pounds
- mother's body fat                 9.0 pounds

Most of this weight is lost during childbirth. The rest can be lost in four to six weeks if the woman is very careful about her diet and exercises according to her doctor's instructions.

A pregnant woman needs to drink plenty of liquids, and so do women who breast-feed. That's because extra body fluids are forming. Six to eight glasses of fluids daily are recommended. Fruit juices, milk, and water are the most healthful. Beverages with caffeine, such as coffee, tea, and colas, and with alcohol are best avoided.

## REST

Pregnant women tire easily as their weight and the demands of the fetus increase. Normal activities such as a job, shopping, or yard work, may be fatiguing, particularly in the last trimester.

Anemia can be another cause of fatigue. An obstetrician can detect this problem if it persists and will have the woman increase her iron intake, possibly with supplemental iron tablets.

To help prevent fatigue, a pregnant woman needs an adequate amount of rest. That means eight to 10 hours of sleep every night, relaxation breaks during the day, and

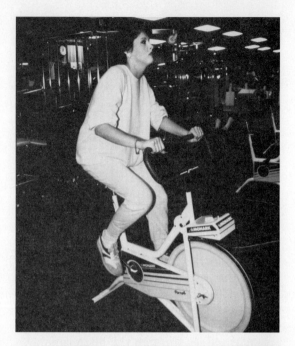

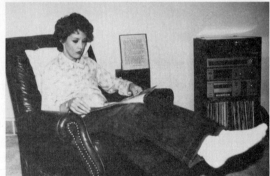

*A pregnant woman needs a balance of activity and rest.*

possibly a nap in the afternoon. The father and other children can help with yardwork and housework.

## ACTIVITY

Exercise in moderation is beneficial during pregnancy. But it shouldn't be carried to the point of exhaustion. Planned sports and exercise should be carefully guided by a woman's doctor. In general, whatever activities a woman has participated in before pregnancy may be continued, with few exceptions.

The best exercise for most pregnant women is walking. It burns calories, exercises the heart, and tones muscles without putting undue stress on the joints. There are specific exercises that strengthen muscles and discipline breathing for delivery. An obstetrician or nurse practitioner can provide instructions for exercises for expectant women.

Travel during pregnancy is generally safe, but women must use common sense. When riding in a car, these are safety tips a pregnant woman should remember:

- Wear a seat belt, fastened below the abdomen. This will protect, not harm, the fetus.
- During long rides, get out of the car and walk around every one to two hours to stimulate blood circulation.
- Stay close to home during the ninth month because exact delivery dates are unpredictable.
- Inform the obstetrician of travel plans.

### EMOTIONAL SUPPORT

Pregnancy brings changes which need emotional support. As a woman's body changes, hormones may affect her moods. She may get upset even when she's normally even tempered. She may feel unattractive, and she may feel somewhat stressed as she tries to plan for changes in lifestyle. During this time, she needs support, reassurance, and time for privacy. A thoughtful husband, relatives, and friends will reassure her about her self-doubts.

A father-to-be may also need to make emotional adjustments. He might feel left out of the changes that pregnancy brings or begin to feel pressured by new responsibilities. A pregnant woman needs to give him support, too, and make him part of the experience of childbearing.

Older children in a family also may undergo emotional adjustments. They will need to realize that a new baby will require more of their parents' time, especially at first. Sharing the time sometimes makes children feel less loved, but talking about these changes will help everyone cope better with the new situation.

## Discomforts of Pregnancy

Over the nine months of pregnancy, a woman has days when she "never felt better." Other days are very uncomfortable. Even in the healthiest pregnancies, there are minor complaints and discomforts.

*Constipation is often a problem during pregnancy. High-fiber foods help prevent constipation.*

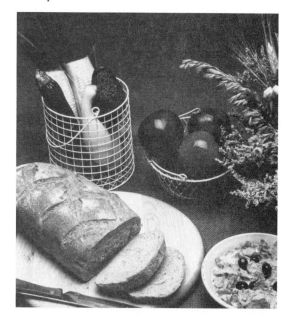

Discomfort during pregnancy can be minimized by following an obstetrician's or a nurse practitioner's advice. When discomfort seems unbearable, there's pleasure in knowing that pregnancy lasts only nine months.

## BACKACHE

Backaches are typical in the later months of pregnancy. A pregnant woman's center of gravity shifts. Pressure from the increasing body weight and growing uterus puts a lot of stress on the back.

## SWELLING

Swelling during pregnancy is normal, especially in the last trimester. In most women, fluid accumulates noticeably in the hands, face, and especially the feet and ankles. Anything that restricts blood flow causes swelling. Summer heat and eating salty foods also cause swelling. Severe swelling can be a sign of a serious problem. All swelling needs to be closely watched and checked by the obstetrician.

## VARICOSE VEINS

Varicose veins are bulging, knobby blood vessels. In pregnant women, they occur in the legs and the rectum. In the rectum, varicose veins are called hemorrhoids.

Varicose veins are caused by pressure on the blood vessels from increasing blood volume and the enlarging uterus. Unfortunately, varicose veins don't always go away after pregnancy.

Hemorrhoids are complicated by constipation which is also common in pregnancy. When a pregnant woman strains during a bowel movement, it further increases pressure of blood vessels in the rectum. Unlike varicose veins of the legs, hemorrhoids are painful, and they also can itch.

## LEG CRAMPS

Cramping muscle pains in the calves and feet are astonishingly painful. Many pregnant women have only a little tingling or numbness in their legs. Leg cramps usually are caused by poor blood circulation to the legs or, less commonly, not enough calcium in the diet. Leg cramps often occur at night.

## STRETCH MARKS

The wavy streaks that develop on a pregnant woman's body are called stretch marks. They are the result of stretching skin over the abdomen, hips, and breasts plus the activity of a pregnant woman's hormones. At first, they have a pale pink or blue color. Later, they take on a silvery, glistening appearance. Stretch marks usually become less pronounced after childbirth but don't disappear.

# Practices to Avoid

Pregnancy is an important time to follow good health habits. This includes avoiding substances and practices that can permanently damage the fetus and the mother.

## WEIGHT-LOSS DIETS

Pregnancy isn't a time to go on a weight-loss diet. Cutting down on calories to avoid too much weight gain is a bad idea. This can harm an unborn baby. When nutrients and calories are deficient, a baby's intelligence can be impaired. The mother's health can be harmed, too.

## SELF-PRESCRIBED MEDICATIONS

Only drugs and medical treatments approved by a doctor should be taken during pregnancy. Sleeping pills, pain pills, laxatives, and antibiotics, for example, can pass to the fetus and cause damage. Even drugs prescribed before pregnancy should be avoided unless the doctor approves.

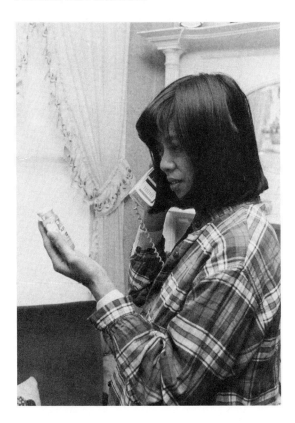

Pregnant women should avoid smoking and smoke-filled rooms. Nicotine inhaled from smoking can retard the fetus' growth. Heavy smoking may cause premature birth and smaller babies.

Alcoholic beverages should be avoided. Alcohol passes through the placenta to the fetus. Even one ounce of alcohol per day, or two beers, is toxic to a baby's delicate body. *Fetal alcohol syndrome* is a condition caused by a woman drinking too much alcohol during pregnancy. The damage to the baby may include mental retardation; facial, heart, and other physical defects; and learning disabilities. Effects of fetal alcohol syndrome cannot be undone.

Illegal drugs such as cocaine and heroin cause serious damage. Prescription drugs and over-the-counter drugs can also be dangerous to the unborn child if not taken as directed by a doctor. Some drugs damage genes, which give directions for physical traits, in the parents' sperm or egg. Damage may cause birth defects. Babies can be born addicted to drugs. Withdrawal symptoms after birth threaten life.

Caffeine is another substance which may cause problems. Caffeinated beverages should be consumed in moderation or avoided. Large amounts have caused birth defects in laboratory animals.

X-rays should be avoided unless approved by the doctor. This includes X-rays at the dentist. If X-rays are necessary, the entire abdomen should be shielded with lead-lined drapes. X-rays can cause birth defects. Immunizations aren't recommended during pregnancy, either.

## Smoking, Alcohol, and Drugs

Nicotine, alcohol, and drugs are hazardous substances that can permanently harm a developing fetus. These substances can cause brain damage and physical deformities. The greatest damage can occur in the first trimester before the woman even knows she's pregnant. Early pregnancy detection can help a woman change harmful practices early before damage occurs.

## High-Risk Pregnancies

High-risk pregnancies are those where one or both parents have a health condition or use substances that could potentially harm the fetus. Some conditions can also be harmful to the mother. A family history of hereditary disease, using dangerous substances, such as illegal drugs and alcohol, and having had diseases, such as diabetes, hepatitis, and STDs are some risk factors. Teenage pregnancies and pregnancies after the mother is over age 35 are also considered to be high risk.

High-risk pregnancies need to be watched closely by a health professional from the very beginning. Most have a healthy outcome. However, some high-risk pregnancies result in complications for the mother and birth defects in the baby.

Lab tests can be performed to detect many birth defects. The most common test is amniocentesis. This involves withdrawal of a small amount of the fluid in the uterus that surrounds the fetus. The fluid can be analyzed for the presence of over 60 defects and disorders and even the sex of the fetus. An

*Physical traits are inherited. What physical traits have you inherited from your family?*

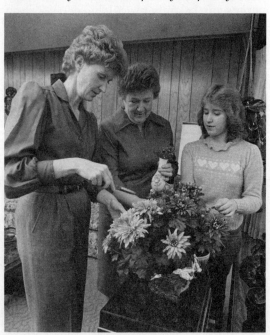

amniocentesis is a good idea for pregnant women over the age of 35, those who have had previous pregnancies with defects, or those who have a family history of defects.

High-risk pregnancies, especially those harmful to the fetus, worry parents-to-be. The pregnant woman often feels emotional stress. Good medical care, good health practices, and the support of others, such as the expectant father, help overcome some problems related to pregnancy.

## Genetic History

Heredity is the major factor in determining the characteristics and traits that a person has. It's typical for children to resemble their parents.

At the moment of conception, the fetus receives 23 chromosomes from each parent, equaling 46 chromosomes. Chromosomes are in the nucleus of each cell. Each chromosome carries thousands of genes. All physical characteristics and traits, such as hair thickness, facial features, and height, develop in the fetus during pregnancy. The code, or directions, came from the genes in the egg and sperm.

The egg or sperm that unite for a pregnancy can carry defective genes. A defect can be inherited, or passed down through many generations. Most genetic disorders, such as hemophilia, are the result of a single defective gene. The tendency to develop certain diseases or conditions, such as certain types of cancer, heart disease, diabetes, and mental illness, may be inherited, too.

Couples who have a family history of hereditary problems can get help from a genetic counselor. The counselor can help predict and prevent tragedies. A genetic counselor might be helpful to prospective parents in these situations:

• The couple has a history of genetic disease in either family.

- The couple already has a child with a genetic disease or a birth defect.
- One or both partners have a genetic disease.
- The woman has been exposed to drugs, X-rays, or a virus before or in the first two trimesters of pregnancy.
- The woman has had several miscarriages. A *miscarriage* is the natural termination of a pregnancy before the fetus can live outside the uterus.

## Environmental Risks

Damage to genes in the egg or sperm may occur from illness or substance abuse by the parents-to-be. Exposure to some industrial wastes may cause gene damage and affect the fetus, too.

## Teenage Pregnancy

Teenage pregnancy is considered to be high risk. The normal demands for growth along with the added physical and emotional demands of pregnancy create hazards for the teenage mother and fetus.

The special concerns of a teenage pregnancy include nutrition, size of the birth canal, and emotional immaturity. An adolescent female already has high nutritional needs because she is still growing. During pregnancy she adds the nutritional demands of the fetus. In a girl who has not completed her own growth, the pelvis may be small, too. Depending on her size, the birth canal may be too small for the passage of a full-grown fetus. The normal emotions of adolescence, coupled with the physical and hormonal changes of pregnancy, may be too much to cope with. The incidence of single motherhood is highest among adolescents. These girls may have less emotional support from the father, her family, and friends than a woman who has a baby at a later and more settled time in life.

Pregnant teens are more likely to experience maternal complications. (These will be discussed a little later in the chapter.) Their babies also have a greater chance of being born underweight or with birth defects.

## Pregnancy Later

While there aren't specifically known causes, pregnant women over the age of 35 have a higher incidence of complications. And their babies have a higher incidence of defects, such as Down's syndrome which causes mental retardation.

With good prenatal care, many women over 35 are having normal pregnancies and healthy babies. Due to a variety of social and personal factors, more women are conceiving and bearing children later in life.

*Down's syndrome is a birth defect more common among children born to women over age 35.*

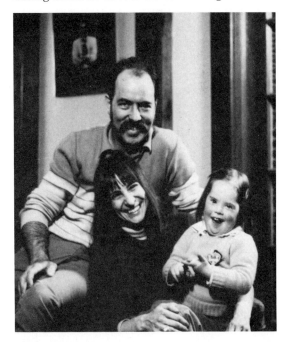

## Maternal Complications

Maternal complications are those that happen to the mother during pregnancy. In turn, they may affect the fetus. Sometimes they result from high-risk pregnancies. Other times the cause is completely unknown or unavoidable. Some maternal complications include miscarriage, ectopic pregnancy, and toxemia.

## Miscarriage

A miscarriage usually occurs before the end of the twentieth week of pregnancy. Some women experience a miscarriage, or even repeated miscarriages, without a known cause. However, there are many known causes including:

- hormone imbalance.
- defect in the egg or sperm.
- infectious disease.
- physical trauma such as a fall or car accident. In most cases, a fetus is well protected from minor mishaps by the amniotic fluid which surrounds it.
- poor environment inside the uterus.

Early signs of a miscarriage are bleeding from the vagina and low abdominal pain. These signs, even in the mildest form, should be reported to the obstetrician immediately. Sometimes a threatened miscarriage can be prevented or at least delayed until the fetus is more mature. The best way to prevent a miscarriage is to practice good health habits prior to and during pregnancy.

## Ectopic Pregnancy

When conception and growth of the fetus occur outside the uterus, this is called an ectopic pregnancy. Ectopic pregnancies may occur in the fallopian tubes which lead from the ovaries to the uterus. The ovaries are the female reproductive organs. An ectopic pregnancy may be caused by faulty reproductive organs, especially the fallopian tubes.

Because the hormone changes of ectopic pregnancy are similar to those of a normal pregnancy, a woman has all the early signs. Even a laboratory test for pregnancy is positive. But as the fetus grows, it puts pressure on surrounding organs, causing cramping and pain. For the safety of the woman, the only treatment is surgical removal.

## Toxemia

Late in pregnancy, some women develop a condition called toxemia. This is a combination of symptoms including high blood pressure, swelling, and protein in the urine. The cause of toxemia isn't known. But many doctors think that poor nutrition is an underlying factor. Smoking and overexhaustion might be, too. Women who already have high blood pressure or kidney disease are at higher risk.

Toxemia needs to be watched closely and treated by a physician. The early stage of toxemia includes frequent headaches and blurred vision. It can usually be kept under control with rest and diet, and a normal birth will result. However, in its later stages, there is a chance of convulsions and coma for the mother. A coma is prolonged unconsciousness. In this stage, toxemia is a life-threatening complication to the mother and fetus. The baby should be delivered as soon as possible for the safety of the mother and baby.

## Childbirth

Childbirth is the big event! After nine months, the time has arrived. Mothers and fathers await childbirth with feelings of excitement, anticipation, and perhaps some apprehension.

## Preparation for Birth

Before birth, many plans need to be made. They include readying the home, making some important decisions, and preparing for the hospital stay.

## PREPARING THE HOME

Before birth, the baby's home and belongings need to be prepared. The nursery should be set up, and baby clothes and a car seat bought. This need not cost a lot of money. Most baby items can be borrowed. And many are received as gifts.

As the mother's third trimester progresses, other children in the family need to be prepared for the arrival of a new brother or sister. Older children should be told as soon as the pregnancy is confirmed. Young children, who have little concept of time, are best told only when they begin to ask questions or a few weeks before the expected birth date. Even with the best explanations and planning, the arrival of a new baby is upsetting to other children in a family. Parents should be prepared for the children's withdrawal, jealousy, or selfishness.

## IMPORTANT DECISIONS

Many important decisions must be made as childbirth approaches. The parents-to-be make choices about where and how to deliver the baby, who the baby's pediatrician will be, and how to prepare for the delivery.

There are many options about where a baby is born. Most couples prefer a hospital because staff and equipment can respond to unexpected complications. Others prefer to deliver at home because they feel secure in familiar surroundings with family and

*Parents can help prepare preschool children for a new brother or sister by reading specially-written children's books about having a baby.*

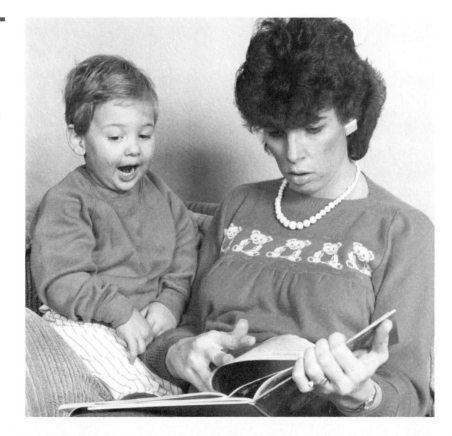

friends nearby. Only healthy women with uncomplicated pregnancies are advised to deliver at home.

At home or in the hospital, there are different methods of childbirth:

- For natural childbirth the mother uses little or no artificial assistance, such as pain-relieving medicines or machines. This reduces problems from heavy medications. Lamaze techniques of breathing and eye-focusing exercises are often used to control delivery.
- The LeBoyer method reduces trauma by allowing the baby to be delivered in a quiet, dimly-lit room and to be immediately massaged and given a warm bath.
- Caesarean section is when the baby is surgically removed through an incision in the woman's abdomen and uterus.

Choosing the new baby's doctor is another important decision. The pediatrician visits the newborn in the hospital, usually on the day of or the day after delivery. So arrangements need to be made in advance. A woman's obstetrician is a good source for referral for a pediatrician.

Classes on childbirth and parenthood are available at most hospitals and from many doctors. Expectant mothers and fathers benefit from the courses by learning what to expect during childbirth and how to safely care for a new baby. This usually gives them confidence and lessens their anxiety. The courses are particularly helpful when the parents are expecting their first child.

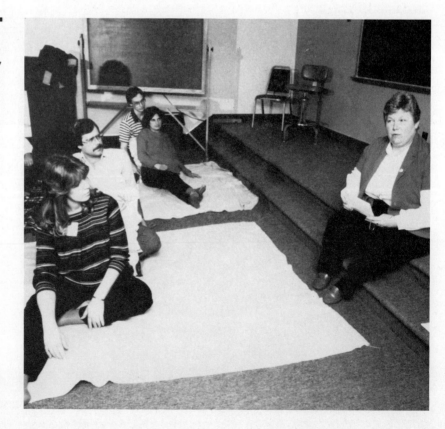

*A few weeks before the pregnant woman's delivery date, she may take classes with her coach. Together, they'll learn exercises and breathing in preparation for childbirth.*

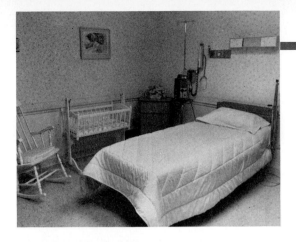

# CHILDBIRTH IN THE EIGHTIES

backache. Women with healthy pregnancies may stay in the labor spa until delivery is near. Then they are carefully transferred to a delivery room.

A Julia bar is a device that assists women in labor. They squat or kneel on a foam pillow while hanging their arms over the bar. Use of the bar eases the discomforts of labor and often speeds the baby's travel through the birth canal. It's different, but it works!

Not long ago, childbirth was treated like a serious illness. Babies were born in a hospital delivery room that looked much like an operating room, and the mother and baby stayed in the hospital for seven to 10 days. Things have certainly changed. Now many women are giving birth at home, in nonhospital birthing centers, and in specially-equipped hospital birthing rooms. Nontraditional devices are also being used to make childbirth easier.

A birthing suite or room is a combination labor and delivery room that has a homelike decor. There are no harsh lights or stainless steel equipment. Instead, the birthing room may have colorfully decorated bedroom furniture, pastel-colored drapes, a wicker basinette, and flowered wallpaper. The bed, however, is adjustable for ease of delivery of the baby.

Some hospitals and birthing centers now have hot tubs! Labor spas, similar to commercial hot tubs, provide relaxation and comfort for women in labor. Soaking in warm, circulating water decreases the discomfort of labor contractions as well as

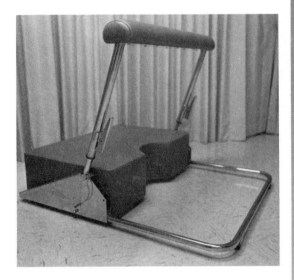

## HOSPITAL STAY

Babies rarely are born on their exact due date, so it's wise for a pregnant woman to be ready to go to the hospital any time in the last month. Knowing the way to the hospital and having all supplies ready saves time and relieves stress when it's the real thing.

A practice trip to the hospital is important for expectant parents. They learn how long the trip takes, the location of the admissions office, the location of the emergency entrance, and where the car should be parked.

Some hospitals offer orientation tours of the maternity department. Seeing the rooms, equipment, and nursery in advance is reassuring. It's also a good time to learn the hospital's policies on visitors and visiting hours.

Pre-packing a bag of the mother's and baby's supplies for the hospital is helpful. Hospitals supply the basics—plain gown, toiletries, and all health supplies. Most women also want personal items, such as slippers, cosmetics, and grooming supplies. The baby needs a complete outfit to wear home from the hospital.

## Birth Process

Birth is an eventful finale to a miraculous process. During pregnancy, the fetus has become a being capable of living outside the mother's uterus. During the last month, the baby moves into position in preparation for childbirth. This is sometimes referred to as the baby dropping.

Labor is the way a woman's body prepares for and delivers a baby. It's not known exactly what causes labor to start. But the mother has clues that labor will begin soon. When this happens, the doctor or nurse midwife should be called. These are clues that labor is about to begin:

• Slight, mucus bleeding comes from the vagina. This may happen a few days before labor begins.

• The amniotic fluid surrounding the fetus leaks out, slowly or in a gush through the vagina. The sac holding the fluid has broken. When this happens, a doctor usually advises the woman to come immediately to the hospital.

• Abdominal cramps get more intense and more frequent. These are called contractions. The doctor will want to know how frequent they are and how long they last. This may mean that labor has started. Most women go to the hospital when contractions are five to 10 minutes apart.

With these signs, the woman might be instructed to go to the hospital immediately. Or it might be a false alarm, and she is told to wait for true labor to begin.

At the hospital, the mother goes to the maternity department where the baby will be born. A health professional, usually a nurse, examines and prepares her for labor and delivery. The length of labor varies from woman to woman, but the average length for all deliveries is 16 hours.

The first stage of labor is marked by frequent, intense, and regular contractions. Eventually these are only minutes apart, and each contraction lasts one minute. Controlled breathing, relaxation between contractions, and diversion help the mother from getting too tense. Tight muscles make labor more difficult. The father or other coach can provide emotional support. Some women need medication to strengthen contractions or to relieve discomfort.

With each contraction the uterine opening, called the cervix, dilates, or widens. It must dilate to about four inches, or 10 centimeters, for the baby to be born.

In most hospitals, a coach is allowed into the delivery room with the mother. Usually

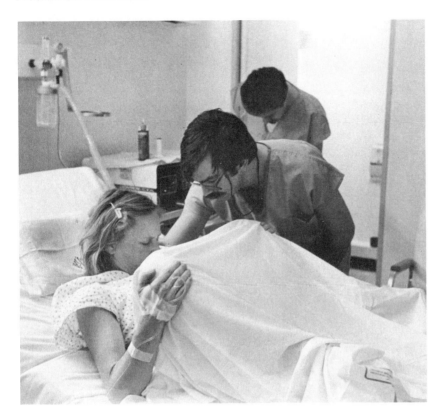

*In the delivery room, a woman gives birth with the help and support of her coach and health professionals.*

the coach is the father but can be a friend or any relative. The coach helps the woman in labor by providing information, comfort, diversion, and the security of sharing the experience with someone special.

As the time for delivery approaches, uterine contractions push the baby into the birth canal. Most babies move through the birth canal head first. The head is soft and flexible so it can move through the birth canal. When the baby's feet or bottom come through the birth canal first, this is called a breech birth.

Delivery of the baby is the next stage of labor. When in a normal position, the baby is delivered in three phases: first the head, then the shoulders, and finally the body and legs. The doctors and nurses attending the delivery don't rush the delivery. The baby comes when it is ready. The mother assists the process by pushing, or bearing down. The doctor may make a small cut in the woman's vaginal opening to make sure it's large enough to let the baby through. This is called an episiotomy. This keeps the mother's tissues from being torn.

The last stage of labor is expelling the placenta, often called the afterbirth. This causes little pain to the mother.

As soon as the baby is delivered, the doctor or nurse midwife checks the baby's breathing and other signs of health. Immediate medical attention is given to the newborn by doing the following:

• The baby is held head down to drain away fluids that might cause choking.

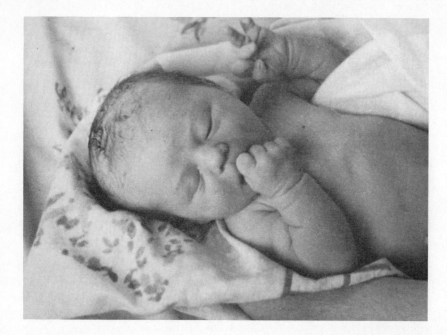

*This is the moment that the parents have waited nine months for.*

- A bulb syringe is used to clear the mouth and nose of mucus which might block the baby's airway. Then the baby can breathe and cry.
- The umbilical cord which provided nourishment and oxygen before birth is tied, clamped, and cut off.
- Drops of antiseptic, such as silver nitrate, are put in the baby's eyes to protect them from infection.

The mother and coach may hold and touch the newborn in the delivery room. This helps begin an emotional attachment, called *bonding*. Bonding grows stronger as time passes.

## Postnatal Care

Immediately after birth, the newborn baby and mother need close monitoring by health professionals. This is called postnatal care. There are risks of complications which can be detected and treated early. Also, the baby and mother need care and support to recover from the stress of delivery.

## Care of the Newborn

The attention to an infant just after birth is called neonatal care. A *neonate* is a newborn during the first four weeks of life.

For the first few minutes after birth, a baby is continuously watched by doctors and nurses. They check the newborn's breathing, muscle tone, reflexes, heart beat, and skin color. These are indications of the baby's health and well-being.

While mother and baby are still in the delivery room, identification bands are put on the baby's wrist and ankle. These bands identify which baby belongs to which mother. Footprints are taken for identification, as well. These steps ensure that babies won't be mixed up.

While the mother is in the recovery room, the baby is taken to the hospital nursery. There, nurses give the baby a thorough examination.

The newborn may stay in the hospital nursery during the mother's stay. However, in most hospitals, the mother may choose to keep the baby in her hospital room. This is called rooming-in. The mother provides for the newborn's needs. The father can visit at any time. Both parents can learn together to handle and care for the baby. The first few days are a time of closeness where the parents' and baby's attachment to each other grows.

## Recovery of the Mother

In the delivery room, the mother is tired. Some women say that giving birth is the hardest work they'll ever do. New mothers need time to recover from the stress of pregnancy and delivery.

The mother spends a few hours in the maternity recovery room. There she is closely watched for signs of complications. Nurses feel the mother's abdomen to determine the condition of the uterus. They may even massage the uterus to slow bleeding. Discomfort from uterine cramps are common. Temperature and blood pressure are checked for signs of infection and bleeding.

If she has no complications in the recovery room, the new mother is taken to her hospital room. Most women stay in the hospital for two or three days to rest after the delivery. They need rest before fully assuming the responsibilities of parenthood. Nurses in the hospital also teach new mothers about breast feeding, baby care, and personal care.

Once home, new parents realize the full responsibility of infant care. It's not unusual for new mothers to have conflicting feelings about motherhood for the first few weeks. Some women feel depressed. Called postpartum blues or postnatal depression, these emotions usually come from hormone changes, the tiring effect of childbirth, and the adjustment in lifestyle. Help and support from the father and other family members help her cope. These feelings usually pass when new routines are established, and she is rested.

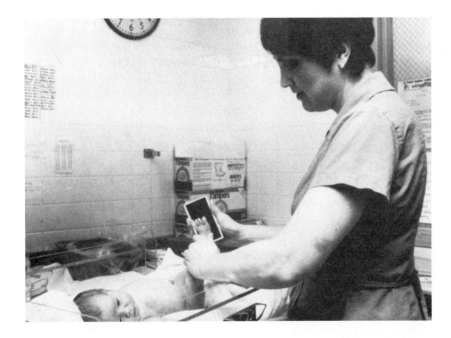

*Footprints are used in the hospital for identification. They are also a keepsake for the parents.*

A few weeks after delivery, women usually have a follow-up checkup with the doctor.

## Infant Complications

Newborn babies have drastic adjustments to make. Immediately after birth, their bodies must begin breathing, eating, and doing many other functions. Sometimes there are complications in these basic body functions. For the newborn's health, complications should be detected and treated as soon as possible. Some complications are prematurity and jaundice.

### PREMATURITY

The longer a fetus grows in its mother's uterus, the more developed it is, and the better its chances are for survival at birth. Prematurity is when a baby is born too soon, before its body systems are developed fully.

Premature babies weigh less than five and one-half pounds. They have their body features, but they're thin with weak muscles. All of their body systems are underdeveloped. They may struggle just to breathe and hold their body heat. Some very tiny babies are put in incubators for protection and careful monitoring. Incubators are enclosed cribs where temperature and air flow can be controlled.

Premature babies have a higher than normal incidence of impairments and infant death. Their development is slower than full-term newborns, but most catch up by the age of two or three. With excellent care, babies born as small as two pounds become healthy children!

Premature babies stay in the hospital after the mother goes home. Expert nursing care is important for the baby's survival. Nutrition, hygiene, protection, and observation are part of the baby's care. The mother and father are encouraged to visit and, if possible, hold the baby often.

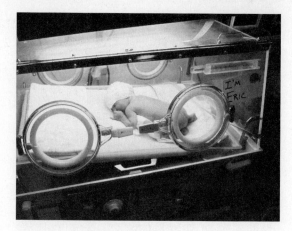

*Premature infants as small as two pounds at birth can survive when they're kept in incubators. All aspects of their health are closely watched until the infants have grown enough to be on their own.*

### JAUNDICE

About one third of all newborns have jaundice. This is a yellow coloration of babies' skin and eyeballs. Jaundice in most newborns is not usually dangerous. It's caused by too much bilirubin in the blood. Bilirubin is a by-product from the breakdown of iron which comes from changes in the neonate's red blood cells. Usually within a few days after birth, the baby's liver handles the problem, and the yellow color goes away. Putting the baby under an ultraviolet light helps the condition, too. There usually are no lasting effects.

In a small number of babies, jaundice is a serious condition, especially among premature babies. Severe jaundice can cause permanent brain damage, so it must be treated quickly. The most effective treatment includes ultraviolet light, blood transfusions, and medicine. A blood transfusion is the transfer of blood from one person to another. About one half of the infants with severe jaundice survive.

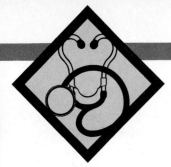

# CHAPTER CHECKUP

## Reviewing the Information

1. What are the signs of pregnancy?
2. Name two changes in the developing fetus for each of the three trimesters.
3. Why is good prenatal care important in the first trimester?
4. What does a prenatal exam include?
5. What are four special nutritional needs of a pregnant woman?
6. What types of activity are appropriate during pregnancy?
7. Why might a pregnant woman need emotional support?
8. Name five substances that can be harmful to a developing fetus.
9. Why are backaches common late in pregnancy?
10. Why isn't pregnancy a time to follow a weight-loss diet?
11. What are four high-risk pregnancies?
12. Why is teenage pregnancy a concern?
13. Name four things that might cause a miscarriage?
14. What can parents-to-be learn from a visit to the hospital in preparation for childbirth?
15. What are the signs that labor is near?
16. Describe the birth process.
17. Describe three things done to a newborn immediately after delivery.
18. What is rooming-in?
19. What is a premature baby?

## Thinking It Over

1. What are the responsibilities of parenthood during pregnancy?
2. How might a father-to-be support prenatal care?
3. What conflicting feelings might parents-to-be have early in pregnancy?
4. How might a pregnant woman change her eating, and exercise habits?
5. How might a health condition of the parents affect an unborn child?
6. How might a coach help a pregnant woman during labor and delivery?
7. What challenges face a pregnant teen?
8. How do nutritional needs for pregnant and non-pregnant women compare?
9. How might chances for birth defects be reduced?

## Taking Action

1. Find out about common wives' tales about prenatal care. Research why these myths are inaccurate.

2. Interview a mother about her pregnancy—about her prenatal care, discomforts, and labor. Write what you learn.

3. Plan a nutritious day's menu for a pregnant woman.
4. Take an orientation tour of the maternity department at your local hospital.

# 9 Infant Care

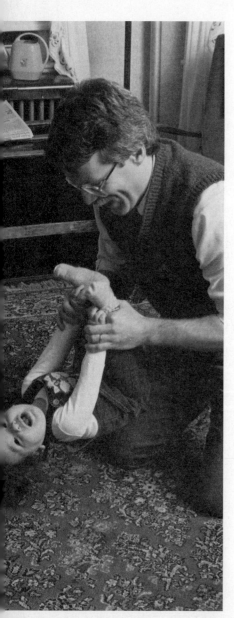

After reading this chapter, you should be able to:

• plan a safe sleep and play environment for an infant.

• explain healthful and safe ways to feed, bathe, and clothe a baby.

• communicate with a baby in ways that promote healthy growth and development.

• propose medical supervision needed for an infant.

## Terms to Understand

| | |
|---|---|
| allergy | diarrhea |
| burping | fever |
| colic | infant |
| cradle cap | sudden infant death syndrome |
| diaper rash | |

Infants are wonderful beings, and taking care of them is a big responsibility. An *infant* is a baby from birth to one year of age. Infants need a safe and healthy environment for their growth, development, and happiness. You may share in the responsibilities of infant care if you baby-sit or have an infant in your family.

A healthy baby:

- has a steady gain in height and weight. The average baby weighs seven to eight pounds and measures 20 inches at birth. By age one, he or she triples his or her birth weight and grows 50 percent longer.
- has an appetite. An infant will eat and drink without much coaxing.
- sleeps well. Newborns spend most of their time sleeping. They wake up seven or eight times a day. By four or five months, they sleep through the night and stay awake longer during the day.
- feels good most of the time.

Part of creating a safe and healthful environment is providing safe surroundings, special handling, the right food, and nurturing activities. Nurturing means caring for a baby or child in a loving and emotionally supportive way. Medical care is also a part of safe, healthful infant care.

## Safe Surroundings

Protecting the baby from harm is an important priority. Infants are totally dependent on others for their safety. Keeping an infant safe means choosing equipment very carefully, being alert to hazards, and being prepared to respond to life or death emergencies.

### Infant Equipment

Cribs, baby seats, toys, and other infant equipment should be chosen with safety in mind.

#### CRIBS

Babies need a safe place to sleep. When they're newborn, they may sleep in bassinets, or small basketlike infant beds, or in a box, a basket, or a dresser drawer if it's padded well. Cribs, which are larger, are

*Keep the rails of a crib up when an infant is sleeping or playing.*

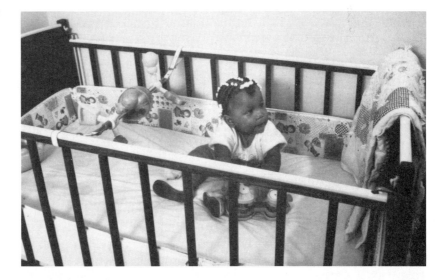

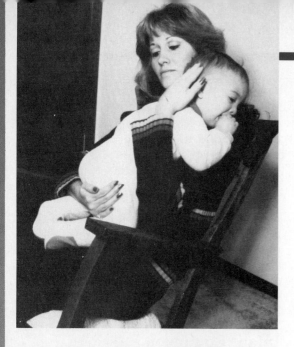

# NEONATAL CARE

A neonate is an infant in its first four weeks of life. During that time, a baby needs special care.

- Don't get the stump of the umbilical cord wet. Before birth, the umbilical cord connected the fetus to the mother's placenta, which provided the fetus with nourishment. At birth, the umbilical cord is severed, and the remaining stump gradually dries up. Sponge bathe the baby until the umbilical cord dries and falls off. This happens within a week or two, leaving a depression called the navel. Sometimes the navel bleeds slightly for a few days. This should be cleaned gently with soap and water or with alcohol. The doctor should be informed if bleeding lasts longer than three days.
- If an infant boy is circumcised, wash the sensitive area gently, and apply petroleum jelly for about two weeks, or until the area heals. Circumcision is the removal of foreskin from the tip of the penis. This is done for hygienic or religious reasons. For uncircumcised infant boys, press the foreskin back gently for cleansing.
- Support the newborn's neck and back. The neck muscles aren't strong enough yet for the baby to hold his or her head up. The picture on the left shows how to hold the infant.
- Protect the two soft areas, called fontanelles, on the head. These are areas where the skull bones haven't yet grown together. One soft spot is in front over the forehead, and the other is at the crown of the head. The soft spots close up as the skull bones grow together. This usually takes a year or more.
- Feed the newborn when he or she is hungry, about 6 to 12 times a day and about two to four hours apart. A newborn usually wakes up two or three times during the night to eat.
- Provide an undisturbed place to sleep. Newborns sleep most of the time. They use up a lot of their energy eating and crying.
- Help the baby establish a schedule for eating and sleeping. This usually takes about a month. Babies benefit from having a rhythm to their lives.
- Keep the newborn warm, dry, and clean.
- Know that a baby's bowel movements are different. The first bowel movements are a sticky green-black color. They turn yellow, green, or brown within a week or two. Often they are very soft. This is normal.
- Develop a sense of trust by giving the newborn plenty of attention and love.

used when the baby is able to turn over. This often occurs around two months of age.

Some cribs are safer than others. A safe crib has:

- sides high enough to keep a baby from falling out. The recommended height is 26 inches.
- slats no more than 2⅜ inches apart so the baby can't put his or her head in between.
- a firm mattress which fits snugly into the bed frame to keep the baby from getting caught between the mattress and the bed frame. If you can place two fingers between the mattress and frame, it isn't snug enough.
- a railing latch which the baby cannot release.
- a bed frame where the mattress may be lowered to make the bed safe as the baby gets older and can stand in the bed.
- bumper pads to protect the infant from rolling into the slats. These pads also may make the newborn feel cozy and secure.

Some parents put a baby into their own bed for sleeping. However, adults may roll onto the baby. A baby is always safer in its own bed.

## INFANT SEATS

A baby needs safe infant seats. A baby carrier, a high chair, and a car seat are important for infant care.

Many parents seat their newborns in reclining baby carriers. A safe carrier is sturdy so that it won't tip easily. It also has a harness to keep the baby in place. A baby carrier should be placed out of the flow of household traffic and in a secure place, such as on the floor near a chair where the mother or father is sitting. A baby carrier is not a safe or suitable substitute for a car seat unless it is specifically designed to also meet this purpose.

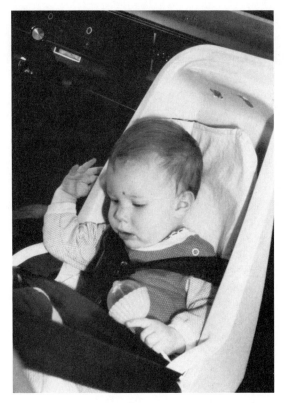

*For safety, young children must be harnessed into a car seat. Newborns are safest in a rear-facing seat, and toddlers face forward.*

A more active baby who sits up needs a high chair for feeding and for play. A high chair should be sturdy and have a safety belt that includes a strap between the legs, and an adjustable footrest. It also should be easy to clean.

A car seat, held in place by the car's seat belt, protects a baby in an automobile. Adult safety belts can't protect babies or toddlers. A newborn is safest in a rear-facing seat which holds him or her in a half-reclining position. A car seat for older babies and toddlers faces forward. A car seat provides the most protection when it is placed in the back seat of an automobile.

All states require that children younger than four years of age or weighing under 40 pounds be restrained in a car seat. Securing a baby in a car seat should become a habit which begins when a newborn first comes home from the hospital.

### INFANT TOYS

Babies need toys for mental stimulation and for muscular development. Although toys may be educational and fun, they can also hurt babies. Check everything you give a baby to play with to see if it is safe. Ask yourself these questions:

- Does it have small parts that can be removed, swallowed, or put in the nose or ears?
- Does it have sharp edges or points that can cut?
- Does it have ropes or loops that can strangle?
- Is the toy fireproof?
- If it breaks, will it injure the baby?
- Does it have toxic, or poisonous, paint?

Most toymakers put an age-group label on toys. Toys can be bought according to these labels, but they should also be carefully inspected for safety before being given to a baby or a child. It is the consumer's responsibility to judge each toy for safety.

## Hazards for Infants

As babies begin to crawl about, they may try to play with things that can be dangerous. Keep harmful objects out of their reach.

- Plastic bags, coins, and marbles are examples of objects that attract babies' attention and can cause suffocation or choking.
- Electric wall outlets should be protected with special plugs or guards so that infants don't stick an object or their fingers in them.
- Cabinets with household chemicals and medicines should be locked. It is best to

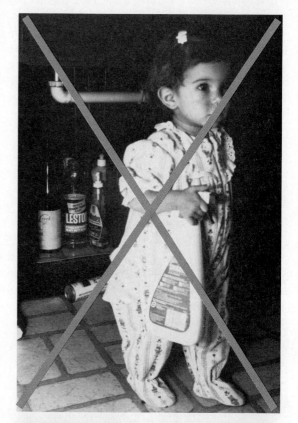

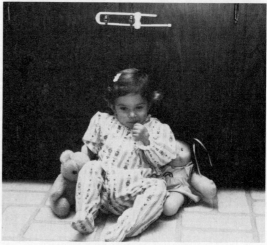

*When infants start crawling, they can get into cabinets containing dangerous household products or medicines. Keep these products in high or locked cabinets.*

keep all household cleaning products and medicines in high, out-of-reach places or in locked cabinets.
- Child-proof gates can be installed so crawling infants don't fall down stairs.
- Wires and cords should be out of reach so that babies and small children don't pull things down on top of themselves.

## Handling a Baby with Special Care

Parents can help provide safety for babies by holding them carefully, by watching them closely when other children are around, and by giving babysitters safety instructions.

## Holding a Baby

The way you hold a baby makes it feel safe and secure. Since a baby's muscles aren't well developed yet, the support you provide is important. When you pick up and hold a baby, support its head, back, and hips. Refer to the illustration below.

## Safety with Other Children

Careful supervision is necessary when children are with a new baby. Young brothers and sisters, who aren't used to competition for their parents' attention, may harm a newborn by overturning the bassinet or by hitting the baby. Curious toddlers may poke at or pull on a baby as a sign of interest. Children can hurt a baby unintentionally with rough play. Preparing young children for a new baby may prevent this.

After a time, most children learn how to act around a new baby, and they learn loving, nurturing behavior. Then close supervision may not be necessary.

## Safety with Sitters

Parents can't be with their baby all the time. Time away from a baby is often good

*Handle a newborn with care:*
- *Turn the baby onto his or her back.*
- *Slip one of your hands under the hips.*
- *Slip your other hand under the baby's head and shoulders.*
- *Raise the baby gently into your arms. Support the head with your hand. When a baby grows strong enough, it will hold its own head without your support.*
- *Don't make sudden movements which may be frightening or may cause injury.*

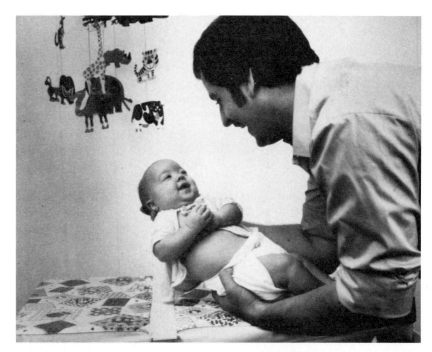

for the parent-child relationship. And time spent with another nurturing person is good because babies learn to relate to and trust others. Other caregivers also can broaden an infant's experiences.

A good, reliable sitter is experienced and mature enough to handle difficulties and necessary care. Infants and toddlers usually respond best when the same sitter stays with them each time since familiarity builds trust and rapport.

## Feeding an Infant

Mother's milk or a specially-prepared formula is a baby's first food. Either food provides nourishment for a baby's normal growth and development.

Both breast and bottle-fed babies should be held, cuddled, and talked to during feeding. This is also important when feeding an infant solid foods. Soft talking or singing provides comfort, love, and a sense of security. It's important for babies to associate eating with pleasant, happy times.

### Breast Feeding

Breast feeding is a natural, easy, and low-cost way to feed an infant. Mother's milk is healthful, it has the nutrients a baby needs, and it also helps the baby build a natural immunity to many illnesses. It's sanitary, pre-warmed, and easy to digest. Breast feeding also promotes bonding, or closeness, between the mother and baby. For mothers who are with their babies during the day, breast feeding is convenient. Working mothers can also breast feed if they manage their personal schedules carefully. Breast feeding has another advantage for the mother. It helps her return to her pre-pregnancy weight more quickly.

A nursing mother must choose her own food carefully to get the needed nutrients. She needs a balanced diet from the four food groups with extra foods from the Milk and Cheese Group and plenty of liquids. Chapter 8 shows a balanced diet for a breast-feeding woman. As during pregnancy, a nursing mother should avoid substances which can be passed to the baby—nicotine, alcohol, drugs, and caffeine.

### Bottle Feeding

Bottle-fed babies may be just as healthy as breast-fed infants. Bottle feeding is the choice of many parents, especially those who work outside the home. Some fathers prefer bottle feeding so that they may share in the feeding responsibility and feel a closeness to the infant. Some babies learn to both breast feed and bottle feed. In this way, a mother is free to work, but she can still give her baby the benefits of breast milk.

Health experts have found that letting babies go to bed with a bottle may cause tooth decay. As they continue to suck on the bottle, their erupting teeth are exposed to the natural sugars in juices or milk for a long time. This leads to decay.

Some bottle-fed babies may become too plump if parents encourage them to always finish the bottle. Breast-fed babies eat only until they are full.

The parents who choose bottle feeding shouldn't give cow's milk regularly until the baby is about one year of age. Formula is more like mother's milk. And it has nutrients not found in cow's milk. Formula is also easier to digest and less likely to cause allergic reactions. An *allergy* is a sensitivity to a substance which can cause a rash, stomach pain, vomiting, or diarrhea.

The baby's doctor will suggest the type of formula and the type of bottles for an infant. Directions for preparing the formula are usually given on the package. The doctor will also advise parents when the baby is ready for cow's milk.

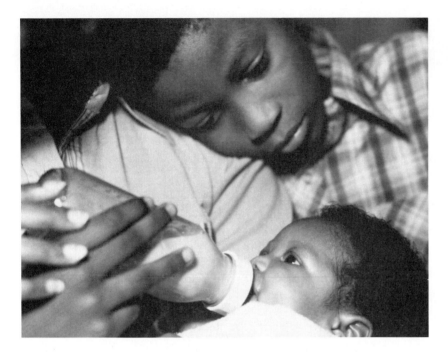

*When feeding a baby, tilt the bottle so the nipple is always full of milk. And always hold a baby while bottle feeding.*

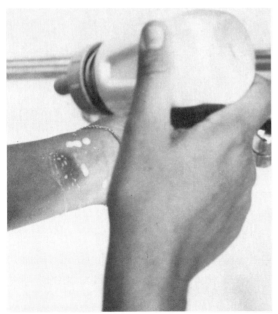

*Check the temperature of the formula before giving a bottle to a baby. It should be neither hot nor cold.*

Bottles must be handled in a sanitary way so they don't transmit harmful bacteria. Bottles and nipples should be cleaned in hot, soapy water, then rinsed thoroughly, dried, and stored in a clean place. The caregiver should avoid touching the point of the nipple, too, so it stays as clean as possible. Unfinished formula left in the bottle should be discarded.

## Burping

When babies suck milk from the breast or bottle, they swallow air. Then they feel very uncomfortable. *Burping* helps babies expel that air.

To burp a baby, follow one of these two procedures:

• Place a towel on your shoulder. Hold the baby up with his or her head against your shoulder. Turn the baby's head to the side. Pat or rub the baby's back until the air is released.

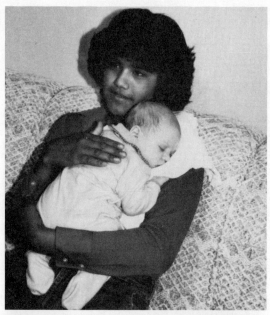

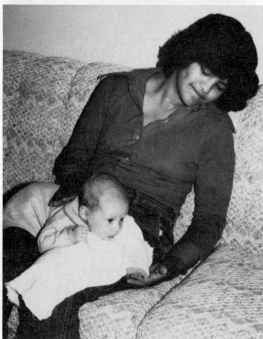

*Either method of burping an infant helps expell swallowed air. Stop every two ounces to burp the baby.*

• Place a towel on your lap. Sit the baby up in your lap, supporting the chest with one of your hands. Lean the baby forward. With your other hand, rub or pat the baby's back until the air is released.

## Solid Foods

A newborn can't easily swallow or digest solid foods. But between three to six months, the digestive system is ready for simple foods, such as baby cereal. Pediatricians tell parents when to begin solid foods. Baby cereal is the first solid food. Fruits, vegetables, and meats are added in progression, as recommended by a health-care professional. Pureed or strained foods are given first, then coarsely ground food, and then chopped foods. This is so the baby doesn't choke.

Some foods should be avoided until a child learns to chew. A baby can choke on nuts, raw carrots, grapes, corn, popcorn, seeds, bites of hot dogs, and other small foods.

Solid foods should be introduced into the baby's diet one at a time. This makes it easier to identify any food that may cause an allergic reaction. Any food that causes a rash, abdominal discomfort, or a change in bowel habits should be discontinued.

A gradual addition of a variety of foods provides needed nutrients. Babies also learn to like many foods as different ones are added to their diet.

Foods should be served at lukewarm temperatures. Hot foods can burn a baby's mouth and tongue.

Baby food shouldn't have salt, sugar, fat, or spices added.

Communicable illnesses may be spread through foods. Don't feed an infant directly from a jar of baby food. Instead, place a small portion in a bowl so the unused portion won't be contaminated by repeatedly inserting the feeding spoon. Bacteria from the spoon multiply quickly in warm food.

Refrigerate any baby food left in the jar immediately. Be sure to use sanitary procedures when cleaning the baby's eating utensils. Wash them in hot, soapy water, and rinse them thoroughly before drying and placing them in a clean place.

Babies shouldn't be forced to overeat or finish a bottle. They let caregivers know when they are full. Infants and children who are overfed may develop weight problems.

## Keeping an Infant Clean and Warm

To feel secure and happy, a baby needs to feel warm and clean. Think of how a baby snuggles under a warm blanket. Warmth and cleanliness make a baby feel comfortable, secure, and happy.

## Bathing the Baby

Bathing a baby can be pleasant for both the baby and the caregiver. It should be a relaxed, unhurried opportunity to give loving care. When possible, bathe the baby at the same time every day.

## Bathing Equipment

A comfortable bath area is warm and free of drafts. A bathinette, a large clean dishpan, or even the kitchen sink may be used for bathing. A bathinette is a bathing table for infants. A towel can be used to line and cushion the sink. A flat surface, such as a cabinet top, is also needed for placing the baby on before and after the bath.

Before beginning, assemble the supplies. These include:
- large and small bath towels
- washcloth
- bath pad
- baby soap
- baby shampoo
- cotton balls
- lotion, or oil and powder
- fresh diapers (and diaper pins, if needed)
- clean clothing

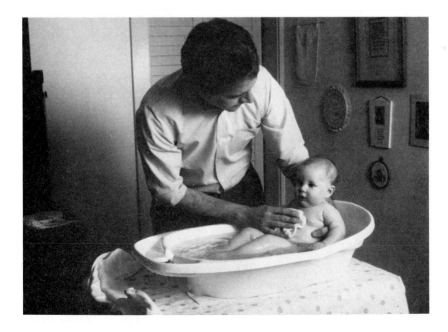

*A baby can't hold its own head up and out of the water. The caregiver must support the baby's back and head while giving a bath.*

## SAFETY IN THE BATH

A baby's bath has many hazards. Take special care to keep a baby safe during a bath.

- Keep a small towel under the infant tub to prevent it from slipping.
- Use bath water that's about 100° F. Hot water might burn baby's sensitive skin, and cold water can cause the baby to get chilled. Test the temperature by lowering your elbow into the water.
- Support the head and back properly while you bathe and dry the infant.
- Always keep one hand on the baby during the bath. He or she could fall out of the tub or drown, even in a small amount of water.
- Use mild soap to prevent skin irritation.
- Do not put soap on the baby's face. It might get in the eyes.
- Wash and rinse the hair with the head tilted down so water and shampoo don't run into the baby's eyes.
- Do not use cotton-tipped sticks to clean ears or nose; a washcloth is sufficient. Cotton-tipped sticks may injure a baby's tender tissue. Don't attempt to clean inside the nose or ears.
- When the baby is older, do not allow standing or climbing in the tub. A youngster can easily slip, fall, and receive an injury.
- Never leave the baby alone in a tub or bathinette. If you can't ignore an interruption, wrap the baby in a large towel. Then take the baby with you, or put him or her in bed.
- Dry the baby carefully, giving special attention to skin folds, where rashes might start. Then dress the baby immediately to prevent chills.
- Gently talk or sing to the baby while bathing him or her to relieve fear of the water.

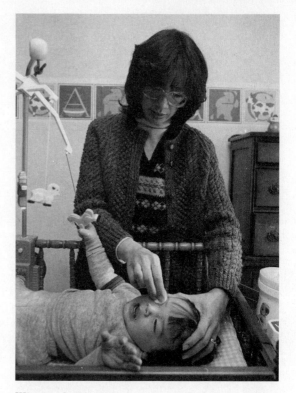

*Wipe each eye with a new and clean cotton ball moistened with warm water and squeezed out. Gently wipe the eyes from the nose towards the ears.*

## Infant Clothing

Babies need clean, comfortable clothing. Lightweight clothing is usually suitable for indoors. Garments worn outside depend on the season and the local climate. In the hot summer, a diaper and shirt might be enough. But in the winter, babies need warm clothes to go outside.

Since babies grow very fast, they don't need many clothes. But they need enough for a change when they soil their garments. Essential items include: diapers, cotton-knit shirts, nightgowns or sleepers, sweaters and caps, socks, small blankets, and bibs.

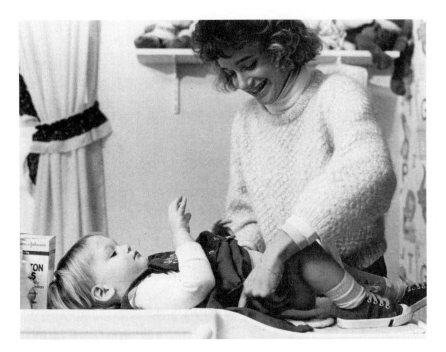

*Changing diapers is a time to talk in a gentle, nurturing way with a baby.*

## DIAPERS

Changing diapers is part of infant care. Change a baby in a secure place where he or she won't fall. Use cotton balls moistened with oil to cleanse the baby after removing a diaper soiled by urine. After a bowel movement, wipe the baby with soft tissue, then a soft, wet washcloth. Rub on a mild lotion to prevent dry skin.

As you change or bathe a baby, you may notice diaper rash. *Diaper rash* is an irritation of a baby's soft, sensitive skin, caused by bacteria and dampness. These rough, often pimply, patches of skin need immediate attention. Frequent diaper changes help since this keeps the baby clean and dry. Usually a mild rash disappears if the baby's bottom is left uncovered for a few minutes after the bath. Air dries the rash in most cases. Rubber pants, on the other hand, aggravate the problem. If diaper rash does not clear up, consult a doctor.

After changing diapers, handle them carefully to prevent the spread of bacteria. Rinse soiled cloth diapers in a flush toilet. Then store the rinsed diaper in a covered container until laundry time. Fill the container with water that has a small amount of vinegar or bleach added.

Cloth diapers must be washed in very hot water and a mild detergent to destroy bacteria and to help prevent skin irritation. A mild detergent is less likely to irritate a baby's sensitive skin. Disposable diapers should be wadded and disposed of in a trash container away from people.

## BABY CLOTHES

Clothing that is easy to put on and to remove helps prevent a baby from becoming fussy. Clothes with front openings, snap crotches, and large neck openings are easier to change. Infant clothing such as those

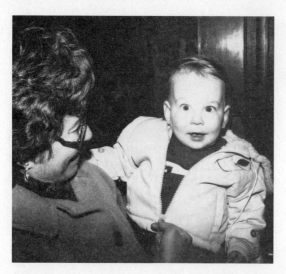

*Zippers and concealed snaps are safe fasteners for baby clothes. Buttons on the front might be pulled off and swallowed.*

made of stretch fabrics allow free movement as well. And wash-and-wear fabrics make parents' or caregivers' work easier!

Infant wear must be safe. Buttons and other details must be attached securely so that the baby won't pull them off and swallow them. Flame-resistant clothing reduces the possibility of burn injuries.

Footwear protects infants' feet from cold and injury. Socks or a sleeping suit with feet help keep the feet of a newborn or crawling infant warm. When babies start walking, shoes offer protection outdoors. They might slip in socks without shoes. And shoes without socks rub and may cause blisters. A good-fitting shoe won't cramp a child's feet or cause pain. Since babies' feet grow fast, their feet should be checked frequently to see if new shoes are needed. Going barefoot indoors helps strengthen foot muscles.

## Clean, Warm Surroundings

A healthful home is quiet, clean, and comfortable. Babies need a quiet place for sleep-

ing, warmth for comfort, and protection from getting chilled. A temperature of about 72° F is right for infants. A clean house protects babies from bacteria which cause infections.

## A Nurturing Environment

A nurturing environment promotes an infant's health and well-being. Communication with the baby and doing stimulating activities are all part of a nurturing environment.

From birth, human contact creates a bond of close emotional ties between parents and their baby. These ties are easily developed between an infant and a successful caregiver—usually the mother or father. Bonding creates trust, security, and love which, in turn, promotes emotional, mental, physical, and social health.

### Communicating with Babies

Communication is a nurturing activity. Parents and other caregivers communicate by giving the baby attention. They may hold, cuddle, and talk to an infant. Their looks and smiles show love. Communication also includes attending to a baby's needs. A baby who is held, loved, and caressed sees the world as a warm, friendly place.

Babies communicate as well. But their approach is quite different. They cry and fuss. They look, smile, and make pleasant sounds. A baby's touch is also a sign of communication with others.

Parents who respond to a baby's cries quickly and consistently don't spoil their children. Rather, their response fosters trust, security, and confidence which lead to independence for the child later.

### Handling Fussy Babies

Sometimes babies are fussy for no apparent reason. This is the way they show their emotions. They whimper or cry and act as if

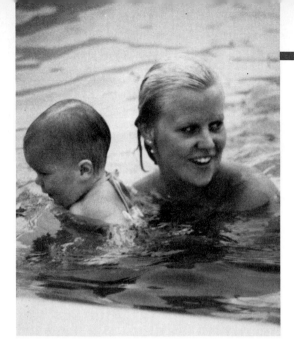

# SUPERBABY!

Imagine babies who are learning to read, work a computer, and play the violin! Today some parents are trying to rear superbabies. Many of these parents are older, well-educated people. They are successful in their careers, and they're financially comfortable. They are using all the information available, including new approaches to child care, to rear their children for successful living.

These parents believe that intelligence can be greatly expanded by involving children in educational activities at a very early age. They believe that infants are like sponges, absorbing everything they are exposed to. This belief in the ability to influence intelligence is so strong that they involve themselves and their babies in special activities.

Mothers may participate in activities during their pregnancy which they believe will influence the baby. For example, they may listen to classical rather than popular music or read classical literature.

After the baby is born, parents use flash cards to teach their babies to read. Some parents enroll their infants in exercise classes to advance muscular development or begin waterbaby classes to reduce fear of water. Other parents start toddlers in violin lessons or begin giving them experience in computer use.

Parents who choose this type of baby care are motivated by love. They want their children to have the skills and intellectual abilities necessary for future success and happiness.

Advocates say that an infant can master simple math at seven months and can recognize words at eleven months. These specialists have developed schools where parents and babies may be enrolled to learn to develop skills for improving intelligence.

Not everyone agrees with the superbaby theory. Critics say that overstimulation actually may be harmful. Early mental development may interfere with a child's social and emotional development. Superbaby activities may foster insecurity, overdependence on parents, and ultimately failure. Some child psychologists have treated young children raised with "super" care for stress.

All child care experts agree that children can learn at an early age. They also agree that an enriched environment is important for infants. Some, however, doubt that any amount of special training can turn normal infants into superbabies.

they are uncomfortable and unhappy. When this happens, don't ignore them. See what's wrong.

- Check for signs of illness or discomfort. See the chart on this page.
- Move the baby to a new place. Perhaps he or she is uncomfortable.
- Pat the baby's back, and sing softly. This is soothing.
- Check to see if the diaper or clothing needs changing.
- Turn the baby on his or her stomach for sleeping. Pressure and warmth on the abdomen may be very comfortable. When babies sleep on their stomachs, the involuntary movement of their arms won't cause them to wake up.
- Perhaps give the baby a pacifier.

## Medical Care for Infants

Medical care is part of infant health care. Parents and caregivers need to understand the importance of regular medical checkups. They need to recognize signs of illness. And, finally, they need skills for caring for a sick infant at home.

The medical care of an infant should be supervised by a health care professional. Even before a baby is born, parents should choose the baby's doctor or locate an appropriate clinic. The family doctor or obstetrician can recommend a pediatrician, or the clinic may refer the pregnant woman to another doctor in the same clinic. Chapter 4 lists points to consider when choosing a doctor.

## Medical Checkups

Regular checkups by a family doctor, a pediatrician, or staff at a health clinic are recommended at one, two, four, six, nine, and twelve months of age. Checkups help monitor the infant's development and identify conditions that need treating. During the first year of life, doctors check certain reflexes that indicate development. Immunizations against certain diseases are given. As you learned in Chapter 7, an immunization builds up the body's resistance to many illnesses.

Record keeping is also an important part of responsible infant health care. Procedures for maintaining the family health record are described in Chapter 4.

## Signs of Illness

Babies often need the care of a health professional when they get sick. Anyone who cares for infants should recognize the signs of illness shown below. Identifying symptoms early, then providing appropriate care, can prevent more serious illnesses from occurring.

### TAKING A BABY'S TEMPERATURE

The average normal body temperature is 98.6° F. A *fever*, or body temperature above 98.6° F, may be a sign of illness. A flushed face, bright glassy eyes, and drowsiness suggest that a baby has a fever. To be sure, a

### Is the Baby Sick?

Look for these symptoms of illness, and report them to the pediatrician.
- Rash
- Runny nose
- Coughing
- Lethargy (drowsy, sluggish, and uninterested in surroundings)
- Fever
- Difficult breathing
- Pain
- Vomiting that lasts more than one day
- Frequent diarrhea
- Lack of appetite
- Excessive crying

caregiver should take the baby's temperature. When a child is ill, body temperature should be checked every four hours.

There are two appropriate methods of taking an infant's temperature—the rectal and the underarm methods. The rectal method is used most often. The underarm, or armpit, method is recommended when the child is too young for taking the temperature by mouth and too active for the rectal method. Chapter 11 describes these procedures for taking body temperatures. The mouth, or oral, method is inappropriate for babies. If an infant's temperature rises above 101° F when taken rectally or above 99.6° F when taken under the arm, contact the baby's doctor.

When the body temperature rises suddenly, a fever can cause a convulsion. Convulsions can cause the clenching and contracting of muscles which come from ab-

normal messages between the brain and the nerves. They usually don't result in permanent damage. If a convulsion occurs, stay with an infant or a child to prevent injury from thrashing about or from inhaling or choking on vomit. Don't try to stop the thrashing. The convulsion will pass quickly. Then call the doctor and start cooling the infant's body down.

To lower a high temperature, remove all unnecessary clothing. Sponge the arms, neck, and face with warm water and let it dry. Cover the body after sponging to prevent chills.

## Calling the Doctor

Doctors respond to a parent's or a caregiver's calls best when the caller gives clear, specific information in a calm manner. This is easiest to do when notes are written before calling.

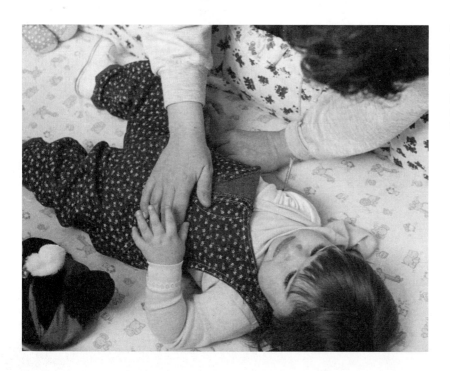

*Never take a baby's temperature by mouth. It's unsafe. Use the skin (underarm) or rectal method described in Chapter 11.*

When you call, give your name and the name and age of the baby. Tell the doctor or nurse what signs of illness you have observed. Be sure to include the baby's temperature. The doctor or nurse will probably want to know about bowel movements, too. Ask for any instructions. Write down the directions and follow them carefully. In Chapter 11, you'll learn more about contacting the doctor and observing and caring for a sick family member.

## Caring for a Sick Infant

Infants are very susceptible to communicable illnesses. Their bodies cannot resist colds and other diseases yet.

A caregiver should follow the advice of a health professional when caring for a sick infant. A sick baby is more comfortable if a normal routine is followed. He or she needs plenty of rest and attention. Infants often need more fluids when they're ill, too, especially if they have a fever.

Medicine should only be given under a doctor's supervision. Aspirins usually aren't recommended to treat colds, flu, or other viral diseases for infants or children under age 12. This is because aspirin usage has been linked to a high incidence of Reye's Syndrome. Reye's Syndrome is a very serious condition of infants and children which usually occurs about a week following a viral infection. Symptoms include violent vomiting, hallucinations, severe headaches, and wild behavior.

As a rule, medicines shouldn't be mixed with baby's milk or food. If all the milk or food is not taken, the baby won't receive the proper amount, or dosage, of medicine. Liquid medicines are usually best for small children. They can be measured into a spoon, then poured into the back of the mouth when the youngster opens his or her mouth. If the taste is too objectionable to the infant, the caregiver may need to mix medicine into a small portion of applesauce or strong-flavored soft food. Formula, water, juice, or perhaps a cracker after the medication is taken will help get rid of the aftertaste.

## Common Health Concerns

Common health problems affect many infants from time to time. For any health concern, caregivers should consult a health professional if they're not sure what to do.

### TEETHING

Babies begin to teethe at different ages. Teething occurs when teeth cut through the gums for the first time. Most infants get

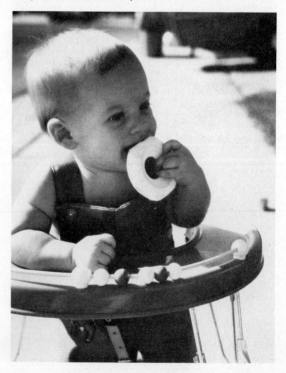

*Chewing on something hard helps relieve the discomfort of teething. What could you give a baby that would be safe?*

their two lower front teeth between the ages of five and nine months. By two years of age, they usually have all their baby (primary) teeth. Some babies experience discomfort when teething, and so they're irritable. Others have no problems at all.

When teething causes babies to get fussy and drool, parents may massage their tender gums for relief. Babies often discover that chewing on a clean, nonshreddable cloth or a teething ring helps.

Teething doesn't cause serious health problems. However, parents shouldn't dismiss signs of illness simply as teething. When a baby has a fever or a digestive problem, a doctor should be consulted.

## COLIC

*Colic* is not an illness, but an uncomfortable condition accompanied by gas pains in the stomach or intestines. A baby with colic cries continuously for several hours at the same time every day, usually after the evening feeding. None of the usual calming behaviors quiets the baby. This crying often lasts from one feeding to the next. Colic may be caused by immature digestive and nervous systems. It begins in the first three weeks after birth and usually ends by three months of age.

Colicky babies are usually quite healthy. Although colic does no real harm, it is uncomfortable for the baby and a worry for the parents.

There is no specific treatment for colic unless the doctor feels the infant needs medication to relax the stomach and intestinal muscles. However, as a caregiver, you may help relieve a baby's colic pains. By placing him or her on your shoulder, then gently patting the back, you can help release the gas. Sometimes laying the baby on his or her stomach on a warm bed pad helps. Some parents think a pacifier helps relieve colic.

Doctors may recommend adding cereal to the baby's diet to reduce a frequent, colicky condition.

## FEAR

Fear is a painful emotion for babies. Infants who are afraid experience stress and feel insecure. These emotions affect health and development if they aren't controlled.

Infants and children often fear being left by their parents. They may also fear strange people, strange situations, and strange objects. Most babies fear loud noises, too.

Babies often express fear by crying, or they try to escape fearful objects by turning away or hiding if they can. A comforting response and reassurance help relieve fear.

At about four months of age, babies begin to notice that there are differences in people. They also fear that their parents or other important caregiver may leave them. The fear is called separation anxiety. It is natural because the key caregiver represents security. These are ways parents can reduce separation anxiety:

- Take the baby with them as much as possible.
- Assure the baby that they'll return. They might use a common phrase to indicate that they're leaving and another phrase to announce their return. For example, "Bye, bye, we'll be back soon," and then, "Hello, we're here again."
- Let the infant spend time with another caregiver so that he or she feels comfortable if the parents must be away.

Strangers may frighten a baby unintentionally. Babies need time to relax in the strangers' presence. Parents should hold babies for a time when meeting new relatives or friends. Then others may hold the baby without frightening him or her.

Babies also fear loud noises. Don't give them loud, squeaky toys or metal spoons to

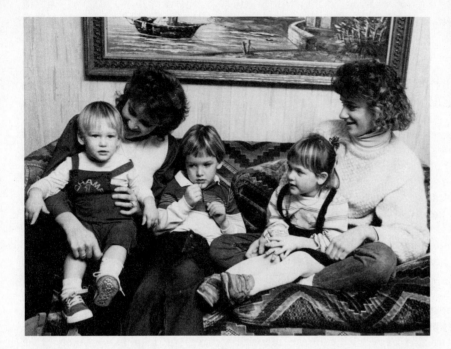

*Babies need the emotional security of consistent care. Using the same babysitter whenever possible provides some sense of security.*

bang. If a loud noise does frighten them, reassure them as you would for any frightening event. Pick them up and hold them.

## HICCUPS, SPITTING UP, AND VOMITING

Hiccups, perhaps caused by gas, are common among infants. If hiccups don't disappear quickly, you can give the baby a bottle of warmed water. If hiccups persist, call the baby's doctor for advice. Hiccups neither bother nor harm a baby.

Many babies also spit up small amounts of milk or formula frequently. This is sometimes called a wet burp and is normal. It differs from vomiting in that a wet burp occurs within a few minutes after feeding, comes up gently, and is undigested. One way to reduce spitting up is to burp the infant halfway through and after each feeding. Another way is to prevent the baby from gulping formula fast. As long as the baby

continues to grow, parents shouldn't worry when a baby spits up.

Vomiting is a sign of illness and can lead to dehydration. If a baby vomits repeatedly or also has a fever or diarrhea, consult a pediatrician.

## CRADLE CAP

Sometimes patches of crusty skin, called *cradle cap*, form on an infant's head. This mild disorder probably is caused by secretions from the oil glands in the scalp. To treat this condition, rub baby oil on the scales at night to soften the patches. Then bathe the head gently but thoroughly during the next morning's bath. If necessary, loosen the patches with a soft brush or washcloth.

## SUDDEN INFANT DEATH SYNDROME

Occasionally very young babies die when they're sleeping, often at night, for no apparent reason. This is called *sudden infant*

## First Aid for a Choking Infant

# Artificial Respiration

Determine consciousness:
- Tap feet or chest.
- Talk loudly near ear.
- Shout for help.

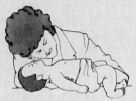

**A**—Airway open.
   Look, listen, and feel for breathing.

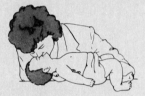

**B**—2 puffs.
   Cover mouth and nose with your mouth.

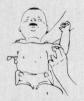

**C**—Check for pulse middle upper arm
   (brachial) and breathing. (5 to
   10 seconds)

If still not breathing, begin artificial
respiration—1 breath every 3 seconds.
Count: 1, one-thousand; 2, one-thousand;
3, breathe.

If possible, continue artificial respiration
while trying to get help; or do not leave for
more than 30 seconds.

# Choking

**CONSCIOUS INFANT**

If infant is actively coughing, just watch
him. DO NOT DO ANYTHING.

If infant is NOT coughing or crying:
- Begin giving 4 back blows between the
  shoulder blades.
- Support body with your arm, keeping head
  lower than feet.

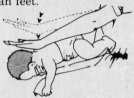

Next:
- Give 4 chest thrusts ½ to 1 inch deep
  1 finger width below the nipples.
- Again, support body with your arm,
  keeping head lower than feet.
- Check the mouth by looking.

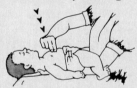

Continue back blows and chest thrusts until
infant coughs, or object comes out, or infant
becomes unconscious.

**UNCONSCIOUS INFANT**

Should the infant become unconscious (limp
and lifeless):
- Open the airway.          If air will not go in:
- Listen for breathing.     • Give back blows.
- Try to give 2 puffs.      • Give chest thrusts.
                            • Check the mouth.
                            • Try to give a breath.

Continue repeating these steps until the
airway clears so you can start artificial
respiration.

*death syndrome* (SIDS), or crib death. These deaths often are unexplainable. Though SIDS doesn't happen often, scientists are studying the syndrome to learn why it happens.

## THUMB SUCKING

Many babies suck their thumbs or two fingers. This practice is often part of an infant's normal development. Sometimes thumb sucking starts with curiosity when babies discover their fingers. Thumbs also may substitute for nipples in the babies' need to satisfy their urge to suck. Thumb sucking or finger sucking often provides comfort to babies.

Thumb sucking is most common in a baby's first year of life. After age one, most children suck their thumbs only when they're under stress.

Moderate thumb sucking isn't harmful. It doesn't change the shape of an infant's teeth or jaws. In fact, for babies and small children, thumb sucking is somewhat like gum chewing for adults. It may provide relaxation, relieve tension, or satisfy boredom.

Parents shouldn't worry when babies suck their thumbs. By ignoring this practice, thumb sucking won't be reinforced. A child who feels secure, relaxed, and loved is less likely to continue this practice.

## DIARRHEA

*Diarrhea* is loose, runny, and frequent bowel movements. Diarrhea is usually caused by a mild intestinal infection. Most cases clear up in two or three days.

Adjusting the diet often can cure diarrhea. Bottle-fed babies may need their formula diluted for a short time. Some babies may need to stop eating solid foods until the condition clears up. Sometimes a certain food can cause a baby to have diarrhea, and the food has to be eliminated from the baby's diet.

If the problem persists, get a doctor's advice. The baby could become dehydrated and malnourished.

## CHOKING

Babies and small children can easily become victims of choking. They may get food or a small object caught in their throat. Choking cuts off the air supply. Brain damage can occur in four to five minutes when the body doesn't get oxygen from breathing. Choking can even cause death.

If an infant starts choking, follow the steps on page **221**. Unless you can easily see the object, don't use your finger to locate and remove the object. You might push it further into the air passage. If the baby stops breathing or becomes unconscious, call for emergency medical help at once.

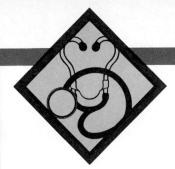

# CHAPTER CHECKUP

## Reviewing the Information

1. What are the characteristics of a healthy infant?
2. What characteristics should a caregiver look for in a crib?
3. What questions should you ask if you are selecting a safe toy for an infant?
4. Why should older children be supervised when they are with an infant?
5. Why shouldn't a baby be put to bed with a bottle of juice?
6. Why should solid foods be introduced to the baby's diet one at a time?
7. Name five safety tips for bathing an infant.
8. List three features in a baby's clothes which promote safety.
9. How should diaper rash be treated?
10. How may a caregiver communicate with an infant?
11. Name three symptoms of illness in an infant.
12. Why shouldn't you give aspirin to a baby or child without a doctor's advice?
13. Name three common health concerns which parents of infants may need to deal with.
14. How might a caregiver help relieve a baby's discomfort from teething?
15. What is separation anxiety, and how might a caregiver help relieve it?

## Thinking It Over

1. Describe a safe sleep and play environment for an infant.
2. Compare the advantages and disadvantages of breast feeding.
3. Name five guidelines for feeding an infant in a safe way.
4. How could you protect a crawling baby from hazards?
5. What could you do if you were babysitting a fussy baby?
6. What would you do if a baby had a fever and diarrhea that persisted for two days?
7. What's the difference between a wet burp and vomiting, and how should a caregiver respond to each?

## Taking Action

1. Write a one-page article on ways to communicate with an infant. Share your article with the class.
2. Interview a parent about the cost of medical care for the first year of an infant's life.
3. Read the feature article, "Superbaby." Then find examples of special programs for infants in your community.
4. Interview a parent on ways he or she has planned a safe environment for a new baby.
5. Spend a half hour playing with an infant. Be a nurturing caregiver.
6. Using a life-sized baby doll, demonstrate bathing and diapering an infant safely.

# 10 Child Care

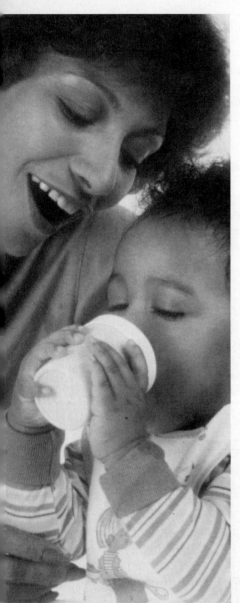

After reading this chapter, you should be able to:

- list the signs of a healthy child.

- describe daily routines which promote good health.

- describe ways to keep children safe.

- describe routine medical care for children.

- describe the appropriate response to a child's health problems.

## Terms to Understand

| | |
|---|---|
| asthma | hyperactivity |
| child abuse | pinworms |
| enuresis | scoliosis |
| fluoride | tetanus |
| food jag | |

Raising healthy, happy, responsible children is the goal of parents and caregivers. Good health care for children includes keeping them well and helping them develop normally, not just caring for them when they're ill or injured.

## Wellness for Children

Wellness is the result of appropriate and loving attention to a child's needs. Successful parents and caregivers enjoy children and make them part of their lives. They work toward providing a healthful environment with activities that promote normal development.

Parents and other caregivers help children develop healthy attitudes and habits by practicing good health behavior themselves. Children generally copy their parents' attitudes and habits. For example, if parents are gentle, happy, and communicative while bathing a young child, the child will look forward to bathing as a pleasant experience. Children also imitate bad health habits, such as smoking, irresponsible use of alcohol, and not wearing seat belts.

### A Child's Health Needs

Every child is a unique individual. Yet every child has the same basic health needs. By meeting a child's physical, emotional, and social needs, caregivers can help ensure a child's well-being. Needs common to all children include:

- wholesome food
- adequate rest
- exercise and play
- safe environment
- good hygiene
- medical and dental care
- love and attention
- security
- sense of belonging
- acceptance
- freedom to develop independence
- moral guidance
- freedom to make mistakes
- mental stimulation
- variety of experiences
- discipline
- friendships
- privacy

## Signs of Health

Recognizing the signs of wellness in a child is an important skill of parents and other caregivers. Common characteristics of a healthy child include: a good appetite, normal physical development, sound sleep habits, a positive attitude, playful behavior

*Happy, playful behavior in children is a sign of good health.*

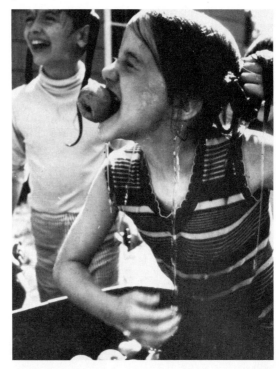

alone and with others, physically active behavior, and the ability to express thoughts and feelings.

## Promoting a Child's Health

Children are nurtured in their homes, in the homes of friends and relatives, at school, and in day care settings. Nutrition, rest, hygiene, play, and emotional support all contribute to a child's health and happiness.

## Nutrition

Eating is a pleasure that starts in infancy and lasts throughout life. The pleasures associated with being held and drinking milk or formula are a baby's first experiences with food. These positive feelings of being secure, well cared for, and well fed help establish good eating habits which should be reinforced as children mature. Good food habits, in turn, result in good nutrition and promote good health.

Food not only satisfies hunger and nourishes children. It also offers learning experiences. Eating with others teaches social behavior. And the tastes, smells, appearance, and textures of food add to a child's eating pleasure.

### NUTRIENT NEEDS

Children need nutrients to help them grow normally, to give them energy to learn and play, and to keep their bodies functioning well. You learned about the specific functions of nutrients in Chapter 1. Everyone needs the same nutrients, but the amount depends on a person's age and sex. Younger children need fewer nutrients than teenagers. In general, boys and girls need about the same amount of nutrients in their

*Children who skip breakfast may not have much energy for school work. This may affect their mental, physical, and social development.*

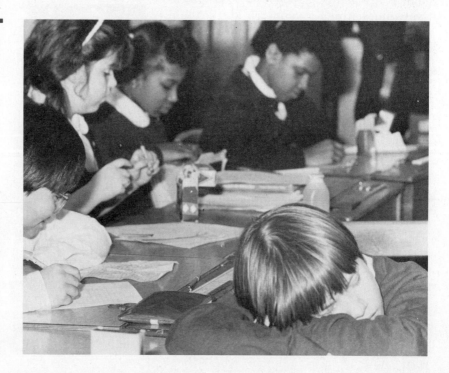

preschool and school years. As teens, boys need slightly more.

Children who don't consume adequate amounts of nutrients may not develop normally. Poor diet affects more than physical development. It lowers resistance to disease. It limits children's energy level; they may not have the energy to fully participate in physical activities. Hungry children also are less alert, so they may not work up to their full potential at school. With extreme nutrient deficiencies, children can experience stunted growth, poor dental and skeletal development, and other problems.

Eating too many calories and often getting too little exercise, can lead to childhood obesity. Obesity affects a child's emotional, social, and physical development. Fat children often are ridiculed unfairly by peers. This may lower their self-esteem. They might experience physical problems such as breathing problems and joint problems. They may feel less able to participate in active play or sports. Childhood obesity often leads to adult obesity, as well. Parents of overweight or obese children should consult a doctor.

**GOOD FOOD HABITS**

Children are more likely get the nutrients they need without consuming too many calories when they follow good food habits. Parents and caregivers concerned about a child's health and nutrition may follow these guidelines to help children establish food habits for a lifetime of healthful eating:

- Provide nutritious meals with daily menus representing the four food group guidelines. Balanced menus help children get the nutrients they need.

## Food Needs of Children

| Group | Recommended Daily Amount | Average Serving Size |
|---|---|---|
| Milk-Cheese | 2 to 3 servings for children under 9 years<br><br>3 or more for children 9 to 12 | 1 cup milk |
| Fruit-Vegetable | 1 serving of foods high in vitamin A<br><br>1 serving of foods high in vitamin C<br><br>2 additional servings of any fruit or vegetable | Approximately 1 tablespoon of food for each year of the child's age; a single serving for a four-year-old would be 4 Tbsp. |
| Meat-Poultry-Fish-Beans | 2 servings | Approximately 1 tablespoon of food for each year of the child's age |
| Bread-Cereal | 4 servings | 1 slice of bread |

- Maintain regular meal schedules when possible. Meals served at the same time each day give children a sense of order and security. At the same time, this promotes good nutrition.
- Provide snacks if children need them. A three-year-old who can only eat small amounts of food at one time may need morning and afternoon snacks. A ten-year-old usually doesn't need a morning snack if he or she eats an adequate breakfast.
- Help children select snacks appropriately. Encourage nutritious snacks, such as fruit, milk, raw vegetables, and whole wheat crackers, which provide servings from the four basic food groups. Discourage snacks just before mealtime because they take away a child's appetite. Instead schedule a child's snacks at the midpoint between meals. Don't encourage frequent snacking, particularly of sticky, sweet foods since this promotes tooth decay.

- Serve foods that children enjoy eating. Preschoolers like simply-prepared foods, finger foods, foods in funny shapes, and foods with bland flavors. School-age children tend to like many foods that adults and older children also enjoy.
- Encourage children to develop preferences for many different foods. Serve new foods periodically, and encourage them to eat at least two bites. A varied diet is healthful since the nutrient values of food differ.
- Don't worry if a two or three-year-old gets on a food jag. A *food jag* is eating one food over and over, such as bread and jelly sandwiches, and perhaps avoiding many nutritious foods. Parents shouldn't worry or make a big deal about this. Food jags pass quickly. The child is just showing independence.
- Be flexible. If children reject a healthful food entirely, simply reintroduce it in another form, such as zucchini served as zucchini bread. Or if a child doesn't like

*Children enjoy eating finger foods. These nutritious snack foods also teach them healthful food habits.*

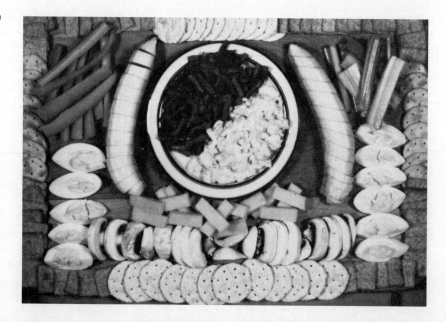

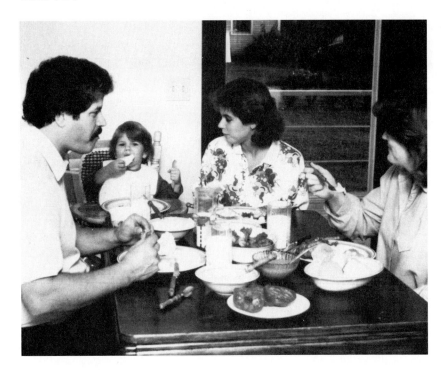

*A pleasant meal environment promotes good eating habits and creates positive attitudes toward food. What are the positive aspects of this meal?*

oranges, you can serve strawberries or grapefruit.

- Avoid using food as punishment or reward. For example, avoid promising dessert if all the vegetables are eaten. This can develop a negative attitude toward vegetables.
- Avoid deciding how much food a child must eat before he or she is allowed to leave the table. A child can't eat as much as an adult can. Requiring a child to "clean the plate" may contribute to overeating and overweight.
- Avoid disciplining children at mealtime. Eating together should be a pleasant time. Stress at mealtime may keep children from eating adequately.
- Allow young children to feed themselves as soon as they show an interest. This may be messy, but it's necessary for normal development.

- Be a role model. Children whose families use pleasant table manners will use good manners, too. If parents enjoy mealtime, children will. And if a variety of food is eaten by parents, children will learn to like many foods.

## Rest

Routine sleeping habits are just as important as routine eating habits for growth and development. Rest gives a child's body the chance to renew itself. Good sleep habits are promoted by a regular bedtime and by preparing the child appropriately for sleep or rest.

After infancy most children take two naps a day and sleep throughout the night. After a child is two years old, the morning nap may be omitted. By school age, the afternoon nap usually has become simply a rest period. As naps become shorter or nonexistent, earlier bedtimes are recommended to promote good sleep habits.

Bedtime should be calm and pleasant. Stimulating play, such as roughhousing or hide-and-seek, is not a good idea just before bedtime because children have a hard time settling down. Before bedtime, a short, quiet play period, followed by a warm bath, may be helpful. Many children look forward to reading for a few minutes in bed. Younger ones may like having stories read to them.

Sleep problems are common. For example, a child may fear the dark. If so, the parent can talk to the child about the dark and perhaps leave a nightlight on. Being sure a child's hunger, thirst, and toilet needs are met before going to bed also reduces sleep problems.

Giving a child special attention just before turning off the lights and being consistent about bedtime rules may be the most important guidelines for putting a child to bed. All children enjoy being "tucked in"!

*Bedtime stories help relax children and help put them to sleep.*

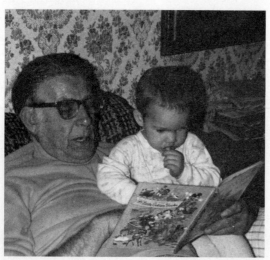

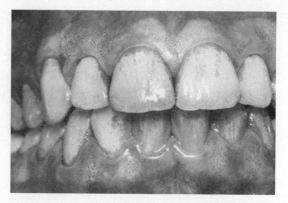

*Children can see if they've done a thorough job of brushing and flossing their teeth using a disclosing tablet. The vegetable dye in the tablet stains the plaque left on the teeth.*

## Hygiene

Good hygiene contributes to a child's immediate health, self-esteem, and life-long wellness. Dental care, cleanliness, and sanitary toilet habits are part of good hygiene.

### DENTAL CARE

Proper dental care should begin at birth. This includes daily cleaning, fluoride use, proper diet, and regular checkups. Preventive dental care protects a child's teeth from decay and gum disease. It establishes habits to help ensure a healthy, confident smile.

Baby teeth and gums need to be cared for to help prevent problems later. Brushing is a habit which begins as soon as teeth come through the gums. Until children can brush for themselves at 4 to 5 years of age, parents should supervise the child's cleaning. A child can begin to floss at about 8 or 10. In Chapter 1 you learned that flossing helps remove plaque and food particles that may cause decay between teeth.

A dentist should check teeth and clean them every six months beginning at about age one. Professional cleaning removes calculus, the hardened plaque that can cause gum disease. Regular dental care given early may eliminate the need for fillings and other serious gum and dental problems as children get older.

*Fluoride*, a naturally-occurring mineral that helps prevent tooth decay, is especially important as teeth are developing during childhood. Fluoride helps make teeth stronger and more resistant to decay. Dentists usually apply a pleasant-flavored fluoride compound to children's teeth as part of a regular dental checkup. Most communities now add fluoride to their water supply. In towns that don't follow this practice, or in rural areas where well water without fluoride is consumed, the dentist might recommend that children use tablets, drops, or bottled water that contains fluoride. Many toothpastes also contain fluoride.

A child's tooth may be knocked out during an accident. If this happens, the caregiver or parent should immediately recover the tooth and take it in a glass of cool water or milk with the child to the dentist, preferably within 30 minutes. Sometimes it can be reset in the jaws.

## CLEANLINESS

Cleanliness contributes to physical and mental health. Body sores, cuts, and punctures are irritated by dirt and can become infected by bacteria. Sticky hands also attract insects. Being clean also feels good!

Responsible caregivers teach children to wash and bathe carefully each day. By age three or four, most children can wash their own hands and bathe themselves.

Children need to establish the habit of washing their hands after using the toilet and before eating. Washing with soap and water removes harmful bacteria from their skin. Young children may need a sturdy stool to stand on so they can reach the sink.

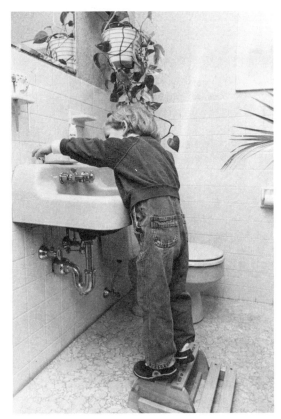

*A handy, sturdy step stool enables a small child to be more independent in personal hygiene.*

Daily bathing is important throughout life. Children should learn to enjoy bathing as a pleasant routine but shouldn't be allowed to spend long periods of playing in the tub. A tub where children can sit is safer than a shower. Many people also stick rough-surfaced mats or appliques on the bottom of the tub to help prevent slipping when getting in and out. Children should be supervised for safety.

By having their own towel, towel rack, comb, cup, and toothbrush, children are encouraged to practice good hygiene habits.

## TOILET HABITS

Pediatricians usually recommend that toilet training begin between 18 months and two years of age. Children who can talk enough to express their desire to use the toilet, who no longer drink from a bottle, and who are mature enough to control their sphincter muscles can be trained easier than younger children. The sphincter muscles control the openings of the bladder and the bowels for elimination of body wastes.

A small potty chair makes toilet training easier. A regular toilet seat may frighten a child who may be afraid of falling in the toilet or falling off. But a small seat can help a child feel more secure. Later, an adjustable seat or a step stool may be helpful. Training pants may be a reward for a child who learns to control bowel movements. Children may cooperate more if they are made to feel more grownup.

When children rebel against toilet training and hold their bowel movement, they may get constipated. The stool, or bowel movement, then becomes hard and painful to pass out of the body.

The parents' or caregivers' attitudes can make toilet training a healthful and pleasant accomplishment. Children need love, understanding, patience, and praise during toilet training. Parents and caregivers who talk freely about toilet habits and who are aware of the child's elimination patterns are usually successful in toilet training.

## Play

Play is the work of children. It is as normal as breathing, and it contributes to physical, mental, and social health. By riding a tricycle, children develop leg muscles. By working a puzzle, they learn to solve problems. By playing "house," they learn to get

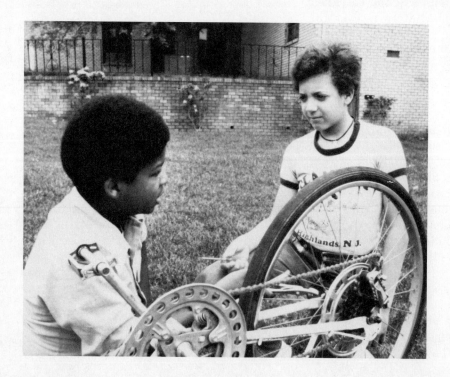

*Through play, children learn to work and cooperate with others.*

along with other children. Play benefits children in these ways:

- It expands knowledge.
- It develops physical skills, strength, flexibility, and coordination.
- It promotes social skills.
- It promotes personal relationships.
- It develops communicative skills.
- It promotes emotional development.
- It helps relieve stress.

Active play provides necessary physical exercise. It contributes to large and small muscle development. Dramatic play may be a part of active play, too. When children act out roles of others, such as pretending to be a fire fighter or a favorite TV character, they learn to express feelings and ideas. This contributes to emotional and social health.

Puzzles, dolls, and trucks are used with quiet play. Quiet play with dolls or trucks promotes creativity and problem solving. It also helps children develop the ability to entertain themselves. Quiet play with puzzles and books promotes mental stimulation. As children grow older, they may be part of organized group activity which is vital to social health.

## Emotional Support

Normal children go through many stages of emotional development. Children as young as six months express fear and anger. Their ability to respond to affection begins at eight months to a year. At age two, they feel sympathy. Preschoolers and competitive seven-year-olds may express jealousy. By 10, children often become big worriers.

Children also learn to express joy, happiness, contentment, grief, and sorrow, among other emotions. These emotions are expressed through body language, behavior, and even play. Parents and caregivers need to learn to recognize different stages of emotional development and the outward signs

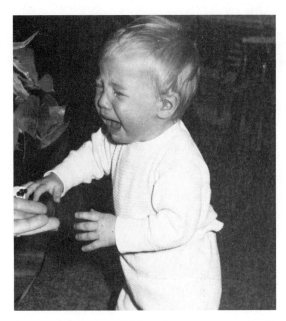

*In a caring home, children learn to express and deal with their emotions in a healthy way.*

of emotions. This enables them to offer better support in troubled times and also to help children express their feelings openly and constructively.

### LOVE AND ATTENTION

Authorities believe that children need love and attention to develop normally. Caregivers who express affection for the child with frequent hugs, kisses, and pats promote a child's emotional health. Children need to be told, as well as shown, that they are loved.

Children need caregivers who are constant and consistent with their expressions of commitment and love. Good parents never withhold expressions of love as punishment. At times, parents don't like the child's behavior, but they still like the child. Love that is constant helps children develop trust, self-esteem, and a sense of security. Children who are secure in their parents' love are willing to take risks which help them develop normally.

Children need friends their own age. Emotional and social health depend on good peer relations, in addition to good family relations. Children first learn social behavior and personal commitment at home. This behavior is later transferred to relationships with friends.

Sometimes children need to be alone. They may need a quiet time to "cool off" if they've been upset. Children also need private time to develop a sense of self, to get in touch with their feelings, and to develop individual skills.

A caring family encourages a child to express grief, anger, and other emotions. Talking about feelings and teaching children to handle them is part of health care. Suppressed emotions may build up stress which, in turn, adversely affects behavior and learning.

## DISCIPLINE

Appropriate and effective discipline promotes both emotional well-being and physical safety. Although each child is unique and styles of parental care differ, the same principles guide effective, loving discipline for all children. These are principles which parents and other caregivers should follow:

- Model firm but loving behavior. Children will follow the examples set.
- Help prevent a problem which might require discipline later. Let children know the rules up front and the reasons for the demands.
- Give instructions in short, clear phrases with one direction at a time. In this way, children learn rules more easily.
- Be consistent with routines, expected behavior, and discipline. Consistency

among parents and other caregivers is important so children aren't confused.
- Set limits and enforce them.
- Give children choices within limits so they feel they have some control. For example, say, "You may take your bath now or after your homework. Which time do you prefer?"
- Respond immediately when a child misbehaves. Children need to link the act with the discipline so they learn what behavior is unacceptable.
- Make the response appropriate for the age of the child and the severity of the act. For example, if a toddler wanders into the bathroom and unrolls all the toilet tissue, simply move him or her to another room, provide other toys, and keep the bathroom door closed. On the other hand, if a three-year-old has used a toy to beat on the furniture, explain why that is inappropriate, and take the toy away for awhile.
- When children misbehave, make it clear that you're unhappy with the act, not with the child. Show love at all times.
- Separate accidents from intentional misbehavior. Be understanding and fair.
- Use praise and rewards to positively reinforce good behavior.
- Treat the child with respect and dignity even as you discipline so self-esteem isn't lost. Never ridicule, speak with sarcasm, or put a child down.
- Provide extra attention for the difficult, hostile child but not immediately following bad behavior.
- Promote self-discipline within the child. For example, help a school-age child plan time to do homework and still enjoy a favorite television program.
- Avoid frequent scoldings. Positive, rather than poor, behavior should get the most attention.

- Do not use the silent treatment. It's always better to let children know why they are being punished or why you are unhappy with their behavior.
- Avoid punishing in anger and yelling at the child. You can be more objective and fair when emotions don't take over.
- Avoid severe punishment. It is an outlet for adult anger that may make the child think that violence is acceptable.

## SOOTHING FEAR AND ANXIETY

Children have different fears at different ages. Three-year-olds are often afraid of storms, animals, and the dark. Six-year-olds with active imaginations might be afraid of ghosts, being abandoned, or the death of a parent. The fears of older children are usually more realistic.

Some fear is useful. Children need to understand the dangers in their world so they learn to be cautious. For example, they must learn the healthy fear of crossing busy streets so they don't get hit by a car.

Some children develop feelings of over-anxiety or phobias. Over-anxiety is unreasonable response, often without cause, to a potentially frightening experience. This response may come from an earlier experience. For example, a child may have exaggerated fears of railroad crossings if he or she has seen a car hit by a train. The fear may continue even though other railroad crossings are perfectly safe. Phobias are long-lasting fears without basis. You learned about them in Chapter 7. Both over-anxiety and phobias prevent children from behaving normally.

Parents can soothe these emotions by talking about them with children. For example, "I know you are afraid of this loud noise. But let me show you what makes it. When those big clouds bump into each other, they make a loud noise. The noise won't hurt you!"

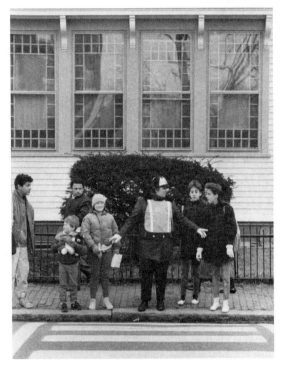

*By learning caution and safe behavior, children can act responsibly in potentially dangerous situations. They don't have to be afraid.*

Some other ways parents and caregivers can help children reduce fears are to:
- set a good example by not being afraid.
- allow children to admit their fears. Don't ridicule or diminish their feelings of fear.
- protect children from fearful things or events until they seem able to handle them.
- stay with children until they are secure in unfamiliar surroundings.
- prevent situations which cause unnecessary fear, such as putting up a gate to prevent falling down the stairs or using a nightlight to help prevent fear of darkness.

## SIGNS OF EMOTIONAL PROBLEMS

By observing children, you may detect emotional problems. Children with emotional problems often withdraw from groups. They may be noncommunicative, hyperactive, destructive, and even self-destructive.

Hyperactivity is more than overactive or restless behavior. *Hyperactivity* is a physical condition identified in children who are much more excitable, active, and distractable than their peers. Although their intelligence is usually normal, they may have a very short attention span and difficulty learning. No one is sure of the exact cause of hyperactivity, but scientists are studying this problem.

Emotional problems get in the way of normal development. They prevent children from developing satisfying relations with others. Emotional problems may affect a child's schoolwork and, in turn, mental development. Emotional problems also may keep a child from participating in physical activities which, in turn, affect the development of the body. A child psychologist can help children who have emotional problems.

Mental health authorities disagree on the causes of emotional problems. Some believe the causes are physiological, meaning there is a physical cause. Others blame environmental factors, such as parental neglect, abuse, rejection, overprotection, severe parental conflict, abandonment by one or both parents, or parents with poor mental health.

## Preventing Accidents

Each year in the United States, more young children are crippled by accidents than by disease. More children die from accidents than die from cancer, birth defects, and pneumonia combined. Automobile accidents, falls, poisoning, drowning, and fire are the most common accidents among preschool children.

*Young children safely enjoy water play when they wear flotation devices to protect them from drowning.*

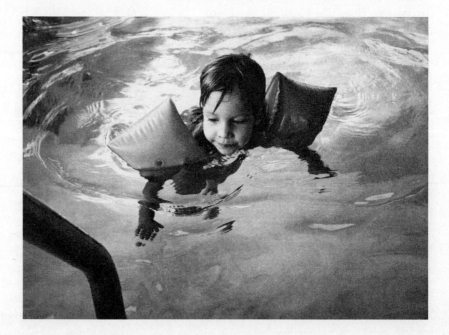

Safety is an important part of child health care. Sensitive parents and caregivers recognize safety hazards and plan ways to eliminate them. They create a safe environment and teach the children safe habits.

## The Child-Proof Home

Many accidents occur at home. To make home a safe place, it needs to be child-proofed. The chart on this page lists characteristics of a child-proof home.

Some other situations increase the risk of accidents at home:
- when children are tired, hungry, or unhappy.
- when the environment is new to the child.
- when caregivers are inexperienced in child care.
- when conditions are overcrowded.
- when children are hyperactive or have underdeveloped perceptual skills. Perceptual skills are those involved with the senses.
- when children are alone.
- when young children play outdoors in unrestricted areas.

## Safe Toys

Children's toys are more complicated than infants' toys, and they also can inflict injury. Toys with certain characteristics are potentially dangerous. These are toys that:
- break easily.
- have sharp edges or points that cut.
- have pieces that can be removed and swallowed.
- are made with flammable materials.
- shoot weapons or missiles that can pierce eyes or other parts of the body.
- are toy weapons that can inflict real wounds.

### A Child-Proof Home

| Potential Dangers | Precautions |
| --- | --- |
| Cleaning products Insecticides Other household chemicals | Placed on high shelves, out of the reach of children, or in locked cabinets |
| Medicines | Labeled clearly, placed out of the reach of children, in bottles with child-proof tops |
| Electric cords | Out of the reach of children |
| Painted surfaces | Free of toxic paint |
| Windows and doors | Secured with latches which small children can't open |
| Small rugs | Securely attached to the floor |
| Traffic paths | Free of toys |
| Table accessories | Removed if they may injure the child or may be damaged easily |
| Furniture | Lightweight furniture removed temporarily from any room where children may tip them over onto themselves |
| Outdoor play yards | Fenced |
| Matches | Out of the reach of children |
| Sharp objects | Out of the reach of children |

• have nails, screws, or wires that can be exposed if the toy is broken.

As stated in Chapter 9, check the suggested age-group label on any toy you consider buying. Even if you think a child is very smart, buy the right toy for his or her age. Then inspect the toy yourself for safety.

## Playing with Pets

Pets provide valuable experiences for children. However, authorities say that children under the age of three are seldom ready for pets. Children must know how to act around animals first.

• Choose a pet with care. Consider the age of the child, the size of the pet, the temperament of the pet, and the care needed. Avoid turtles and birds as pets since they may carry diseases.
• When you give a puppy, a kitten, or some other pet, show the child how to treat the animal. For example, say, "Pat Rover gently; we don't want to hurt him."
• Explain that unknown or wild animals are not pets and should not be handled. These animals can be dangerous.
• Help children through loss and grief when a pet dies. Many guidelines for accepting the death of a relative or friend, described in Chapter 14, also apply to the loss of a pet.

## Safety Rules

Safe habits are learned. Responsible parents teach children rules for safety as early as possible so they become habits.

Parents should teach very young children these safety rules:

• Leave wall plugs and electric cords alone.
• Handle sharp objects with care.
• Look both ways before crossing a street.
• Hold rails when climbing stairs.

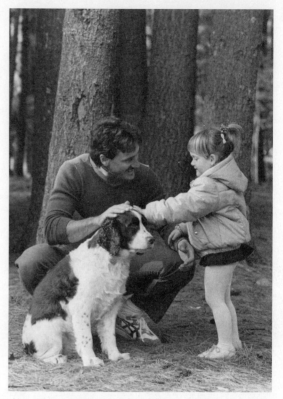

*By your example, show a young child how to pet a dog or cat gently. Your calm behavior will keep the animal from biting.*

• Never leave toys, clothes, books, or other objects on the stairs.
• Avoid playing near a street. Never run into a street to retrieve a ball or other toy; ask a grown-up to get it.

As young as possible, children should learn how to tell their name, their address, and their telephone number in case of emergency. They also need to know how to contact parents at all times. A safe home has a special place where parents post their telephone numbers when they're away.

Children should know what to do in case of fire. For example, they should recognize the sound of the home's smoke detector alarm and know various escape routes. Children need to know that they can extinguish a fire involving their own clothing or hair by rolling on the floor or ground.

Teaching children to use safety restraints in cars is also very important. Chapters 5 and 9 discuss these safety devices.

Effective communication between parents and children is vital for safety. Parents or caregivers need to know where children are at all times. Children need to develop the habit of telling them where they will be. Parents who communicate clearly with their children and who encourage children to share their experiences are better able to protect them.

Children who come home from school and and have no caregiver need safety guide-lines. These children, often referred to as latchkey children, should know what they can and cannot do when they're home without adult supervision. Set guidelines such as never letting strangers know they are alone or not using certain kitchen or workshop equipment, to protect them from potential dangers.

School-age children need to recognize dangers outside their homes. For example, children should learn that getting into a car with a stranger is dangerous.

Parents can protect children from sexual abuse by helping them understand inappropriate behavior with adults. Parents may explain that people don't expose private parts of their bodies to others and that children shouldn't allow others to handle those parts of their bodies.

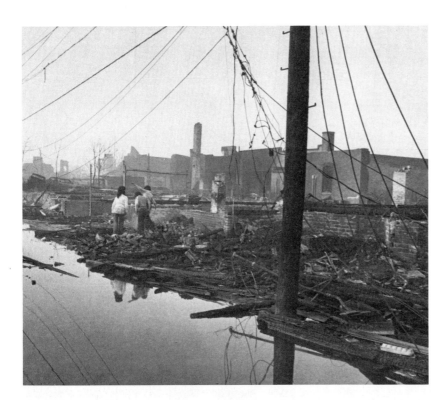

*Caregivers need to know where children are. Children may become so involved in play that they wander into unsafe places.*

# CHILD ABUSE

A neighborhood child is found with cigarette burns all over his or her body. A baby is scalded in steaming bath water. Emergency room staff report a child with welts and bruises over 30 percent of his or her body. These are examples of child abuse.

*Child abuse* is neglect or mistreatment which results in physical or emotional injury. A child who is beaten, burned, left neglected and unfed, or not given medical care is physically abused. Emotional abuse may be caused by repeatedly putting the child down or withholding emotional and social expressions of love and caring. Sexual abuse includes fondling, incest, or rape.

Child abuse is found all over the country among all socioeconomic groups. Recently it has gained widespread public attention. No one knows how extensive child abuse is, but estimates show at least one million cases in the United States each year!

Abuse affects a child's physical and mental health as well as intellectual, emotional, and social development. The results reach far into adulthood. Poor self-concept, the inability to love, lack of trust for others, violent behavior, low achievement in school, physical deformity, and even death can be caused by child abuse.

Who abuses children? Parents, friends, relatives, or day care workers—all may become abusive. Some reasons are related to drug and alcohol use, ignorance, severe emotional problems, immaturity, personal problems, and inability to control emotions. Many abusive adults were abused as children.

Victims are often identified by medical personnel when parents bring children for emergency treatment. Parents may at first say that the child was injured in a fall or other accident. They often won't admit the problem. Bruises, welts, burns, broken bones, withdrawal behavior, neglected appearance, disruptive behavior, and nightmares suggest possible abuse.

Children may be protected by teaching them to leave dangerous situations and get help. They should know:

- how to say "no" to adults and friends if inappropriate or questionable activities are suggested.
- that their bodies belong to them and that no one has the right to touch them in uncomfortable ways.
- who can help. This includes teachers, counselors, police, and neighbors, as well as parents and relatives.
- how to get emergency help.
- how to avoid strangers who offer treats or car rides.
- that they should always walk with someone else, never alone, and only in lighted areas. They should also avoid going into public restrooms alone.
- how to communicate openly and freely with parents.
- that they're not guilty of wrongdoing if they are abused.

An individual who suspects child abuse should first be sure of the facts and then act. Sources of help are police, school nurses, school counselors, local welfare workers, children's protective services, and child abuse hotline workers. Laws require medical and school personnel to report suspected cases of child abuse to the appropriate authorities. Child abusers can also get help to change their behavior.

## Routine Health Care

Routine visits to the doctor and dentist help prevent health problems. This also helps children establish a lifelong routine of medical checkups and care.

The frequency of medical checkups depends on the child's age. Between age one and two, checkups are recommended every four months. From age two to six, a checkup every six months is advised. After six, children should have an annual checkup. Medical checkups may be given by the child's pediatrician, by the family physician, or at a well-baby clinic.

During checkups, the doctor assesses a child's overall health and development. The doctor checks the child's heart, lungs, reflexes, vision, hearing, weight, height, and speech. Urine and blood tests may be done to check for signs of health problems. Immunizations, taken orally or by injection, are also part of regular checkups. Doctors and parents should keep records of a child's immunizations. The chart on page **242** shows an immunization schedule.

During routine checkups, health professionals also may give parental advice on a variety of child-rearing practices. Diet, physical activity, discipline, and expectations are other topics they might discuss with parents.

Once the child enters school, a school nurse screens, or checks, for growth, hearing, vision, and scoliosis. *Scoliosis* is curvature of the spine, which can often be corrected when diagnosed early.

A dental visit every six months is preventive health care, too. Teeth are cleaned and inspected for cavities. X-rays are taken to see how the teeth are developing. If necessary, cavities and other corrective work is done before dental problems become major. Braces may be recommended during puberty or adolescence to straighten teeth and create a pleasing smile.

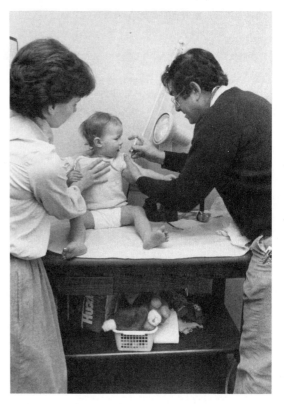

*Calm, reassuring talk reduces a child's fear of being immunized.*

Visiting the doctor or dentist frightens some children. But calm, confident parents can help children relieve fears. Talking to the child about medical and dental visits reduces fear. For young children, parents or caregivers might take toys or books for entertainment during waiting periods. Holding the young child during much of the examination also helps. Reading a book about doctor or dentist visits to the child before the actual visit may help, too.

## Childhood Health Concerns

Sickness and injury are part of growing up. Parents and caregivers who understand childhood health problems can help keep

## Schedule for Immunizations

| Age of Child | Type of Immunization | Sequence |
|---|---|---|
| 2 months | Diphtheria-Pertussis-Tetanus<br>Polio | First<br>First |
| 4 months | Diphtheria-Pertussis-Tetanus<br>Polio | Second<br>Second |
| 6 months | Diphtheria-Pertussis-Tetanus | Third |
| 15 months | Measles-Mumps-Rubella | |
| 18 months | Diphtheria-Pertussis-Tetanus<br>Polio | Fourth<br>Third |
| 4–6 years | Diphtheria-Pertussis-Tetanus<br>Polio | Fifth<br>Fourth |
| 14–16 years and<br>every 10 years<br>after that | Diphtheria-Tetanus | |

*Source: U.S. Department of Health and Human Services*

*Doctors can help relieve children's fears by teaching them about their bodies. Here children examine the internal organs of a doll in a pretend doctor's office. The physician answers questions.*

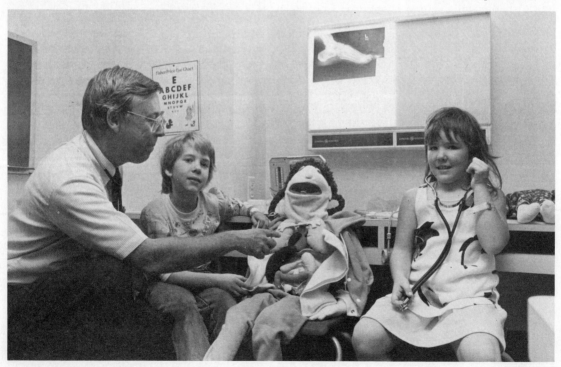

their children well and can help speed recovery. Infectious diseases and allergies are among the health problems which concern parents.

## Infectious Diseases

Several infectious diseases are common during childhood. In Chapter 7 you learned how many infectious diseases are prevented and treated. The chart on pages **244** to **247** describes the symptoms, spread, and treatment of common infectious childhood diseases.

Some childhood diseases can be prevented with immunizations. Either oral or injected immunizations protect children from diphtheria, pertussis (whooping cough), polio, red measles, German measles, and mumps. Adults, as well as children, need regular immunization against tetanus. *Tetanus,* sometimes called lockjaw, is a serious, and often fatal, disease that occurs when certain bacteria that live in the soil get into a deep wound. Tetanus is likely to occur when a person who hasn't been properly immunized is wounded by a piece of rusty metal or receives any type of deep puncture wound. When children run barefoot they can get wounds easily.

## Allergies

An allergy is an extreme sensitivity to something. Children may be allergic to certain foods, such as milk, wheat, eggs, or strawberries, or objects, such as household dust, mold, pollen, and feathers.

Allergic reactions may be sneezing, itching or watering eyes, rashes, difficult breathing, or other health problems. When an allergy is suspected, the problem should be discussed with the child's doctor. Tests can be given, and treatments may be prescribed to relieve the reaction. If possible, the child should avoid the allergy-causing substance. The allergy may disappear eventually.

Sometimes an allergy can trigger an asthma attack. When a person has *asthma,* the bronchial tubes that lead from the windpipe to the lungs become partially obstructed. This results in difficult breathing, wheezing, and coughing. Asthma is a chronic condition. It cannot be cured, but an attack can be relieved by special treatments. Asthma occurs in school-age children, and some children outgrow it by puberty.

## Breath Holding

Children sometimes hold their breath when they are frightened, punished, or denied their requests. This may frighten parents, especially if the child holds his or her breath long enough to turn slightly blue around the mouth. Children can't hold their breath long enough to damage their health, however. Very quickly, the child naturally gasps for air.

## Enuresis (Bedwetting)

Bedwetting, or *enuresis,* among children age four and five is a common problem that may result from a physical or an emotional problem. Stress from parental demands or disciplinary methods may be the cause. Or the cause may simply be too much liquid or not going to the toilet before bedtime.

If parents relax their standards or change their habits of giving evening beverages, the bedwetting often disappears. Punishment, however, usually aggravates the situation. If enuresis continues, parents should discuss it with the child's pediatrician. The doctor will test for physical causes and prescribe treatment, if appropriate. If not, enuresis may require more time to correct itself.

# Communicable Childhood Diseases

| Disease | Incubation Period | Symptoms | Source of Contact | Period of Communicability | Home Health Care |
|---------|-------------------|----------|-------------------|---------------------------|------------------|
| Chickenpox | 13–17 days. | Fever and headache, followed by appearance of rash within 24 hours. Rash starts as small pink spots which turn to tiny blisters. New pox may appear for 3 or 4 days and may spread over entire body. Blisters turn to scabs in 4 days. | Contact with diseased case; droplets from nose and throat; or airborne spread of secretions of respiratory tract of infected person. | As long as 5 days before the eruption of chicken pox; not more than 6 days after the first crop of blisters. | Confine for 6 days following first symptoms; apply baking soda and water paste or allow to soak in a tub of baking soda and water. Trim fingernails to prevent breaking blisters. |
| Common Cold | 12–72 hours. | Runny nose; sneezing; overly tired; usually no fever, or sudden high fever for a short duration. | Contact with infected person; discharge from nose and mouth; sneezing and coughing. | Usually 24 hours before onset of symptoms and 5 days after onset. | Keep comfortable; plenty of rest and liquids; confine until symptoms disappear and child feels well. |
| Diphtheria | 2–6 days. | Sore throat and fever; symptoms become severe rapidly. Occasionally affects other mucous membranes or skin; lesions marked by patch or patches of grayish membrane with surrounding dull red inflammatory zone. | Contact with a diseased person or a carrier of the disease; discharge from nose and throat; or lesions. | Usually 2 weeks or less; seldom more than 4 weeks. | Contact doctor; confine until released by doctor or health department. |
| Dysentery (Bacillary) | 1–7 days. | Diarrhea; malaise; toxemia; fever; cramps. | Bowel discharge of infected person or carrier; contaminated food or drinks; flies. | During acute infection and until infectious agent no longer present in feces; usually within a few weeks. | Sanitary conditions necessary. Consult with doctor or nurse. |

# Communicable Childhood Diseases (continued)

| Disease | Incubation Period | Symptoms | Source of Contact | Period of Communicability | Home Health Care |
|---|---|---|---|---|---|
| (Infectious) Hepatitis Type A | Variable 10–50 days. | Early signs are abrupt onset of weakness, loss of appetite, fatigue. Then fever, nausea and abdominal discomfort, followed within a few days by jaundice. | Person-to-person contact between infected individuals; water contaminated with human excretions. Spreading is primarily through infected feces, urine, and/or diapers. Outbreaks related to contaminated food, milk, raw or uncooked clams or oysters. | Probably from two to three weeks before onset of disease and throughout the illness. | Isolation during first 2 weeks of illness and at least 1 week after onset of jaundice. Sanitary disposal of feces and urine; controlled handwashing before and after meals and toileting. Gamma globulin* for family contacts but not for contacts at day care center. |
| Impetigo | 4–10 days. | Vesicular (blistering) and crusting skin lesions, commonly on the face and often on the hands. | From skin lesions of infected persons; from carriers' nasal secretions. | As long as purulent (containing pus) lesions continue to drain. | Avoid common use of toilet articles; keep the surrounding skin clean; avoid contact with infants and debilitated (weak) persons. Consult a doctor. |
| Influenza | 24–72 hours. | Fever; chilliness or chills; discomfort; aches or pains; general malaise; sore throat; cough. | Discharge of nose and throat from infected persons, possibly airborne. | Probably limited to 3 days from clinical onset. | Consult with doctor or nurse. |
| Red Measles (Rubeola) | Varies from 8–13 days. | Fever, cold symptoms; sneezing and inflamed eyes; hard and dry cough; runny nose 3 to 4 days prior to rash, beginning on the face, becoming generalized; blotchy, dusky red color. | Contact with someone who has rubeola; discharge from nose and throat early in the illness before symptoms appear. | From beginning of the warning symptoms to 4 days after appearance of rash. | Confine for 7 days after appearance of rash; follow doctor's advice for care. Vaccination; gamma globulin* must be given within 2–3 days after exposure for effectiveness. |

* Gamma globulin is a fraction of blood plasma rich in antibodies and used against measles, hepatitis, etc.

# Communicable Childhood Diseases (continued)

| Disease | Incubation Period | Symptoms | Source of Contact | Period of Communicability | Home Health Care |
|---|---|---|---|---|---|
| Meningitis (Meningococcal) | 2–10 days. | Sudden fever; intense headache; nausea, often vomiting; stiff neck. | Direct contact with diseased person; nose and throat droplets of person carrying disease but not sick. | Until meningococci are no longer present in discharge from nose and mouth; usually disappear within 24 hours after start of treatment. | Isolate until 24 hours after start of doctor's medication. Confine until released by doctor or health department. |
| Mumps | 12–26 days; ordinarily 18. | Fever; vomiting; aching glands near ears and jaw line; painful swelling of salivary glands. May affect testes or ovaries. | Contact with someone who has mumps; droplets from nose and mouth of infected person. | 48 hours before swelling commences. Urine positive as long as 14 days after onset of illness. | Confine to bed until fever and swelling subside; remain indoors unless weather is warm. |
| Pediculosis (Lice) | Eggs hatch in 1 week; maturity in 2 weeks. | Infestation of the scalp, hairy parts of the body, or of clothing, especially along the seams of inner surfaces, with adult lice, larvae, or nits (eggs). Crab lice usually infest the pubic area. They may infest the eyelashes. | Direct contact with infected persons or with clothing containing lice. | While lice remain alive on the infected person and until eggs in hair and clothing have been destroyed. | Follow doctor's orders. |
| Pinkeye (Conjunctivitis—Acute Bacterial) | 24–72 hours. | White of eyes redden and are runny with matter; swollen eyelids; develops about 48 to 72 hours. | Contact with items used by infected person—fingers, towels, handkerchiefs, etc. | During course of active infection. | Remain away from others until recovered. Use a separate towel and washcloth. Local application of prescribed medical treatment. |
| Ringworm (Skin Infection) | 10–14 days. | Dry, circular splotches on skin and bare spots on scalp. | Direct contact with others who have the disease; contact with clothing and items of infected persons; lesions of animals. | As long as lesions are present. | Thorough bathing—soap and water; application of prescribed medicine. Remain under medical treatment until cured. |

# Communicable Childhood Diseases (continued)

| Disease | Incubation Period | Symptoms | Source of Contact | Period of Communicability | Home Health Care |
|---------|-------------------|----------|-------------------|---------------------------|------------------|
| Rubella (German Measles) (3-day) | 14–21 days; usually 18. | Mild fever; headache; sore throat; symptoms similar to a cold; rose rash; inflamed eyelids and eyes (conjunctivitis). | Contact with someone who has rubella; droplets from nose and throat, especially before rash appears. | About 1 week before and 4 days after onset of rash. | Contact doctor and follow instructions. |
| Scabies (Itch) | 2–6 weeks before onset of itching. | Severe itching and scratching; mite burrowed under skin between fingers, bends of body, and in folds of skin; small lesions like pinholes in a line. | Direct contact with infected person or clothing items of person, particularly undergarments and soiled bedclothes. | Until mites and eggs are destroyed by medical treatment. | Application of prescribed medical treatment by doctor. Confine until symptoms are no longer present. |
| Sore Throat (Simple) | 2–5 days. | Scratchy throat, sore, swallowing difficult; may have fever. | Upper respiratory discharges from infected persons. | As long as fever (if present) persists. | Consult doctor or nurse. |
| Streptococcal Infections (Including Scarlet Fever and Strep Throat) | 1–3 days. | Sudden infection; nausea; possibly vomiting; headache; fever; sore throat; glands of neck swollen; with scarlet fever, rash appears within 24 hours with fine, "grainy" touch—neck, chest, folds of elbow, and groin. | Contact with case of carrier of disease; discharge from nose and throat; may be spread through mild and unrecognized case. | 10–21 days for untreated cases; 24–48 hours with treatment. | Confine until symptoms disappear. Continue therapy for 10 days. Penicillin is normally used for treatment. |
| Whooping Cough (Pertussis) | Within 10 days. | Low fever; gradually worsening cough (over 1 to 2 weeks) limiting inhalation and ending with whoop, vomiting. Lasts 1 to 2 months. | Contact with case; discharge of nose and throat; articles freshly soiled with discharge. | 7 days after exposure to 3 weeks after onset of typical paroxysms. | Primary immunization during early childhood; follow with routine booster shots. |

## Heat Rash

During very hot weather, children may get a heat rash, or prickly heat. A heat rash consists of many pinhead-size red pimples that burn, tingle, and itch. To treat heat rash, bathe the child in cool water, apply powder to relieve the rash, and dress the child in lightweight, clean clothes. This treatment usually provides quick relief.

## Nosebleeds

Nosebleeds are common when children bump their nose or get a sore in their nose. A simple nosebleed usually stops within a few minutes. To treat a nosebleed, have the child sit quietly with the head tilted forward. Pinch the fleshy part of the nose for about 10 minutes, and ask the child to breathe through the mouth. Apply cold pads to the bridge of the nose and forehead. If the bleeding doesn't stop within 20 minutes, call the child's doctor or an emergency medical service.

## Pinworms

*Pinworms* are white, threadlike worms which can live in the digestive tract. Many children get pinworms from time to time. Good hygiene is the best way to prevent them. Handwashing before meals and after using the toilet is especially important because pinworms may be carried under unclean fingernails. A common symptom of pinworms is rectal itching especially after going to bed at night. Pinworms may be eliminated with medication provided by a physician.

## Responding to a Child's Health Problems

When children become ill or injured, caregivers must know how to respond. This includes being able to identify signs of possible illness:

- drowsiness during normal playtime
- sore throat
- persistent cough
- difficulty breathing
- vomiting
- diarrhea
- lack of appetite
- earache
- runny nose
- pain
- prolonged irritability

## Home Care

Patience, understanding, and certain home nursing skills are important when a child is recovering from illness or injury. Very small children require more attention than school-age children. By checking on them often, they are reminded that they're being cared for. They usually need a quiet and comfortable place to rest and sleep, nutritious food, and clean surroundings.

Children need quiet activities when they are sick or injured. Books, puzzles, scrapbooks, quiet hobbies, and television offer entertainment without physical exertion. Many children relax when a parent or caregiver reads to them. When a child misses school, the caregiver might need to get schoolwork for the child to complete at home.

Giving medication correctly is often vital to a child's recovery. Some guidelines for giving medicines are:

- Follow the physician's instructions closely.
- Make a written schedule of medication showing when each dose has been given.
- Never tell a child that medicine is candy. A child might get into the medicine on his or her own and take an overdose thinking it really is candy.
- If a child has difficulty swallowing pills, crush and dissolve them in a small

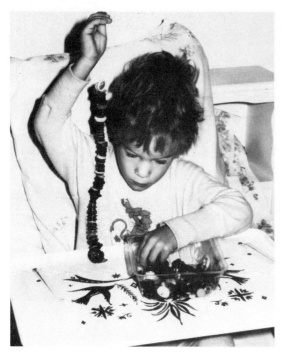

*When children are sick, quiet play rather than strenuous activity promotes recovery. They may not need to stay in bed, but frequent naps are important.*

amount of juice, applesauce, or peanut butter. Ask a doctor before doing this because it may change the way the medicine is absorbed into the body. If this is done, a child must eat all the food so he or she gets all the medicine.

- Remember not to give children under age 12 aspirins for colds or flu. This may lead to Reye's Syndrome, described in Chapter 9.
- If you must leave a sick child in the care of others, leave carefully-written instructions for the type, amount, and schedule of medication.
- Follow additional guidelines for administering medicine given on page **248.**

## Emergency Care

Accidents are common when children play, and injuries are inevitable. Most are minor, but some require emergency care. When you react to a child's emergency, respond calmly, and reassure the child in a quiet manner. Follow standard first aid procedures when you treat a child's injury.

When a serious accident happens, determine if the child is conscious. Next check for bleeding, burns, and broken bones. Move the child as little as possible, but do make him or her comfortable. Maintain the child's body temperature with a light coat or blanket while help is on the way. If you are baby-sitting, call parents, a neighbor, or a doctor if you cannot provide all the help needed or if you're not sure what to do. Get emergency help if the injury is serious.

If you call a person by telephone, give this information in a calm voice:

- your name
- child's condition
- facts about the accident
- exact location
- what help the child is being given

Refer to Chapter 6 for a complete description of emergency and first aid procedures.

## Hospitalization

Hospital care may become necessary if an illness or injury cannot be treated at home or if surgery is required. Hospitals can frighten a child. A hospital is an unfamiliar place, and a stay there usually involves separation from the family.

In non-emergency situations where parents know in advance that a child is to be hospitalized, they can prepare the child for the hospital stay. This reduces anxiety and speeds recovery. These are ways to prepare the child:

- Talk about the experience and explain the medical treatment and how it will

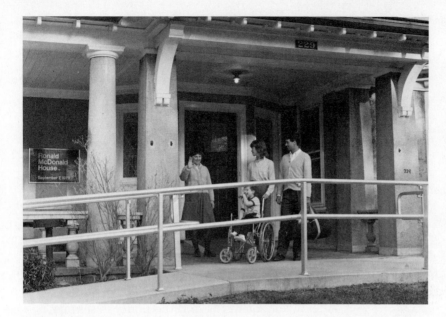

*The Ronald McDonald House® provides a homelike environment for families of children who are getting hospital care. Sometimes the sick children stay there, too, if they are getting outpatient care. There are more than 100 Ronald McDonald Houses around the world.*

help. Encourage the child to talk about the visit with you.

- Have the child participate in a children's hospital tour.
- Visit someone who is having a comfortable hospital visit.
- Obtain a storybook about hospital visits, and read it to the child.
- Purchase something fun for the child's stay at the hospital, such as new pajamas, funny house slippers, new books, or a new toy.
- Ask the doctor to talk with the child in a reassuring manner about the visit.
- Stay with the child in the hospital as much as possible. Some hospitals allow parents to stay overnight.
- Using a doll for a patient, let the child be a nurse or doctor and play act a hospital visit.

## Selecting Day Care

When both parents work outside the home, they may need day care for their chil-

dren. Infants and preschoolers may need part-time or all-day care. Grade-school children may need after-school or summer programs.

Day care may be at home, at a friend's or relative's home, or at a day care center. Some parents prefer that a caregiver comes to the home, particularly for a young infant or toddler. In this way, the child's normal routine isn't changed. The child isn't exposed to extreme weather or to other children's illnesses. Other parents prefer a day care center that offers special learning programs, play equipment unavailable at home, and a chance to learn social behavior by spending time with other children.

Parents need to evaluate programs carefully. Before they make a choice, they need to be sure that the facilities are safe and that the program contributes to the child's overall health and well-being. Usually parents can observe day care centers in operation. The chart on page **251** lists points to consider.

## Selecting Day Care

| Points to Consider | Questions to Ask |
|---|---|
| Schedule | • Does the center operate during the hours the child needs care? |
| Facilities | • Does the center have necessary safety features?<br>• Is adequate space provided for the number of children served?<br>• Are rooms bright and cheerful?<br>• What play areas and equipment are provided?<br>• What outdoor facilities are provided for play? |
| Staff | • How have the staff been trained?<br>• What safety and emergency training have they had?<br>• How many children does each staff member care for?<br>• Are staff members patient, caring, and communicative? |
| Activities | • Do activities promote social, physical, and mental development?<br>• Are activities supervised at all times?<br>• Is nap time scheduled?<br>• How are children disciplined? |
| Food | • Is the food appropriate for the child's age?<br>• Is the menu adequate for a child's nutrient and calorie needs?<br>• Does the food look appealing? |
| Visitation | • Are drop-in parent visits welcome? |
| Illness | • Will the center keep the child during an illness?<br>• What medical services handle emergencies? |
| Transportation | • Is there transportation to and from the center, if needed? |
| Licensing | • Does the center have the licensing required by law to operate? |
| Affiliation | • Who operates the program?<br>• Is the organization's philosophy consistent with the family's? |
| Cost | • What is the weekly and monthly charge?<br>• What is the family's monthly day care budget? |

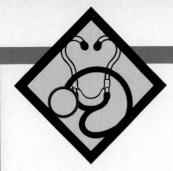

# CHAPTER CHECKUP

## Reviewing the Information

1. What are five health needs common to all children?
2. List five characteristics of a healthy child.
3. Why is a nutritious diet important for children?
4. What might happen if a child does not get adequate amounts of nutrients?
5. What are five guidelines for helping a child establish good food habits?
6. How does fluoride contribute to a child's dental health?
7. How could a parent make it easier for a child to wash his or her hands?
8. How does play promote health?
9. What are five guidelines for disciplining children?
10. Describe four ways to help a child deal with fear.
11. Explain five ways to child proof a home.
12. Describe characteristics of a potentially dangerous toy.
13. What are three ways parents or caregivers can help children who fear a visit to a doctor or dentist?
14. List five infectious diseases common during childhood.
15. How could a parent reduce the fear of a hospital stay?
16. What are five points to consider when selecting a day care center?

## Thinking It Over

1. Make a list of healthful snacks from the four basic food groups for children.
2. How might you discipline a seven-year-old who spilled grape juice on the rug?
3. Plan a bedtime routine for a preschooler.
4. What fears did you have as a child, and how did you overcome them?
5. Explain how you might help a child express anger in appropriate ways.
6. What animals might be good pets for a five-year-old and why?
7. How might you calm a child's fear of a hospital stay?
8. How might you recognize a victim of child abuse?

## Taking Action

 1. Read a magazine column on child care. Summarize the article in an oral report to the class.
 2. Select a book about children's health. Write a two page report and share it with the class.
 3. Find a safe toy in a children's store for a five-year-old. Write a child safety report on that toy.
4. Prepare a healthful snack for a school-age child.
5. Interview your mother to learn how you expressed your emotions as a child.
6. Find out what communicable childhood diseases you have had and which ones you have been immunized against.
7. Call a hospital or clinic to find out what special services they have for children.

# Managing Illness or Injury at Home

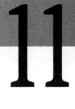

After reading this chapter, you should be able to:

• explain the importance of proper home health care.

• discuss the needs of a sick or injured person.

• identify the characteristics of a good caregiver.

• describe the care of a sick or injured person in the home.

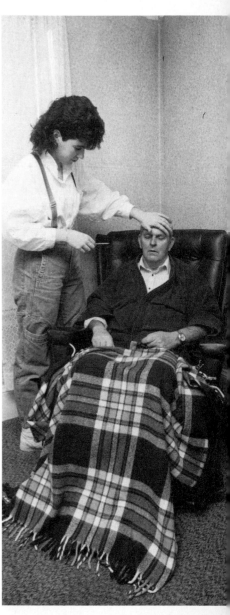

## Terms to Understand

| | |
|---|---|
| bedpan | sanitation |
| documentation | sick room |
| physical therapy | urinal |
| pulse rate | vital signs |
| respiratory rate | |

Hospitals and nursing homes are the usual places for treating sick or injured people. Both provide good medical and personal care. Not everyone who's sick or injured needs or wants to be hospitalized.

Illnesses, such as a cold or chickenpox, aren't serious enough to require hospitalization. People with chronic, or ongoing, diseases, such as Alzheimer's Disease, or disabling conditions, such as arthritis, don't need the highly-skilled medical care available in a hospital. However, they may need daily attention and assistance. People with many health conditions can be cared for at home if a family member or friend can be trained to give appropriate care.

Home health care is defined as meeting the physical and emotional needs of a sick or injured person at home and, if possible, restoring him or her to health. For each illness and injury, the prescribed care differs. Someone with the flu needs bed rest, plenty of fluids, and perhaps distraction from the boredom of being in bed all day. Someone disabled by a severe stroke may need help with everyday activities—eating, dressing, walking, and bathing.

What are the advantages of home health care? At home, a sick or injured person has more freedom. There are no rules about visiting hours, lights out, or meal hours. Families don't need to disrupt their schedules to visit the hospital or nursing home. At home,

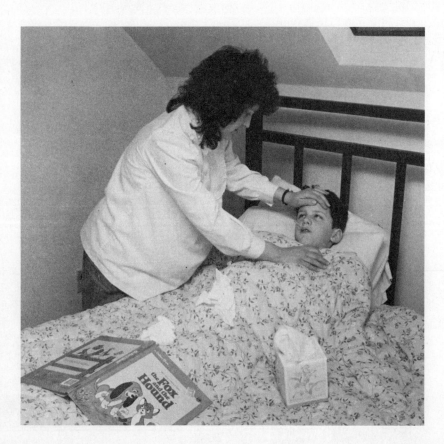

*Many people prefer being cared for at home when they are sick or injured.*

the "nurse" has only one "patient," so the sick or injured person usually gets more attention.

Home health care is less costly than hospital or nursing home care. With medicine and treatment, a one-day stay in a hospital might be $500. A typical nursing home fee can be $1500 per month or more.

Some people feel and eat better in their own home. Familiar surroundings are more comfortable. Patients may prefer home-cooked food. They like being surrounded by loved ones. This positive environment promotes emotional well-being which in turn helps the healing process.

Home health care requires a family commitment, perhaps friends' assistance, and skilled nursing services. A well-devised schedule for care, a carefully-arranged and clean environment, and appropriate medical and personal care are aspects of good home health care.

## Patient's Needs

Good home health care promotes not only physical health. By supporting emotional well-being and independence, when possible, the caregiver supports the healing process, too.

## Physical Health

The goal of home health care is to restore, as much as possible, the physical health of the patient. In some cases, however, the goal is to maintain, for as long as possible, the patient's current state of health and provide comfort.

Some conditions require only temporary care until the disease is cured or the injury is healed. Fractures, flu, and childhood diseases such as mumps need temporary care.

Some people never recover, however, no matter how good their care is. An injury may cause permanent damage, or a disease

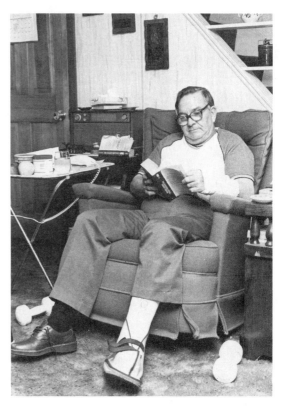

*Injuries, such as fractures, require temporary home health care.*

may never be cured. For example, a victim of a car accident might be permanently paralyzed. People with diseases, such as leukemia or Alzheimer's Disease, may become steadily worse, even with good care. In these circumstances, home health care lasts a long time, perhaps indefinitely. Home care must provide physical comfort and the care required to maintain the patient's current state of health as long as possible.

## Emotional Well-Being

Physical illness or injury often take an emotional toll on the patient causing anger, anxiety, sadness, and withdrawal. These emotions can drain the patient's energy away from the healing process.

Sick or injured people may worry about the effects of an illness or injury on schoolwork, their job, their involvement in sports, their family life, or their appearance. Adults often worry about mounting medical bills and lack of income while they're sick. If the condition is permanent, they may worry about the future.

Each person reacts to illness or injury in a different way. Emotional support as part of home health care can help lessen emotional stress.

## Need for Independence

Illness and injury bring limitations. Imagine that you suddenly became ill or injured and couldn't go to school, participate in school sports, go on a date, fix a snack, or turn on the television. Or worse, what if you couldn't walk, eat, or even bathe by yourself? Your family and friends would need to do everything for you. Dependence on others can be discouraging and hard to accept, particularly for a person who is used to being independent.

The amount of independence a patient can have depends on the illness or injury. People, for example, with heart disease or mononucleosis require a great deal of rest and shouldn't exert themselves. They must depend on others for most of their needs. On the other hand, people who have had a mild stroke or a broken bone don't need bed rest. The more they can do for themselves, the better.

When you care for others, encourage them to be as independent as possible. They'll feel better about themselves.

## Caregiver's Characteristics

The person who cares for a patient is called a caregiver. Caregivers may be family members (a parent, spouse, child, or other relative), friends, or skilled health professionals. For the patient's health, it's usually best to designate one person as the primary caregiver. This person takes the major responsibility for the patient's medication, therapy, and other care.

Some personal qualities are important to being a good caregiver. Good caregivers have a caring personality, time management skills, and careful grooming.

## Caring Personality

Caregivers spend more time around the patient than anyone else. Their personalities and attitudes affect the sick or injured person's outlook and often how quickly he or she recovers. Cheerfulness, gentleness, and tolerance are all important traits of a good caregiver.

Cheerfulness fosters a positive outlook in the patient. It also encourages cooperation and an "I can do it" attitude. Cheerfulness should be sincere, not overdone. False cheer is worse than none.

Gentleness is appreciated when people are sick or injured. A gentle touch is the safe way to handle someone. It also conveys a message of caring.

Tolerance, patience, and courtesy are important even when the patient is being difficult. Could you be tolerant in these situations?

- No matter what you do, your grandfather still complains of pain.
- Your sick baby brother won't stop crying while you try to dress him.
- Your aunt takes ten minutes to walk to the dining room; meanwhile dinner is getting cold.
- Your sister gives every excuse in the world not to take her medicine.

## Time Management

A caregiver needs to manage time carefully because patient care requires a lot of

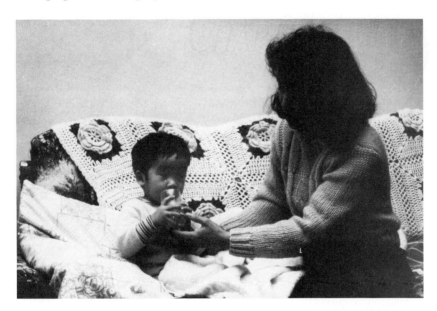

*A caring personality is an important characteristic of a caregiver. What specific qualities would make you a good caregiver?*

time. Usually the caregiver has other personal and family responsibilities, too. Without careful management, caregivers may become exhausted and even ill themselves. And they can no longer give quality care. And the whole family suffers from the stress of a family illness or injury.

Good home health care is both time and energy efficient. Caregivers can use these time management guidelines to plan patient care:

- Plan the day's schedule on paper with the help of the patient, if possible. Then he or she will more likely cooperate. This may include scheduling time for homework, a doctor's visit, or physical therapy.
- Plan tasks in an efficient order. For example, plan a bath after a messy activity like a meal. Or schedule the grooming activities together while a bedridden patient gets up to use the bathroom.
- Allow sufficient time to complete tasks. People usually need more time to do things when they're sick or injured. Being rushed is stressful.

- Keep routines flexible in case the person's health condition changes. For example, delay a physical therapy session if the person becomes nauseated.
- Gather all equipment necessary for a single task of medical care in one trip, if possible.
- Allow time for rest—for the patient and the caregiver. Illness or injury exhausts everyone!
- When possible, dovetail tasks as a caregiver with personal and family responsibilities. For instance pick up medicine during trips to the grocery store. If at all possible, prepare foods that both the patient and other family members can eat. Adjust recipes slightly for the sick, if necessary.
- Ask family members to help, perhaps by doing more chores or running errands.

## Personal Grooming

To someone who's bedridden or housebound, a caregiver who looks fresh and well groomed is refreshing. Follow these personal habits when you give home care:

**THINGS TO DO**

Date _today_

Done

✓ 1. 9:00 *Drop off Anne*
   2. *at therapist*
   3.
   4. 9:15 *Go shopping for*
   5. *groceries*
   6.
   7. 9:45 *Pick up dry*
   8. *Cleaning*
   9.
   10. 10:00 *Pick up Anne*
   11. *from therapist*
   12.
   13. 10:15 *Get prescription*
   14. *filled*
   15.

- Bathe and wear fresh clothes daily. Wash your hands before offering care so you don't pass germs.
- Avoid heavy scented perfumes which may be offensive or cause an allergic reaction.
- Brush your teeth often to avoid bad breath when you're in close contact.
- Keep your fingernails short so you don't accidently scratch the patient.
- Don't wear heavy or dangling jewelry that might hit the patient.

## Patient's Physical Environment

The physical arrangement of a home can make health care more efficient, more pleasant, and easier to manage. The sickroom should be arranged carefully to provide comfort and privacy and to allow space for proper care and equipment. Cleanliness is

*By dovetailing tasks, a caregiver can use time and personal energy more efficiently.*

important to control the spread of disease. With some illnesses and injuries, special medical equipment may be needed for care and treatment.

## Sickroom

The *sickroom* is the place at home where the patient is cared for. A separate room isn't necessary unless the patient is contagious, but it is more relaxing. The sickroom should allow quiet and privacy, but usually not isolation. If possible, it should be near a bathroom. This saves time for the caregiver and makes getting up easier for the patient who can get out of bed.

Natural light will make the sickroom more cheerful. But direct sunlight on the patient's face can be annoying. Partly-closed blinds or shades let in light without harsh glare. Recovery from some diseases though, such as measles, requires a darkened room.

At night, a small light is a good idea for safety. If caregivers check the patient in the dark, a night light will let them see without turning on overhead lights.

Temperature and ventilation should be controlled for comfort. Weather permitting, fresh air from outdoors is best. Otherwise, adequate ventilation helps remove odors. Room temperature should be warm enough to prevent getting chilled, usually between 68° F and 72° F.

For convenience, safety, and pleasure, patients often like these items at their bedside within easy reach: a bell to call the caregiver, tissues, wastebasket, water pitcher, a glass and straw, mirror, toiletries, reading light, clock, calendar, radio, remote control for television, telephone, books, magazines, pencil and paper.

## Special Equipment

Someone who is severely ill or who has a disabling injury may need special equipment. Common equipment includes a hospital bed, urinal, bedpan, and wheelchair.

A hospital bed is good for patients who must stay in bed for a long time and must have their position shifted often. The level of a hospital bed can be raised and lowered. This gives the caregiver comfortable access to the patient and prevents strain on the caregiver's back. The patient can get in and out of bed or change position more easily, too. For example, by pushing a button the head of the bed raises, bringing the patient into a sitting position.

Some patients cannot get out of bed to go to the bathroom, so they use a urinal or bedpan. A *urinal* is a container a man can use for urinating into. A *bedpan* is a container for a woman to use for urination, or a man or woman may use it for a bowel movement. Patients may need some help getting on and off of the bedpan. Using a bedpan or urinal in bed isn't comfortable or pleasant. The caregiver can make it easier by following the guidelines on page **260**.

Some patients can get out of bed, but they can't walk all the way to the bathroom. For them, a bedside commode, which is a chair with a drop-away seat, is best. Under the seat is a bedpan. A homemade bedside commode can be made by putting a bedpan on top of a chair with arm rests. The bedside commode is used like a toilet. Privacy is appreciated by the patient.

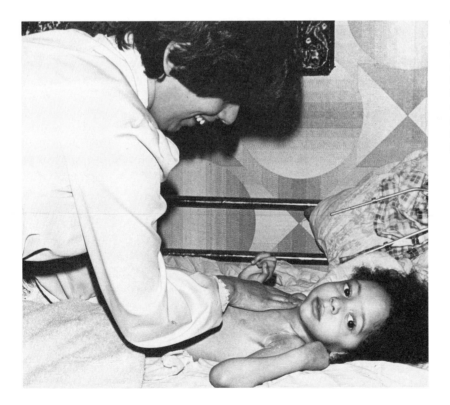

*A hospital bed can be raised and lowered so a patient can get in and out and move about easily in bed. Side rails keep children and the severely ill from falling out of bed.*

## How to Help with a Bedpan or Urinal

- Warm the bedpan or urinal by running warm tap water inside. Empty the water out and dry the outside.

- Put talc or cornstarch on the seat of the bedpan. This will make it easier for the person to slide on and off.

- Sit the person in an upright position. This is most natural.

- Put a soft pad between the buttocks and rim of the bedpan. It will be more comfortable, especially for elderly and thin people.

- Leave toilet tissue where the person can reach it.

- Place a pad underneath the urinal or bedpan, just in case there are spills.

- Be natural and understanding. It can be embarrassing for the patient to have to use a urinal or bedpan.

- Provide privacy by leaving the room or standing behind a partition.

- Offer the patient a wet, soapy cloth for handwashing when finished.

- Eliminate odors immediately with room freshener.

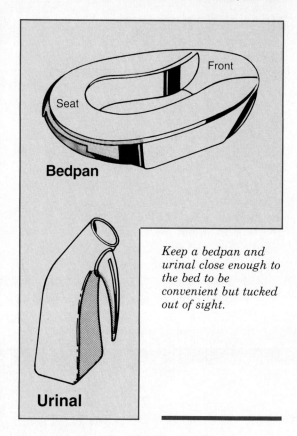

*Keep a bedpan and urinal close enough to the bed to be convenient but tucked out of sight.*

A wheelchair is important for those who can't walk but need to get around. A wheelchair is just that—a chair with wheels. It allows immobile people, or those who can't walk, to go to shopping centers, restaurants, the doctor's office, and just about any place they want to go. If you help someone with a wheelchair, follow these safety guidelines:

- Lock the wheels when you get the person into or out of the wheelchair.
- Be sure you're strong enough to transfer the person into the wheelchair. Get help, if necessary.

- As much as possible, only take the wheelchair over smooth surfaces. Look for wheelchair ramps on curbs and at steps.

Special equipment can be bought or rented. A local health department, community hospital, or physician can help locate what the patient needs.

## Sanitation

Proper sanitation is an important part of a patient's physical environment. *Sanitation* means keeping germs from multiplying. In home health care, this is done by keeping the patient, the sickroom, and the bedding as clean as possible. Caregivers must keep themselves clean as well.

If you're a caregiver, prevent the spread of contagious diseases by following these sanitary practices:

- Keep the sickroom clean and the air fresh.
- Change bed linens regularly, and immediately when they're soiled.
- Use clean towels daily.
- Help change the patient's clothing when it becomes soiled.
- Disinfect bed linens, towels, and patient's clothing by washing them in bleach or other laundry disinfectants.
- Wash your hands before and after handling the sick person.
- Provide routine hygiene care for the patient.

A sick person must also stay away from people with communicable diseases, such as a child with a runny nose. Sick people are less resistant to other diseases. The contagious patient should also stay away from the rest of the household.

Refer to Chapter 7 for other practices to use to prevent the spread of communicable diseases.

## Monitoring the Patient

Caring for a patient at home requires the caregiver to monitor, or carefully observe, the patient's condition. Often the caregiver must write down these observations and talk with the doctor.

### Signs and Symptoms of Medical Problems

Signs and symptoms of illness are changes from a person's normal state of health. They indicate whether or not a person is ill or injured.

To detect medical problems, caregivers first must know what is normal and healthy for the patient. Home caregivers have advantages over doctors or nurses. Because family caregivers know a patient's normal eating habits, skin color, mood, and daily

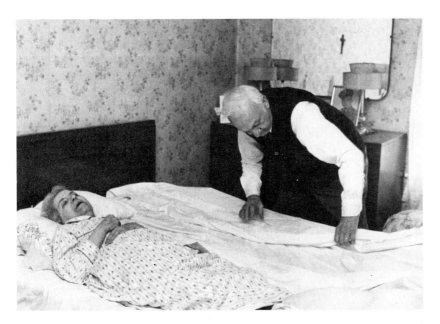

*If you have to change a patient's bed linens, carefully roll the patient to one side of the bed. Change the linens on one side. Then roll the patient to the other side and finish changing the linens. Be sure there are no wrinkles.*

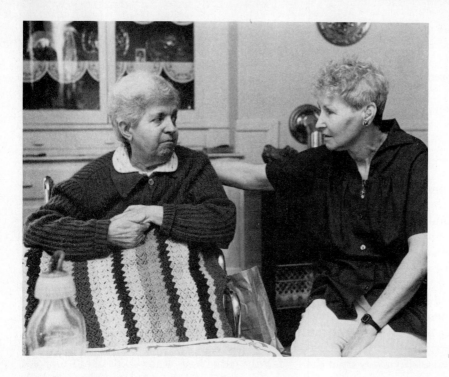

*A good caregiver uses all five senses to observe a person's health condition. What might be observed here?*

habits, they can detect something abnormal more quickly.

By using their senses, caregivers learn about the person they're caring for.

- Look for anything abnormal or unexpected. You can identify many things by observing a person's body and activities. You can see a rash which might indicate that the person has had an allergic reaction. Heavy perspiration could alert you to a high temperature. Or drowsiness could mean the person had too much medicine.

- Listen for signs that something is wrong and perhaps getting worse. Does the person have a cough, and is it getting worse? Is the voice becoming strained? Is the person talking louder than normal? Or do you have to talk louder before the person seems to hear and understand you? Is the stomach growling so loud you can hear it?

- Unusual odors are a sign that something could be wrong. Does the person have bad breath? Have you smelled an unusual body odor? An odor doesn't have to be bad to cause concern. For example, someone with severe diabetes has a sweet, fruity breath odor.

- Don't be afraid to touch the person. Just by touching the skin you can tell if it's warm, dry, or puffy. By feeling the person's forehead with your hand you can often detect the presence of a fever, or abnormally high body temperature. Touching may cause pain. Although you don't want to purposely cause pain, you do need to know if there are any tender spots. Touching can indicate how tense the person is.

- Use the patient's sense of taste, not your own, to detect signs and symptoms. Take note if he or she says that a familiar food tastes unusual.

Now that you know how to check on a sick or injured person, these are the signs and symptoms of medical problems:

- General appearance: Have there been changes? If so, what were they? Notice in particular how the face looks. Is it pale or flushed? Look at the skin for color and swelling. Overall, does the patient seem weaker or sicker?
- Mood: Is the person awake and alert as usual? Has the amount or tone of talking changed? Do you detect a mood change? Do the answers you get make sense? Can the person make eye contact with you?
- Sleep: Have the person's sleeping habits changed? Watch how long the person sleeps and if sleep is restful. Are there changes in the breathing pattern during sleep? What wakes the person up?
- Appetite and thirst: Is the person's appetite increased or decreased? How about thirst? Is he or she asking for water a lot and complaining of a dry mouth? If you suspect a health problem, keep a record of what and how much the sick or injured person consumes.
- Pain: Pain is always a sign that something is wrong. Learn as much as you can about the pain. Exactly how does the person describe the pain? Where is it? Is it severe or mild, sharp or throbbing, continuous or periodic? What causes the pain? Does anything make it go away? Did the doctor prescribe medicine for the pain? Does it help?
- Daily activities: Is there a change in what the person is able to do alone, such as dressing, feeding, or walking?

Note the important signs and symptoms of illness regularly, but don't be too conspicuous. You don't want to disturb or worry the person you're caring for unnecessarily. When you're at the bedside, be alert. You'll detect more signs and symptoms than you think.

# Vital Signs

*Vital signs* are a person's body temperature, pulse rate, breathing rate, and blood pressure. They indicate whether a person is healthy or sick. They're also signs and symptoms of illness.

## BODY TEMPERATURE

A person's temperature is the amount of heat produced in the body. As you learned in Chapter 9, no one temperature is "normal" for every person. Instead, there is a normal range which also varies with the way the temperature is taken—in the mouth, in the rectum, or under the armpit. See the chart below.

Normal body temperature is affected by time of day, age, and individual differences among people. Body temperature tends to be slightly higher in the afternoon and slightly lower in the morning. Infants and young children have slightly higher normal temperatures than teens and adults. Older people tend to have lower normal temperatures.

An abnormally high body temperature, or fever, indicates that something is wrong. But a person may be ill without having a fever. An infection is the most common cause of fever. A fever is often accompanied by chills, a headache, thirst, or loss of appetite. Very high fevers can cause temporary mental confusion.

## Normal Ranges for Body Temperature

| Method | Fahrenheit | Centigrade |
|---|---|---|
| oral | 97.6°–99.6° | 36.5°–37.5° |
| rectal | 98.6°–100.6° | 37.0°–38.0° |
| skin (underarm) | 96.6°–98.6° | 36.0°–37.0° |

Body temperature should be measured when a person complains of feeling sick and when someone looks ill. This is especially important for infants. During an illness, the temperature should be taken every four hours or at the interval recommended by the doctor.

A thermometer is used to measure body temperature. Every home should have at least one thermometer in a first aid kit. A thermometer is a glass tube filled with a heat-sensitive chemical called mercury. Proper handling ensures that thermometers measure temperature accurately and don't break. The chart on this page describes the way to take a person's temperature.

There are three different types of thermometers: oral, rectal, and stubby. The shape of the bulb end of the thermometer differs for each. The oral thermometer is used for taking mouth and underarm temperatures. The rectal thermometer is used for taking rectal temperatures. The stubby thermometer can be used for taking temperatures in the mouth, rectum, or under the arm. Mark the thermometer so you know which way it is to be used.

The oral method of taking a temperature is most common and easiest for adults. It's taken with a thermometer that has a long bulb on the end. The bulb end of the thermometer is placed into the patient's mouth under the tongue. The patient must keep the thermometer in place for five minutes by closing the lips around it. It's then removed and read.

A rectal temperature may be taken for several reasons. It's the most accurate method. It's best for patients with mouth sores, frequent coughing, stuffy noses, or sneezing spells who can't keep their lips closed long enough to take an oral temperature. It's also appropriate for babies and young children who might bite and break a thermometer in their mouths.

If you take a rectal temperature, use the thermometer with the short, rounded bulb. Ask the person to lie on his or her side. You'll have to hold young children in this position. For babies, it's easiest to hold them on your lap on their stomach. Lubricate the bulb end of the thermometer with petroleum jelly and insert it about one inch into the rectum. Hold it in place for four minutes. Then remove the thermometer, wipe it with a tissue or cotton ball, and read it.

## How to Take Body Temperature

- Wash your hands before taking someone's temperature.

- Shake down the mercury level below 96° F.

- Avoid taking temperature for three minutes after the patient drinks something hot or cold.

- Have the patient sit or lie down, in a comfortable position.

- Use the appropriate procedures for taking an oral, rectal, or skin temperature.

- After reading, evaluate the temperature. Is it within normal range for the method being used?

- If the temperature is abnormally high or low, take it again. Use a different thermometer if possible, just to make sure that you are using a thermometer that is working properly.

- Call the doctor for temperatures above the normal range. Ask the doctor for specific guidelines.

- After each use, clean the thermometer. Wash with soap and a soft cloth. Rinse with cool water and dry.

- Store the thermometer in a protective case. Keep it out of the reach of children.

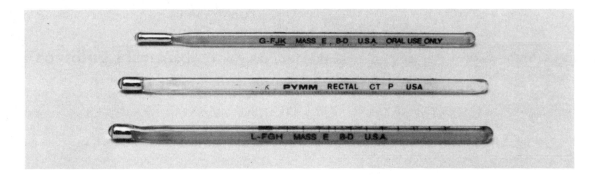

## How to Read a Thermometer

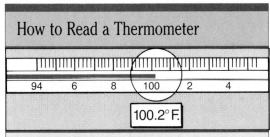

1. Grasp the thermometer on the opposite end of the bulb.
2. Hold it at eye level in good light.
3. Turn the thermometer around slowly until you can clearly see the column of mercury.
4. Notice the lines. Each long line is one degree. In a Fahrenheit thermometer, each short line is one-tenth of a degree. (In a Centigrade thermometer, each short line is two-tenths of a degree.) Most thermometers have an arrow pointing to the average normal body temperature. In Fahrenheit, this is 98.6° F (in Centigrade, 37° C).
5. Notice the line where the column of mercury ends. Read the line that's closest to the point.
6. Record the temperature.

Having a rectal temperature taken can be uncomfortable and, for some people, embarrassing. Be as pleasant as you can. If you seem comfortable with what you're doing, the sick person will be, too.

Temperature in the armpit, called skin temperature, isn't as accurate as other methods. However, it sometimes is the only way you can get a temperature reading, especially with a wriggling child. Dry the armpit well because moisture affects the temperature. Place the bulb end of an oral or stubby thermometer into the center of the armpit, but don't press it sharply into the skin. Ask the patient to hold it in place for seven minutes by pressing the arm tightly against the body. (It takes a long time for skin temperature to register on a thermometer.) Then remove the thermometer and read it.

To read a thermometer accurately, refer to the chart on the left.

### PULSE RATE

*Pulse rate* is the rate of the heartbeat felt in a throbbing blood vessel just under the skin. Normal pulse rate varies among people. Usually men, babies, obese people, and nervous people have a higher pulse. Women, athletes, and people who are asleep have a slower pulse. A pulse of 70 to 90 beats per minute is considered normal for teens and adults at rest.

Find your own pulse. Use the flat side of your pointer and middle fingers on your left hand. Press them on the palm side of your right wrist at the base of the thumb. Feel around the bone but stay near the wrist.

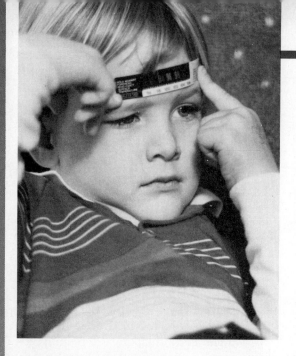

Electronic thermometers are the ultimate in temperature measurement. They're fast, accurate, and even sound a beep when the temperature has registered. It usually only takes 10 to 15 seconds. The temperature is read from a lighted digital display.

When a baby is so squirmy you just can't get a temperature with a thermometer, try a pacifier—a temp-pacifier, that is. It's the latest gimmick in temperature taking. After the baby sucks on the pacifier for a few seconds, body heat registers as a color on the outside of the pacifier. It's quick and easy to read.

# HIGH-TECH TEMPERATURES

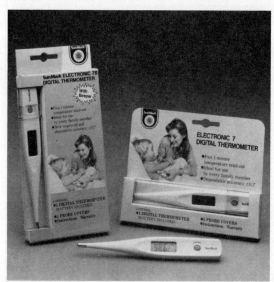

Today you can measure body temperature in some unusual ways. Thanks to modern technology, electronic and chemical equipment is replacing the old, reliable, glass thermometer. According to recent studies, these nontraditional methods are not only quicker than the glass thermometer but just as accurate.

Skin temperature strips are made of a light plastic. To use them, press the strip to your forehead for a few seconds, and watch the numbers appear! The highest number shown indicates your skin temperature. The strip is quick and easy to use on people of any age. Since it won't break, it's great for traveling or camping. Some are even shaped like the latest cartoon characters to delight youngsters.

You'll find your pulse. You can also find your pulse in your neck as learned in Chapter 1.

Take the pulse rate every three to four hours for adult patients. For children with a rising temperature, measure the pulse every hour. Count the beats for a full minute. Use a watch or clock with a second hand. Don't take the measurement for at least five minutes after physical activity. Call the doctor if the pulse rate changes suddenly.

### RESPIRATORY RATE

*Respiratory rate* measures how fast the person is breathing. Breathing rate is easy to measure. Watch and count how many times the patient's chest rises and falls for one minute. Each time the chest rises and falls equals one respiration, or complete breath. The normal adult rate is 12 to 18 respirations per minute. This rate is faster for children and even faster for babies. As with the pulse rate, take the measurement for a full minute, using a watch or clock with a second hand. Do not take the measurement for at least five minutes after physical activity. It's a good idea to measure pulse and respiratory rates while a patient's temperature is being taken.

### BLOOD PRESSURE

Like temperature, pulse rate, and breathing rate, blood pressure helps indicate how healthy a person is. As you learned in Chapter 7, this measurement indicates the force at which the heart is pumping blood through the body. Blood pressure is a technical measurement, usually done by doctors and nurses. It can be done at home with special equipment and training. If someone in your home needs his or her blood pressure checked, learn how to take blood pressure readings.

## Documentation

Caring for someone often requires keeping track of medical information. *Documentation* means writing down everything you need to remember about caring for someone or for sharing with the doctor or nurse. Keep it simple but complete.

## Communicating with the Doctor

After watching and documenting information about the signs and symptoms of health problems, caregivers need to decide when and why a doctor should be called and what to report.

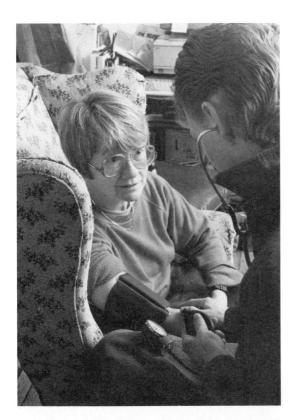

*With training and special equipment, blood pressure readings can be taken as part of home health care.*

## Sample Documentation Sheet

Date _____

| Time | Body Temper- ature | Pulse Rate | Respir- ation Rate | Signs and Symptoms | Care Given |
|------|---------------------|------------|---------------------|--------------------|------------|
|      |                     |            |                     |                    |            |
|      |                     |            |                     |                    |            |
|      |                     |            |                     |                    |            |
|      |                     |            |                     |                    |            |

Doctor's Orders

## WHEN TO CALL

Knowing when to call the doctor isn't easy because some signs and symptoms are significant and others aren't. For example, complaints of pain can be routine, or they can indicate trouble. A little bleeding may not be anything to worry about. How much is serious? What temperatures should be a concern? Usually, the decision to call the doctor comes from a combination of symptoms, not just one.

When you care for a patient at home, you need specific, easy to understand guidelines from a health professional, probably a doctor. These guidelines help you feel secure with your patient care. The doctor identifies the signs and symptoms serious enough to call about. For example, you might be told to call if a temperature goes over 100.6° F or if the pulse rate goes over 100.

A doctor may also give instructions about how to treat common signs and symptoms of health problems. For a high temperature, you may be told to sponge the patient with cool water. For complaints of pain, you may be instructed to give aspirin or massage the area. For an itching rash, the doctor might prescribe an ointment to apply. You can perform many simple treatments with advance instructions from the doctor. Then you don't need to call the doctor every time these signs and symptoms appear.

Based on your observations and the doctor's guidelines, call if necessary for the safety and health of your patient. The time of day or night should not stop you. Your responsibility as a caregiver is to care for someone's medical needs, no matter what time of day.

Two general guidelines may help determine when to call—if the signs and symptoms last for a long time or if the signs and symptoms get worse.

Before you call the doctor, keep these thoughts in mind. Sick children often overdramatize their symptoms to get attention. Bored adults might exaggerate their discomfort or complain more than necessary. A teenager who really wants to go out might try to hide signs of illness.

**WHAT TO REPORT**

When you call a doctor or when the doctor or nurse visits, report what you know. Have your documentation handy. The doctor will ask:

- What sign or symptom concerns you? How severe is it? How long has it lasted? The caregiver might explain, "The patient has complained of a stomachache for the last hour. It's so bad that she's crying."

- What is the temperature, pulse rate, and breathing rate? For example, "The temperature is now 101.4 degrees and was 99.8 just four hours earlier. The pulse is 92, and the breathing rate is 18."

- Is there any bleeding? If so, how much, what is the color, and where is the bleeding coming from? For example, the caregiver might report, "The bandage over the laceration, or cut, on the leg is soaked with bright red blood."

- Especially with babies, the doctor will want to know about bowel movements. You might report, "The child has had two, watery bowel movements in the last hour."

- How is the patient acting? Is this different than before? What is the patient's mood? For example, "The patient seems drowsier than yesterday, but is restless at times."

- Do you notice anything unusual?

Signs and symptoms are clues to a medical problem. The more accurate and thorough you are in your description of them, the more accurate the doctor's diagnosis can be.

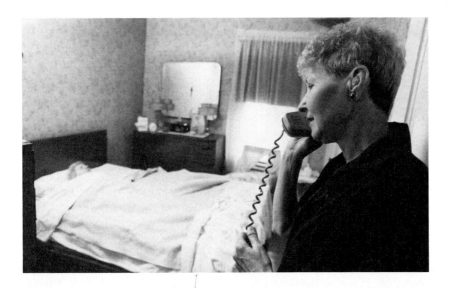

*When you talk to the doctor on the phone, be calm. Don't alarm the patient with the tone of your voice.*

Over the phone, you are the eyes and ears of the doctor.

## Support and Care of the Patient

Caregivers are responsible for many aspects of patient care at home. Adequate rest, activity, nutrition, personal hygiene, pain relief, medicines, and emotional support are part of home health care. Sometimes professional health services are also required within the home.

## Rest and Relaxation

Sick or injured people often feel weak, and they usually want and need bedrest. Rest helps restore health as the body uses its energy to fight off infections or replace damaged body cells.

Bedrest is sometimes prescribed by the doctor as a treatment. People with sudden or severe illnesses, such as hepatitis or flu, need plenty of rest to recover. Those with broken legs may be temporarily immobilized. Some terminally-ill people are permanently confined to bed.

The caregiver's responsibility is to see that the patient stays in bed and rests comfortably. When youngsters are the patients, this isn't always easy!

- Provide plenty of time for rest and relaxation each day. Let the person's body give clues to how much sleep is needed.
- Darken the room during the day to help the person sleep.
- Don't interrupt sleep by checking vital signs and giving medications unless the doctor requires this.
- Create a quiet, non-stressful environment. Ask others to be quiet while the patient is sleeping.

## Activity

For most people who are ill, activity, in the form of exercises or daily routines, promotes health and recovery. The more people can do for themselves, the better they feel about themselves. The patient's independence makes the caregiver's workload easier.

Encouraging the patient to take part in daily care is good for morale. Even if he or she takes longer to dress or bathe, being independent reinforces the patient's self-esteem. The physical exercise required to do things alone can help a patient regain strength, keep muscles loose, improve circulation, and prevent bedsores.

As a caregiver, you may need to help with some activities that a patient can't do alone. Can the person get into and out of bed alone? Can the person walk alone? If not, you need to help. Remember, patient safety is important. You don't want him or her to fall or get too tired.

People who are confined to bed are limited in their activity level. In-bed exercises can provide physical exercise if the doctor approves. Encourage these patient activities:

- Gently rotate the head from side to side, and then completely around.
- Shrug the shoulders up and down.
- Swing the arms out from the shoulders and bend the elbows. Then drop the arms and straighten the elbows.
- While sitting in bed with the palms of the hands against the mattress, roll from one buttock to the other, back and forth.
- One at a time, tuck the knee to the chest and return the leg to the bed.
- One at a time, raise the feet from the bed and rotate the ankles.

*Physical therapy,* or special exercises to restore normal movement, is often part of home health care. Someone with arthritis, a stroke, or broken bones, for example, might need physical therapy. A doctor, nurse, or therapist will demonstrate to caregivers how to provide this therapy.

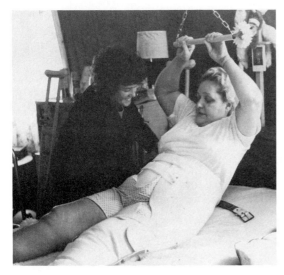

*Exercise for bedridden patients helps prevent bedsores, muscle weakness, and boredom. It also gives a sense of well-being and increases blood circulation.*

## Nutrition

Like you, sick and injured people need nutrients from a balanced diet. Food can contribute to a patient's physical, emotional, and social health, and so it must be part of the home health care plan.

### SPECIAL DIETS

The treatment of some health problems requires a special diet prescribed by the doctor. Extra liquids may be required to prevent constipation and dehydration. Dehydration, an excess loss of body fluids, may be caused by long bouts of vomiting or diarrhea, excessive perspiration, and severe burns. Nutrient requirements may be increased to help rebuild body tissues. The consistency of some foods might be changed for people with digestive problems. Or the diet may be modified with less salt, fat, or calories.

Some chronic diseases require special diets for the person's entire life. Diabetics must follow a rigid menu plan which adjusts the calorie and carbohydrate content of their diets. People with heart disease often restrict dietary fat and cholesterol. Those with hypertension often restrict sodium.

Other conditions require special diets for only a short time. For example, someone with a fever needs extra liquids to prevent dehydration. A person with digestive problems needs foods that won't irritate the digestive tract. And people who have oral surgery might need a liquid diet until they can chew again.

The following describes some types of special diets:

- Bland diets are often prescribed for people with digestive problems. Foods are cooked simply, usually by baking or boiling. Highly-seasoned, high-fat, and gas-forming foods are eliminated.
- Soft diets are also recommended for some types of digestive problems or for people who have trouble chewing. A soft diet often includes semi-solid foods, such as pudding, mashed potatoes, ground meat, pastas, and soups. Foods with a lot of fiber are eliminated.
- Liquid diets are prescribed for very ill patients or those who have trouble chewing and swallowing. These diets consist only of liquids, such as soup, milk, juices, gelatin, or strained vegetables. Getting all essential nutrients is difficult on a liquid diet, so most patients follow it only for a short time.

Preparing special diets can be inconvenient if the foods are different from what the rest of the family eats. And sometimes patients don't like foods prescribed on the diet. However, special diets are an important part of medical treatment which caregivers must follow.

A registered dietitian can help caregivers and patients understand special diets. Together, they can plan menus which include

## Soft Diet

| Breakfast | Dinner |
|---|---|
| ½ cup orange juice | 3 oz. ground or |
| ½ cup cream of | pureed turkey |
| wheat, enriched | ½ cup mashed |
| 1 slice soft white | potatoes |
| bread, enriched | 2 tablespoons gravy |
| 1 egg, soft | ½ cup pea puree |
| scrambled | 1 slice soft white |
| 1 cup milk, whole or | bread, enriched |
| non-fat | 1 custard |

*Patients who have trouble chewing need to eat a soft diet. What other nutritious and soft foods might they be able to consume?*

foods the patient likes and which the caregiver can prepare easily.

### MEALTIME

Illness or injury often affect a person's appetite. Pain, anxiety, sadness, indigestion or nausea, weakness or exhaustion, dry mouth, and boredom can all affect a person's desire to eat.

As a caregiver, try to make mealtime pleasant. Here are some suggestions to help a patient take interest in eating:

- If possible, let the patient join the rest of the family at the table.
- Serve small portions that don't look overwhelming. You can offer seconds.
- Serve mostly hot foods because the aroma may be enticing.
- If nausea is a problem, serve mostly cold foods because they don't have as strong an aroma.
- Serve food at the proper temperature so it's more appealing.
- Make the food look good. Serve foods with a variety of colors, shapes, and textures together. Serve food neatly on colorful dishes.

If the family member must eat in bed, create a special atmosphere at mealtime:

- Remove all unpleasant sights, such as a bedpan.
- Decorate the tray with a flower, a home-made ornament, or, for a child, a small toy.
- Eat your own meal in the sickroom, too, so mealtime is a social time.
- Play music in the background.
- Have the room as bright as possible.
- Make the family member comfortable. Place pillows behind the person's back so he or she can sit up straight.

### FEEDING

A caregiver may need to feed weak people or those who can't use their hands. Adults and teens may have a hard time accepting help, however, because they want to feel independent.

If you must help feed someone, be pleasant. Let him or her know that you enjoy helping and that you like sharing your time. Follow these guidelines if the person you're caring for must be fed:

- Help the person wash his or her hands, and offer mouth care before and after every meal.
- Serve finger foods which are easier to eat without help.
- Never hurry. Offer reasonably sized bites. Allow time between bites.
- Sit down while you feed a patient. You will feel more comfortable, and it creates a more relaxed, social atmosphere. You will also be less likely to rush the patient's eating and less likely to spill.
- Feed the person with a spoon. A fork might stab the person's tongue. Food tends to dribble or fall more easily from a fork.
- Be careful not to spill food. But if you do, wipe the person quickly.
- Except for infants and young children,

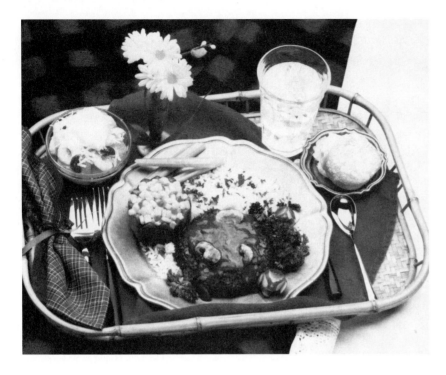

*Cheer up patients by planning to serve food attractively. You might want to serve this meal to an injured teenager.*

let the sick family member decide which foods to eat first.

- Serve beverages with a straw to make drinking easier.
- Talk while you feed someone, but don't expect too many answers. Your patient will have a mouthful of food.
- Document the person's appetite so you can report to the physician or nurse.

## Personal Hygiene

Good hygiene contributes to recovery from illness or injury. Not only does good hygiene help control germs, but most people feel better when they're clean and fresh. Those who haven't been able to rest comfortably may relax and sleep better after a warm bath. Sometimes sick people are concerned about body odors caused by perspiration, bacteria, and wounds. Routine hygiene, including bathing, mouth care, and hair care, helps prevent odors from building up.

**BATHING**

Besides removing dirt and germs from the skin, bathing serves several purposes in home health care, especially for those confined to bed. It promotes comfort, provides relaxation, stimulates blood circulation, prevents bedsores, and helps the patient maintain a positive self image.

A complete bath is not necessary every day. Some sick or injured people prefer to just wash their hands and face a few times a day, then completely bathe two or three times a week. Someone who tires easily may prefer to have a different part of the body bathed each day.

Sometimes people need help bathing when they're sick or injured. Those with broken arms or legs, for example, may not be able to shower or bathe without help. They mustn't get their casts wet. Open wounds shouldn't get wet with bath water because bath water contains many germs.

Bedridden people may need to bathe in bed. Others may need help at the bathroom sink or in the tub.

If you're helping someone bathe, gather these items before you start: a wash cloth, face towel, bath towel, soap and soap dish, clean clothes or a bed gown, and perhaps lotion or powder. You'll also need a basin with warm water if the family member must bathe at the bedside.

If you are helping with a bath, work efficiently and make the patient as comfortable as possible.

- Have the patient help you as much as possible.
- Wash one part of the body at a time and dry it completely. Keep all other parts covered with a towel, blanket, or robe so the patient doesn't get chilled.

*People need different amounts of assistance bathing depending on how sick or injured they are. Encourage a patient to be as independent as possible.*

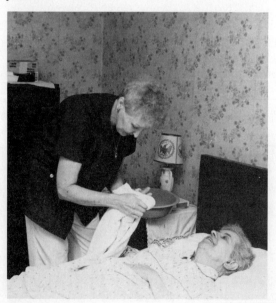

- Keep soap in the soap dish when not in use. This way the water won't get soapy, and the soap won't get mushy.
- Provide as much privacy as possible.
- If bathing at the bedside, change the water in the basin as it gets cold, soapy, or dirty.
- After drying, apply powder, lotion, or cologne if the person requests it.

Bath time can be enjoyable for the caregiver and the patient. Play background music. Talk about the day's activities. Avoid letting bath time become a tedious routine. Go slowly. Sick or injured people usually appreciate the time and individual attention.

## MOUTH CARE

Have you ever had a bad taste in your mouth when you wake up? Or have you had a very dry mouth? Neither is very pleasant. Some diseases and medicines leave a bad taste in the mouth or dry it out. Frequent opportunities for mouth care are a welcome relief to sick people.

If the sick or injured person is confined to bed, you need to bring these items to the bedside: toothbrush, toothpaste, mouthwash, water in a rinsing cup, spit basin, dental floss, and a face towel. Help the person, if necessary.

How often should you offer mouth care? That depends on the person's habits, preferences, and health. Offer mouth care before and after meals, at bedtime, and more often if you see the need. People with braces on their teeth must be especially careful to keep their mouths clean.

For those with chapped, dry lips, apply a small amount of petroleum jelly or a commercial lip balm. For a dry mouth, offer a mouth rinse with a mixture of equal parts of lemon juice and glycerin. Sucking on a clean, cool, moist washcloth or ice chips can also relieve a dry mouth.

Dentures and false teeth require special care. They should be washed with a denture brush and denture cream. Rinse them with warm water; hot water can damage the dentures. Store dentures overnight in a cup of water or a special cleaning solution to prevent drying.

### HAIR CARE

Hair care provides cleanliness, stimulates circulation to the scalp, and improves morale. Daily hair care includes thorough brushing and grooming in a way that the person likes. For a woman, this might include curling the hair.

Hair needs shampooing when it gets dry or oily. For a bedridden family member, use a dry shampoo. This is a special type of shampoo that doesn't have to be applied or rinsed with water. Dry shampoos come in liquid, powder, and spray form. Apply the shampoo, rub it into the hair and scalp, and then brush or towel it out.

A regular shampoo can also be given in bed with a makeshift arrangement. Place cotton balls in the patient's ears to keep water out. After washing, dry the hair quickly so the person doesn't get chilled.

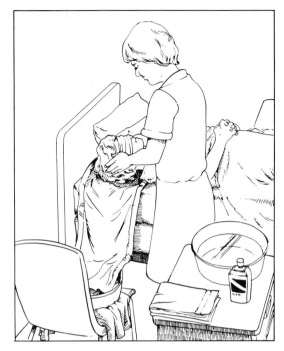

*Using a plastic sheet, which is rolled up on the sides, a patient's hair can be efficiently washed in bed. The pillow should be removed from the head, and the person should be moved so his or her head is close to you.*

## Personal Appearance

Don't you feel better when you know you look good? Looking and feeling attractive is important to the patient's personal attitudes and self esteem. Encourage the patient to take an interest in his or her overall appearance. Suggest that teenagers and adults keep makeup or shaving equipment, brushes, combs, and a mirror handy to use.

Encourage the person you're caring for to dress everyday in daytime clothes. Help him or her dress if necessary. Even a person who is bedridden doesn't have to wear pajamas all the time. As long as clothing doesn't interfere with any medical treatments, your family member can dress in a sweatsuit, jeans, or whatever is comfortable.

## Comfort

Pain is probably the most personal and distressing symptom of illness. Only the sick or injured person really knows what it feels like. And of course, only he or she has to endure it. As a caregiver, you can help relieve pain.

There are many methods of pain relief. Injecting special medicine into the vein requires a doctor's prescription and skilled nursing care. Other methods, such as distraction, massages, and oral medicines, are simple and easily used at home.

Distracting the sick or injured person won't make pain go away. But it will lessen his or her awareness of pain. People notice pain more when their attention is focused on it. So encourage the person to read, watch television, or listen to music. Have games, magazines, and books on hand. Distract your patient with good conversation. Invite visitors over if the family member isn't contagious. If the diet isn't restricted, serve a fun meal, such as pizza or a Chinese dinner.

A massage often relieves pain, promotes comfort, and relaxes. It even stimulates blood circulation, which is especially good if the person is confined to bed. A massage is good for most parts of the body—arms, legs, neck—as long as there are no injuries in the area being massaged. A back rub is usually the favorite massage.

When giving a massage, lubricate your hands with lotion. This moisturizes the skin and makes your hands move more smoothly. Don't use rubbing alcohol. It dries and hardens the patient's skin, causing it to crack.

Be careful of tender places when you massage. Red areas of skin are often caused by poor circulation and pressure. Massage these areas gently with lots of lotion. If the skin is very red and almost broken, don't touch it. Nearly broken areas of reddened skin indicate the beginning of bedsores.

Bedsores are sores that occur when a person must stay in bed for a long time. They are caused by the continual pressure of the body rubbing against the bed or bed clothes. The most common sites of bedsores are the elbows, knees, shoulder blades, heels, hips, and buttocks. Besides massaging, encourage the patient to move and bend the body more or move the person yourself if necessary to prevent bedsores.

## Medicine

Medicine is often part of the treatment for illness or an injury. Medicines ordered by a

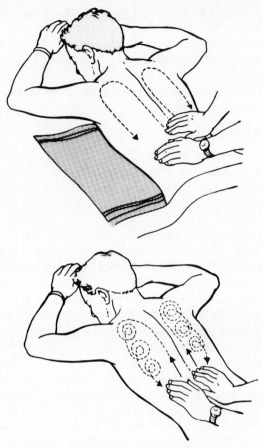

*Use a variety of massage strokes to give a soothing massage.*

doctor are called prescriptions. Those you buy without a doctor's order are called over-the-counter (OTC) medicines. When someone is sick, always get advice from a doctor about taking medicines. Tell the doctor about any allergies to medicines. For some illnesses, the best medicine is none at all!

Some drugs can be purchased in both name brands and generic brands. Generic drugs are the same medicines as brand name drugs, but generic drugs cost less. Brand name drugs carry the name of the manufacturer; generic drugs don't. Ask the doctor or pharmacist about them.

Administer medicines exactly on time and in the proper dosage. Pain-relief medications are usually given as needed, within a specified time interval. For example, the prescription might read: "Codeine, two tablets for pain, every four hours, as needed." When people don't take drugs as prescribed, they're less effective. Give the medicine, as prescribed, until the supply is gone. For example, an antibiotic drug to treat an infection may not completely destroy the bacteria for days, even weeks, after the patient is already feeling well.

Medicines, even OTC drugs, should be handled and taken as directed by the doctor, pharmacist, or product label.

- The recommended dosage should be followed and never increased—an overdose is often hazardous.
- Some drugs should be taken with meals so they don't irritate the stomach. For example, aspirins should be taken with food or a full glass of water.
- Some drugs should be taken without food. Food may interfere with the work of a drug. Certain antibiotics are better absorbed on an empty stomach.
- Some medicines interfere with each other or have a combining effect that isn't healthful. For example, aspirin and anticoagulants thin blood so taking both might cause hemorrhaging, or excessive bleeding.

Medicines have expiration dates that indicate when they are no longer effective. For safety, medicines should be discarded after the expiration date or when they're no longer needed, even if a few pills are left. Prescribed medicines should never be saved for another illness or given to another sick family member even if that person has the same symptoms. Used incorrectly, medicines can be ineffective, and even hazardous!

Medicines should be kept out of the reach of children and away from toxic substances.

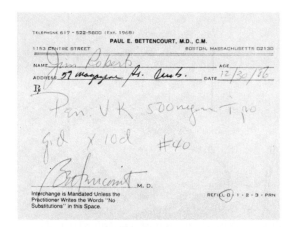

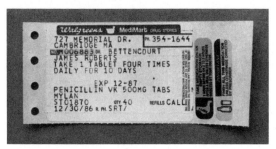

*A prescription for medication is written by a physician. A pharmacist fills the prescription for the medicine. It's the patient's responsiblity to follow the recommended dosage and directions.*

Read more about the safe handling of medicines in Chapter 5.

## Emotional Support

Emotional support is part of good home health care. Be considerate of a patient's emotions. Be an empathetic and understanding listener. Give the person time to talk. Don't take his or her anger, lack of interest, or other emotions personally. Provide things of interest to divert attention from emotional issues. Know that you can't solve all the person's problems, but do what you can to help.

Encourage the feeling of independence by giving the patient the chance to make his or her own choices, "Would you like to watch TV now?", or "Tell me when you're ready for a snack."

A good way to improve the emotional outlook of sick or injured people is to instill hope. Point out small improvements in health. Hope promotes emotional well-being which reduces anxiety. This, in turn, has a positive effect on the healing process.

## Home Services

Special services are available to help families and friends care for patients. These services include home-delivered meals, visiting nurses, and private duty nurses. Community home health care agencies can also provide transportation to the doctor, various types of therapy, blood tests, homemaking services, and other services.

### HOME-DELIVERED MEALS

Home-delivered meals may be important when caregivers can't be home all the time, perhaps because they work. Sick or injured people as well as the elderly and the physically or mentally impaired may not be able to cook for themselves.

Home-delivered meals are nutritionally balanced, ready to eat, and often served hot. Many services offer special diets.

The cost of home-delivered meals depends on the organization providing the service. Usually, the cost is based on the person's ability to pay.

### VISITING NURSES

Visiting nurses periodically visit patients in their homes, but they don't stay. They provide specific care or treatment, and then they leave. They help caregivers in the home with technical or specialized care such as blood pressure measurement, bandage changes, or injections of medicine. Visiting nurses can be arranged through private agencies or the public health department.

### PRIVATE DUTY NURSE

A private duty nurse may be the caregiver. He or she comes into a home and stays with the patient, providing all the care a patient needs. Private duty nurses may be scheduled just for the day, for the night, or around the clock. Having a trained nurse in the home gives the family a lot of freedom.

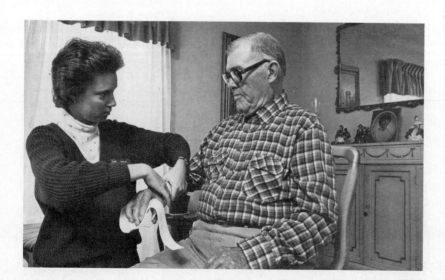

*Injured people can't always change their own bandages. They need the help of a skilled nurse.*

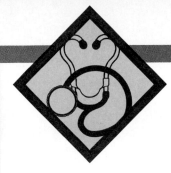

# CHAPTER CHECKUP

## Reviewing the Information

1. What are four advantages of home health care?
2. How can a caregiver support a patient's emotional needs?
3. What are the characteristics of a good caregiver?
4. Describe four guidelines that might help a caregiver efficiently manage the care of a patient at home.
5. Describe the features of a sick room.
6. What special equipment might be required for home health care?
7. Describe four sanitary practices that help prevent the spread of disease in the home.
8. How can you use your senses to detect signs and symptoms of health problems?
9. What are the vital signs, and what does each tell about the patient?
10. How do the different methods of taking body temperature vary?
11. Why is documentation important in home health care?
12. What should you report to a doctor?
13. Why is bathing an important part of health care?
14. How could you help relieve someone's pain?
15. What guidelines should be followed when taking medicines?
16. What outside services might be used to assist with home health care?

## Thinking It Over

1. What problems might a family face if someone is ill for a long time?
2. Consider your own home. What room would make the best sickroom, and how would it have to be changed?
3. What would you wear to care for a sick person?
4. What would you do if your eight-year-old sister's forehead seemed very hot?
5. Suppose the doctor called to find out if a family member was recovering from the flu. What should you be prepared to say?
6. What special care should you give an elderly person who can't get out of bed?
7. Describe a meal you might fix for someone on a soft diet.

## Taking Action

1. Price equipment for a sick room at a medical supply store. Figure the cost of setting up a sickroom, including a hospital bed, wheelchair, and bedpan, for one month.
2. Develop a typical day's schedule for taking care of a ten-year-old who has a broken leg.
3. Take your own and someone else's temperature, pulse rate, and breathing rate. Compare your findings as a class.
4. Prepare a soft meal at home.
5. Go to a drugstore and look at all of the OTC medicines. Make a list of ten of them, including price.

# 12 Managing Special Needs

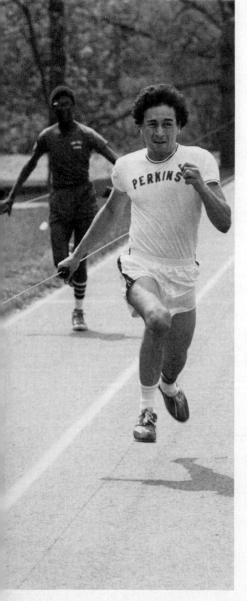

After reading this chapter, you should be able to:

• suggest ways that families and friends can provide emotional support for the impaired.

• identify major types of impairments.

• explain how a home might be altered for a physically impaired person.

• list community services for people with special needs.

## Terms to Understand

| | |
|---|---|
| amputation | mainstream |
| blind | mobility impaired |
| braille | rehabilitation |
| dyslexia | signing |
| learning disabilities | |

People with special needs are just that—special people who are physically, emotionally, or mentally impaired. You may know people with impairments. Perhaps they are blind, mentally retarded, or unable to walk, or perhaps they have trouble learning. All of these people require special, but different, support from family members, friends, and sometimes community organizations. The nature of the impairment determines what special care, support, and management are needed.

## Attitudes Toward Special Needs

People with special needs often live healthy, happy, and successful lives when they view their limitations as challenges to overcome. Family members and friends who show acceptance, love, and respect and who encourage independence help the impaired live a high-quality life.

## Public Attitudes

Today, many Americans with physical, mental, and emotional limitations lead productive lives. Positive attitudes about the abilities of these people have opened many opportunities for education, jobs, and recreation that previously had been closed. Their capabilities are recognized and rights respected and upheld in the world of work. In the community many accommodations have been made in buildings and transportation so that impaired people can be more independent. Schools are now much better equipped to handle impaired students.

Positive public attitudes are dramatically demonstrated in the sports world. In 1984, for the first time, disabled athletes were recognized in the Summer Olympic Games.

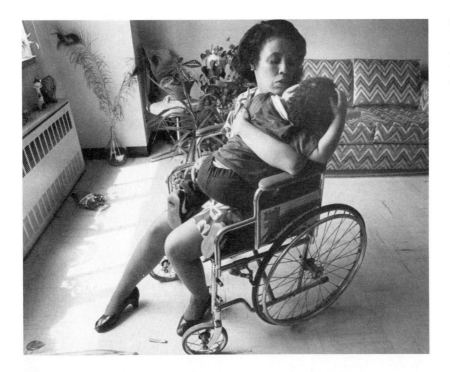

*With support at home, an impaired person can enjoy the pleasures of a happy, healthy, family life.*

Two official events were sanctioned—the women's 800-meter and a men's 1,500-meter wheelchair race!

## Family Attitudes and Support

Each family member plays an important part in helping an impaired person live a high-quality life. Together, they function as a healthy family unit. Families usually provide support in at least these ways:

- Establish a family environment that offers love, nurturing, patience, respect, support, and guidance.
- Communicate openly with the impaired person about his or her condition.
- Involve the impaired person in family activities and decisions.
- Encourage the impaired person to experience the realities of life without being overly protective.
- Encourage as much independence as possible.
- Encourage outside interests.
- Provide privacy within the home as an individual need.
- Accept occasional frustration, depression, and anger as normal.
- Reinforce each success, no matter how seemingly small.
- Help the person see his or her limitations as special challenges.

Parents with impaired children face enormous responsibilities. Child care methods may require major adjustments, such as constant supervision and the use of special equipment. Household schedules may include regular visits to therapists. Families can adjust well if they view these responsibilities with positive attitudes.

Having an impaired child in the family may be stressful. Parents who have trouble accepting the limitations of their child may be disappointed, bitter, resentful, even abusive. They may become frustrated, tired, and irritable with the added care. Parents may have difficulty bonding with an infant who cannot respond in normal ways. Or they might unfairly blame themselves for the impairment. Other children, who are competing for the attention of caregivers, may unjustly resent the time and money spent on an impaired brother or sister. Or they might feel embarrassed by some aspects of the impairment. These are real feelings that need to be overcome so the family unit can be healthy for everyone.

Support groups outside the family help parents, caregivers, brothers and sisters, and the impaired person accept the challenges of impairment. As you learned in Chapter 3, a support group is a group of people with similar concerns who join together to help one another. For example, Recovery, Inc. is a support group of former mental patients. Health professionals, day care providers, and babysitters provide support, too.

## Attitudes and Support of Friends

Social and emotional health depends on people outside the home. Like anyone else, people with impairments need friends. Friends offer support by showing respect, acceptance, and a willingness to help when needed. Friends also include the impaired person in normal activities of daily life.

People with impairments usually want to be viewed as part of a normal world and to make their own place in society. How might you support impaired family members or classmates?

- Be patient if they take longer to accomplish tasks.
- Give them opportunities to be with people who don't have impairments.
- Promote self-esteem by allowing them to be independent when possible.

- Be ready to assist when necessary. Ask what the impaired person would like you to do.
- Encourage them to do things they may be reluctant to do for fear of failure or because they're self-conscious.
- Reinforce their achievements and things they do well.
- Don't feel sorry for them. Be understanding and offer your encouragement instead.
- Don't make assumptions about their lives. Talk about everyday things. You'll probably have a lot in common.
- Talk to the person directly, not through a companion.
- Be natural. Don't be afraid of saying or doing the wrong things.

## Attitudes of the Impaired Individual

Positive attitudes about themselves help impaired people lead healthy, satisfying lives. An impairment is a challenge that people often overcome. They may even excel far beyond expectations because their personal determination is so great. For example, teenagers who have lost one leg have learned to be excellent skiers!

When impaired people understand their condition and potential, they often accept an impairment better. Successful people with similar impairments can serve as role models for them.

A supportive environment fosters positive attitudes. Impaired people usually feel a sense of self-worth when others recognize

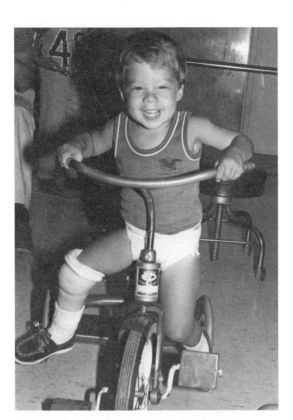

*Artificial arms, hands, and legs, made of lightweight aluminum and plastic, are fitted so well that people using them can lead active lives. Artificial limbs work almost like real ones by using transistors to power them.*

their family contributions and when they share household responsibilities, family decisions, and family activities. When others have high expectations of them, the impaired are more apt to have high expectations of themselves. Home surroundings also can be adjusted to help an impaired person feel success.

People with impairments can establish positive attitudes if they:

- accept limitations that can't be changed.
- develop strengths. Often intellectual pursuits become more interesting when someone is physically disabled.
- consider limitations as challenges, not roadblocks.
- avoid wallowing in self-pity.
- set realistic goals and work toward them without giving up too soon.
- expect other people to be curious without being overly-sensitive to their questions.
- accept help graciously.
- develop interests at school, at work, in people, and in leisure-time activities.
- join a support group to share common problems and solutions.
- find ways to make a unique contribution to others.

## Special Needs

A person with special needs may be physically, mentally, or emotionally impaired. Impairments may be permanent or temporary. They may be present at birth or result from an accident or disease at a later point in life. Each requires unique care.

## Mobility Impaired

People who are *mobility impaired* have difficulty moving part of their body normally. Mobility impairments have many causes.

- Some people are born with impairments, such as being born without part or all of a leg or arm.

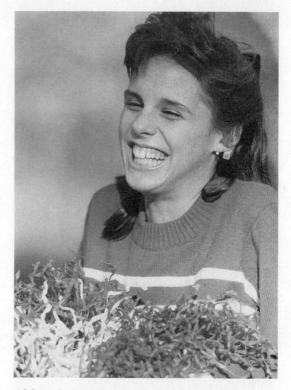

*Although deaf, this high school cheerleader shares an enthusiastic spirit with other students. She can sense the roar of the crowd by feeling the vibrations of sound.*

- Accidents may cause paralysis or amputation. *Amputation* is the surgical removal of an arm, leg, hand, or foot. Paralysis involves the loss of feeling in and the inability to move the affected part of the body.
- Arthritis is a crippling disease that causes pain in the joints. It may be so severe that movement is restricted. It usually affects older adults.
- A stroke may damage the brain and may leave a person partially or totally paralyzed.
- Cerebral palsy causes people to have less control of voluntary muscles due to abnormal brain development prior to birth

or brain damage before, during, or shortly after birth.

- Multiple sclerosis is a disease of the nervous system that causes paralysis or weakness of muscles.
- Muscular dystrophy is a gradual degeneration, or wasting and weakening, of the muscles which makes it hard to move and to maintain posture.
- A fracture, burn, incision, or bad sprain might be the cause of temporary immobility.

Families with a mobility impaired individual can encourage independence and self-esteem by allowing him or her to do things alone and not rushing to help all the time. For example, pushing the person's wheelchair may hurt the person's pride if he or she wants to live as a self-reliant individual.

Often mobility impaired people require more time to move about and to accomplish tasks than other people do. They may need more rest if they're physically weak. As a family member or friend, allow them time, and plan flexible schedules to meet their needs.

What should you do to support a person at home or in public who has a mobility impairment? Be considerate, patient, and knowledgeable about the limitations. Offer help when needed. Don't show visible curiosity. Don't stereotype or ridicule them. Respect facilities such as parking places and bus seats designated for the mobility impaired.

Many other things can be done to help a mobility impaired person have more freedom of movement and independence. The home can be altered and equipment acquired to accommodate the person's needs and provide comfort. Special equipment can be rented or bought to increase mobility both in and outside the home. Proper equipment and planning can help an impaired person do household tasks. Clothing can be

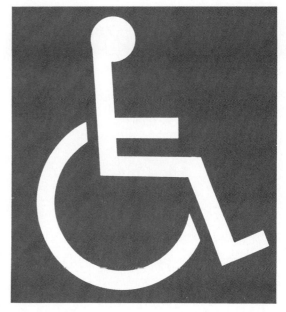

*Never park or sit in places where you see this international symbol. These places are provided to allow easy access for the physically impaired.*

chosen to make dressing a less frustrating task that can be accomplished alone.

## HOUSING ADJUSTMENTS AND EQUIPMENT

Physical barriers present challenges for mobility impaired people. When crutches, walkers, or wheelchairs are required, people with long-term immobilities may need to have their homes altered to allow freedom of movement and personal independence. The frustration of short-term immobility can be accommodated, in part, by minor adjustments. The chart on page **286** suggests more permanent household alterations for the mobility impaired.

Easy-to-use kitchens are convenient and well organized. A small, compact kitchen is appropriate for a person with limited mobility and energy. More space for movement is needed in a kitchen to accommodate a

## Housing Alterations for Mobility Impaired People

| Area | Alteration |
|---|---|
| Pathways | • Widened pathways to permit free movement with crutches or wheelchairs<br>• Nonskid floor finishes; no throw rugs<br>• Doorways widened for crutches and wheelchairs<br>• Ramps in addition to stairs<br>• Lowered light switches and electric outlets<br>• Elevators in multi-level housing |
| Kitchen | • Counters and other work surfaces low enough for someone who is sitting<br>• Continuous counters for sliding utensils<br>• Full-length, shallow storage for easy reach<br>• Pull-out shelves<br>• Turntables or pull-out bins in storage cabinets<br>• Storage near work spaces |
| Bathroom | • Raised bathtub and toilet for ease of transfer from a wheelchair<br>• Spacious bathroom with space for free movement with crutches, a walker, or a wheelchair<br>• Low dressing table with undercounter knee space for a wheelchair or chair<br>• Nonskid floors and bathtub surfaces<br>• Easy-to-reach storage |
| Living Room | • Nonskid floors<br>• Easy-to-open windows and doors<br>• Lowered electric outlets and light switches |

wheelchair, or perhaps, a walker. A walker is a piece of equipment that a person holds on to and moves as he or she walks; it gives support. A four-foot allowance between cabinets is needed for passage.

Countertops should allow a person to work without stooping or without raising the arm above elbow level. Lowered work surfaces and pull-out boards are more convenient for seated people and those in wheelchairs. For seated work, an under-the-counter opening is necessary for knee space. This opening should be 2½ feet wide and 2½ feet high for a wheelchair. A shallow sink (6 inches deep) with knee space underneath and a retractable spray hose is helpful for people who must sit to work at the sink. Pipes should be insulated so they don't burn the legs. For most people with a mobility impairment, the increased ease and use gained from these altered features is worth the cost.

Equipment and supplies need to be stored within easy reach. Magnetic racks, pegboards, open shelves, turntables, pull-out baskets, and roll-out drawers provide easy access and storage. Dishes stacked vertically are easier to pick up. Experts recommend these storage places in a kitchen designed for the mobility impaired:
• tableware—left of sink
• serving dishes—near cooktop
• coffee/coffee pot—near sink
• dishwashing supplies—near sink
• cookware—near range top

Many companies make appliances that are convenient for mobility impaired people. A side-by-side refrigerator-freezer enables someone in a wheelchair to reach frozen foods. Controls for appliances, such as dishwashers and ranges, placed on the front, allow easy reach for persons in a wheelchair. Touch-control panels are easier than dials for people with limited use of their hands. And range burners placed in a single row, rather than front and back, allow people to

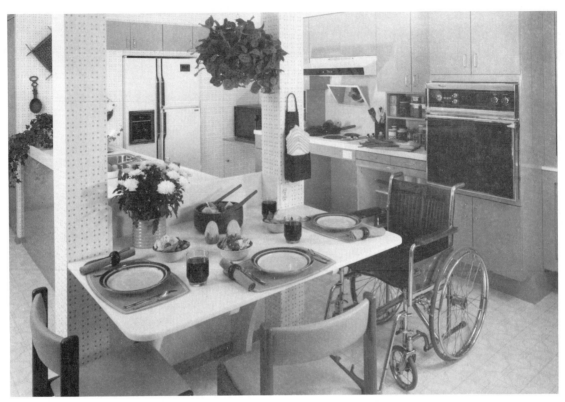

*This living space has been specially designed for someone in a wheelchair. Can you identify the adjustments?*

cook without having to reach over hot burners.

Appliances can be installed for easy access. Electric outlets and switches which are placed low on the front of cabinets enable a seated person to reach them. Wall ovens and countertop burners can be installed at a lower height.

Bathrooms also can be modified for the mobility impaired. A three-foot-wide door and spacious bathroom floor plan enables a wheelchair or person with crutches or a walker to get through easily and to have freedom of movement. Low electric plugs and light switches are easy to reach from a sitting position. Towels and other bathroom items may be stored on low, open shelves for easy reach. Grab bars by the toilet and a non-slip floor make the bathroom safe.

Bathroom fixtures may need adjusting. Toilet seats may be raised by adding a removable elevated seat. For mobility impaired, as well as elderly people, a shower is often easier to use than a tub. In the bathtub or shower, seats, grab bars, and non-skid mats provide safety. A faucet with one handle is easier to use. For people who use a wheelchair or sit for grooming, lowered counters with knee space are essential.

Besides equipping the kitchen and bathroom, a home can be more convenient and accessible to mobility impaired people by choosing furniture, phones, and other equipment selectively. The chart on page **288** offers a partial list.

## Household Equipment for Mobility Impaired People

| Equipment | Characteristic |
|---|---|
| Furniture | • Seats higher than standard<br>• Firm cushions<br>• Arms for support<br>• Furniture arranged to free traffic paths<br>• Remote control for television |
| Kitchen Equipment | • Rolling chair to fit under work space<br>• Holding devices such as pegged boards and bowl holders in easy reach<br>• Lowered range with controls on the front<br>• Side-by-side refrigerator-freezer<br>• Salad spinner, rocker-blade knife, and jar with chopping blades for someone with the use of one hand<br>• Cutting board with two projecting rustproof nails to hold vegetables and fruit in place for someone with the use of one hand while cutting or peeling<br>• Front-opening dishwasher for easy loading and unloading<br>• All-in-one knife, fork, and spoon for someone with the use of one hand<br>• Lightweight, nonbreakable dinnerware |
| Bathroom Equipment | • Seats in the bathtub and shower<br>• Shower nozzles on hoses<br>• Grab bars beside the toilet and the tub |
| Other Equipment | • Intercom to talk with people in other parts of the house<br>• Remote phone to carry<br>• Chairs that lift up and tilt forward so arthritic or stroke victims can get up and down easily<br>• Lifts or chairs that go up and down stairs electrically<br>• Wooden tray across the handles of a wheelchair for doing tasks and carrying things<br>• Long-handled tongs to increase reach<br>• Suction cups to hold bowls, cutting boards, and other equipment in place for someone who can use only one hand<br>• Ramp instead of stairs |

## HOUSEHOLD TASKS

Many mobility impaired people can do a variety of household tasks successfully if the work space is well organized and the proper equipment is available. When an impaired person prepares to do a task, it is important he or she studies the job first. The steps and the needed equipment must be considered. Then a plan can be devised to do the work with the most ease. These are some steps an impaired person can follow:

• Arrange work areas for each job with all equipment for the task in easy reaching distance, particularly if a person must remain seated.
• Be sure the work area is adjusted to the proper height. For example, if the person is in a wheelchair, the work area should comfortably accommodate someone in a sitting position.
• Select the right tool for the job to make work more efficient.

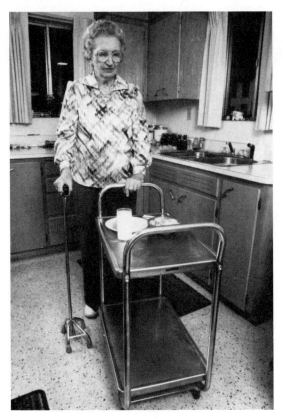

*This older woman considers a tea cart an essential tool for meal preparation. It saves her many steps and allows her to keep her hands free for handling her cane. What suggestions could you offer to make real preparation easier for a physically impaired person?*

- Choose equipment for multiple uses.
- Use the body efficiently. For example, a jar can be held between the knees to open it with one hand.

Consider adding special equipment to make work easier. The chart on page **288** lists many devices for the mobility impaired.

## CLOTHING

Being able to dress oneself is important to a person's feelings of self-worth and inde-pendence. Clothing can be selected to make independent dressing easier for people with limited body movement. There are easy-on, easy-off garments with large openings and fasteners that are easy to close. Fasteners may be magnetic, large buttons, or velcro. Velcro is attached to two pieces of fabric so they stick together firmly.

Some garment styles are easier to put on and wear than others:
- capes instead of coats
- dresses without waistbands
- lined skirts that don't require slips
- pull-on slacks that have an elastic waistband
- slip-on shoes or shoes with velcro fasteners
- sleep shirts or nightgowns instead of pajamas
- clothes with front closings instead of back closings
- non-bulky clothing

For someone who wears leg braces, slacks or pants with full-length side zippers may be better than regular pants.

Special attention must be given to select-ing safe clothing. Skirts or pants that are too long, sleeves that are too full, and dan-gling ties may cause accidents.

## TRANSPORTATION DEVICES

New transportation devices provide inde-pendence and improve the quality of life for the mobility impaired. Electric wheelchairs, computer-controlled chairs, electric lifts, and specially operated cars and vans in-crease mobility. Wheelchairs now can be propelled by a person who is paralyzed from the shoulders down. The chair is activated by a control on the headrest. You may have seen a bus, taxi, or van with a wheelchair lift and a ramp. Controls inside a van or car may be hand-operated so a person with no legs, artificial legs, or paralyzed legs can drive.

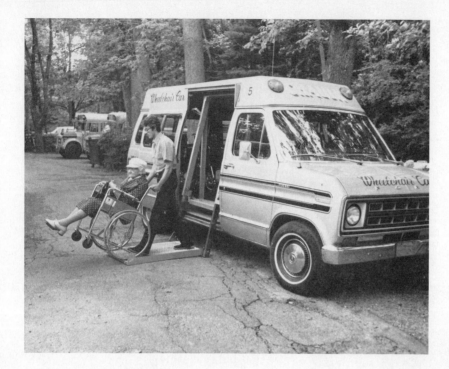

*A bus or van with an elevator lift provides easy access to public transportation for someone in a wheelchair.*

## Visually Impaired

Visually impaired people have trouble seeing. However, they may not necessarily be blind. Many people don't have perfect vision, but eyeglasses or contact lenses correct their sight. The sight of a visually impaired person cannot be corrected with glasses. The person who is partially-sighted has limited vision. Someone who is *blind* has such limited sight that he or she cannot depend on sight for movement and learning.

Imagine the challenge of learning without being able to see. Your eyes probably have helped you learn 80 percent of all you know. People with visual impairment have many difficulties to overcome as they learn. They can't read with their eyes, watch television, or learn by watching the world around them. People born blind need help in learning about colors, forms, and shapes they will

never see. On the other hand, people who lose vision as teenagers or adults already know what most things look like so they adjust more easily. They still need help in adapting to their surroundings and in coping with everyday life, however.

Visual impairment also affects emotional and social health. If people feel they lack control of themselves and their environment, as some visually impaired people do, they may have a poor self-concept. Often visually impaired people feel uncomfortable with unfamiliar people and places. Because they can't see, they can't make eye contact with normally-sighted individuals. Eye contact is an important tool of communication. It allows you to see how the person to whom you are talking is responding to you. Both the visually impaired person and the person with whom he or she is communicating need special sensitivity and perhaps the sense of touch to communicate.

The visually impaired can adapt well and live healthy and enriching lives. Blind people can read by learning to use braille. *Braille* is a system of reading and writing with raised points on paper that the person can feel. Partially-sighted readers can use large print books and magazines. Records, tapes, and people who volunteer as readers are also helpful.

In their homes, visually impaired people need consistent order. Furniture, household items, and personal belongings should be in the same place all the time to prevent frustrations in daily living. Clothing must be carefully organized and perhaps marked with a code that can be felt. Then visually impaired people can dress independently in garments that match. Medicines and household chemicals need special marking and storage so they aren't mixed up and mishandled.

The kitchen can be adapted so a blind person can prepare meals. Braille controls can be placed on ranges and other equipment. Cookware, utensils, food, and dishes must always be put away in the same location. The visually impaired can be somewhat independent outside their homes, too. A specially trained seeing-eye dog or a cane helps guide them.

Parents and other caregivers need to identify visual problems early in a child's life. Then treatment or special training can be obtained before poor sight or lack of sight severely limits educational, emotional, social, and physical development.

## Health Impaired

People who are health impaired have a chronic condition that limits their activities. The condition may be arthritis, heart disease, diabetes, or asthma, among others.

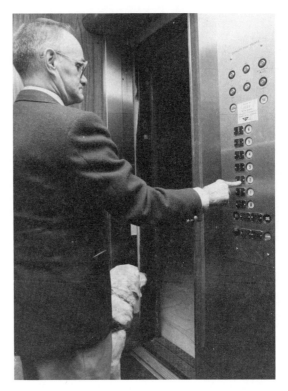

*In many public places, information is written in braille so blind people can be independent.*

People with chronic conditions need to keep their bodies functioning as normally as possible. But their condition may cause limited strength and energy, frequent absence from school or work, and slow achievement in learning or personal tasks.

Family members, other caregivers, and friends can provide positive support when they understand the health condition. Many household tasks can be adapted so people conserve physical energy. For example, lightweight equipment requires less physical strength. Equipment, such as garbage cans with wheels use less energy than lifting and carrying. A well-organized home with few belongings requires less energy to clean. A home without steps is less demanding. Many appliances, such as a microwave oven, electric can opener, and electric garage door opener help conserve physical energy.

Health impaired people may also need help with medical treatment. To learn more about chronic diseases and how to manage illness within a home, refer to Chapters 7 and 11.

## Hearing Impaired

People who are hearing impaired are partially or completely deaf. Partially deaf people may hear certain sounds, but they may not be able to distinguish words. Completely deaf people cannot hear any words, but they may feel the vibrations some sounds make through their sense of touch. For instance, they may touch a stereo speaker and feel the vibrations the music makes. This allows them to experience and enjoy music.

Hearing loss has many causes. Sometimes it's present at birth. Or diseases, such as measles, mumps, and certain viral infections, may be the cause. Physical damage to the ear, high fevers, and loud noises may cause loss of hearing, also.

Hearing impaired people communicate in many ways. They might use sign language, read lips, and write their messages. Sign language, or *signing,* is talking with hand and finger movements. Partially deaf people may supplement limited hearing with lip reading. Speaking is difficult if a person has never heard the sounds of words and cannot hear his or her own speech. Some deaf and partially deaf people may be able to talk, particularly if they lost their hearing after they had learned to speak. Their voices may be loud or very soft, however, because they can't perceive the volume.

Hearing impaired people may face some social and learning problems. They may

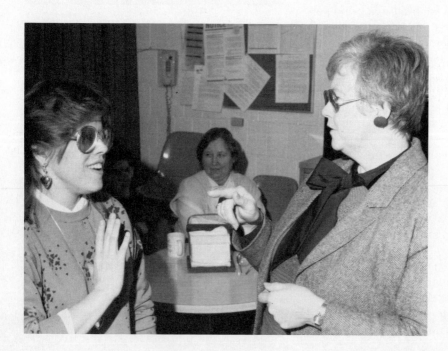

*By signing, deaf people can share lively conversations with others who are deaf or who have normal hearing.*

have difficulty following oral instructions and directions. They may be happier working one-to-one than in groups where communication is widespread and ongoing. They may be reluctant to join groups and establish friendships because it's difficult to communicate.

Many people who are partially deaf have strong visual ability. When one sense is diminished, other senses often become more acute. They may compensate for their disability so thoroughly by lip reading and mastering speech that others aren't aware of a hearing loss. Hearing aids provide help for many hearing problems. Surgery, too, may restore some forms of hearing loss.

Some devices, such as flashing-light systems for doorbells, kitchen timers, and smoke alarms, allow hearing impaired people to function better within the home. Phones also can have built-in amplifiers for those with partial hearing. And a special phone attached to a computer allows people to type messages back and forth to each other.

Sensitive and patient family members and friends can reduce frustrations for the hearing impaired:

- Be aware that they can't hear background noises.
- Know that hearing aids have a limited range of pick-up.
- Learn sign language.
- Face the person when you're speaking.
- Speak loudly if the person is only partially deaf, but not too loud for the hearing aid.
- Take time to be a good listener.

## Speech Impaired

Some people have difficulty speaking clearly and succinctly. This causes others to have trouble understanding them. This problem is called a speech impairment.

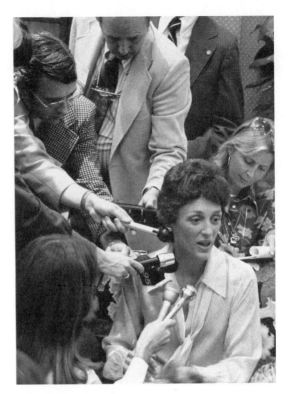

*Joan Mondale overcame her stuttering problem to give speeches and television interviews in support of her husband Walter Mondale's campaign for the 1984 U.S. presidency.*

Many speech problems, such as stuttering and lisps, among children can be corrected with speech therapy. Stroke victims with partial or total speech loss sometimes can be rehabilitated. *Rehabilitation* means restoration back to a normal condition. Hearing impaired people often have speech problems, too, because they can't even hear to monitor their speech. They need special training, but even completely deaf people can learn to talk.

Other impairments can't be corrected by therapy. Cleft palate is a severe impairment that affects speech. This is a condition in which the roof of the mouth, or palate, did not form properly during fetal development, leaving a gap in the palate that often can be corrected surgically. There may still be some speech impairment requiring therapy.

Speech impairment makes communication more difficult. Family and friends must be patient and listen carefully. They might rephrase the person's words to be sure they're understood.

People, especially children, with speech impairments may become shy and withdrawn. They may be embarrassed to talk in class, with peers, or with strangers. Thus their social development and self-concept may suffer. For these reasons, speech therapy or surgery to correct the problem early in life is important to their emotional and social well-being.

## Mentally Impaired

People who are mentally impaired have a lower intellectual capacity than normal. This may be a mild or a severe deficiency. Intelligence is often measured by a test. The score is called the intelligence quotient (I.Q.). You've probably taken this type of test at school. A score of 90 to 110 is considered average, or normal. Seventy or less is considered mentally retarded.

People may be born mentally impaired or retarded. It can also be caused by a severe injury to the head or by certain diseases.

Retardation affects behavior and the ability to learn. Mentally impaired people respond and learn more slowly than others do. They may have impulsive, immature behavior and often have a short memory and poor coordination.

Mildly retarded people often can work at some skilled and unskilled jobs. Schools provide special programs for educating them. Severely retarded people lack self-help skills and often have problems with social adjust-

ment. The degree of impairment determines if they can live independently or if they require complete protective care.

Raising a mentally impaired child is a special challenge. It's often hard for the family to see the child progress slowly while others develop normally. Mentally impaired people make their own unique contributions to family life, however. They often are affectionate, loyal, and responsive when they're shown love and respect.

If you know people who are mentally impaired, focus on their strengths. Praise them for the things they do well. Include them in group activities. Be patient with their efforts to contribute and learn. Mildly retarded students may be mainstreamed in your classes. *Mainstream* means being included with normal individuals. Look for ways these students contribute to your classroom experiences.

## Emotionally Disturbed

Emotionally disturbed people see the world in a distorted, confused way for prolonged periods of time. They may lack ability to get along with others. They may be unproductive yet quite intelligent. Their behavior may be inappropriate. They may have limited skills in handling stress. Often they have a negative self-image. They may be abusive or hostile at times. Emotional problems affect their jobs, their families and friends, and their personal happiness.

Emotionally disturbed children may be withdrawn, show destructive and aggressive behavior, show anxiety, and act in a self-destructive way. Emotional illness hinders a child's development.

Severe stress can cause emotional disturbances. Emotional problems can also have physical causes. Sometimes body chemicals are out of balance, and people are treated with medication.

Professional help is necessary for people with severe emotional problems. The caring family seeks such help when signs of emotional disturbance appear. The family physician can recommend appropriate health professionals to offer needed help. In addition, family and friends can offer patient, understanding support and follow the recommendations of the health professional. Many emotionally disturbed people recover.

## Learning Disabled

*Learning disabilities* are disorders that cause a person to have difficulty reading, speaking, listening, thinking, writing, or all of these. Learning disabled people may have difficulty following directions. Some may have short attention spans, impulsive behavior, and social problems. Some may be awkward, listless, and easily distracted. Some learning disabled people have dyslexia. *Dyslexia* causes people to reverse letters and numbers in their mind when they read and write.

Learning disabled people usually have normal or above average intelligence. In fact, many brilliant people, such as Thomas Edison and Albert Einstein, were learning disabled.

Special teachers work with learning disabled children. They assess their abilities and recommend educational experiences which may help overcome the problems.

Having a learning disability is frustrating for students who see their friends progressing faster or more easily than they do. Low self-esteem is common when students have trouble competing with others. As a family member or a friend, you can help. Praise the accomplishments of someone with a learning problem. Tutor him or her in schoolwork you understand. Be patient and accepting.

*Children with learning disabilities often need special tutoring at home from a parent, a brother, or a sister.*

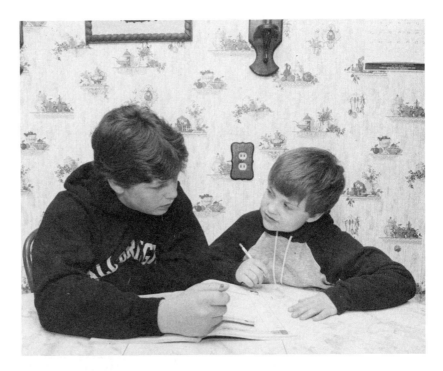

# Assistance for the Impaired

Support within the family and from outside sources helps the impaired live healthy, happy, useful lives. Support is much more than medical assistance. People must also learn how to live with an impairment. They may need educational assistance and emotional support from others with similar problems.

The Decade of Disabled Persons from 1983–1992 has brought public attention to impaired people. The decade was organized by the United Nations, and President Reagan highlighted it with a White House Ceremony in 1984. This observance is designed to make people more aware of the unique needs that impaired people have and to encourage new services and research on their behalf.

## Support Organizations and Services

Many national and international associations offer assistance and support to the impaired and their families. Each organization has specific objectives for different groups of people. Some private, nonprofit associations are:

- The Arthritis Foundation
- Association for Retarded Citizens
- Braille Institute of America
- Epilepsy Foundation
- March of Dimes Birth Defects Foundation
- The Multiple Sclerosis National Society
- Muscular Dystrophy Association
- National Society for Crippled Children and Adults

Government agencies to help the impaired include:

- President's Committee on Employment of the Handicapped
- Social Security Administration
- U.S. Bureau of Family Services
- U.S. Children's Bureau

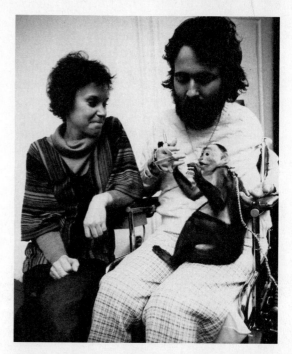

In a new program, **Helping Hands: Simian Aides for the Disabled**, simian monkeys are being trained to help quadriplegics become self-reliant and more independent. A quadriplegic can't use his or her arms or legs. The monkey can open and close doors, turn lights off and on, turn book pages, change tapes in a recorder, and even bring snacks from the refrigerator!

- U.S. Vocational Rehabilitation Administration

Services from both private and governmental groups include:

- financial aid for medical treatment, education, personal services, research, and job training
- specially equipped schools with specially trained teachers
- vocational and job training
- assistance in finding jobs
- aides who provide assistance with physical care and daily activities
- special services, such as braille and "talking" books

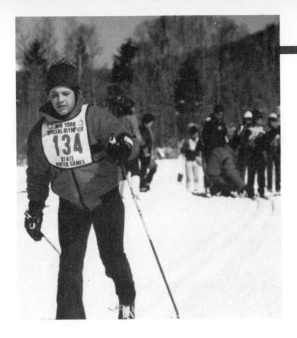

# THE SPECIAL OLYMPICS

"**I** can never forget the crippled boy who ran his race on crutches, or the blind boy who followed the voices of his coach down the track, or the little girl who stopped just before the finish line to wait for a friend, or the young man who loved running so much that he didn't stop at the finish line but tried to run another lap around the track." These are the words of Eunice Shriver Kennedy as she described her feelings while watching competition in the Special Olympics events.

Special Olympics are organized competitive events for mentally retarded children, youth, and adults. This program was organized in 1968 by the John F. Kennedy Foundation. Anyone who is eight years of age or older and has an I.Q. of 75 or below can participate. These special athletes compete in 16 sports, including the one-mile run, the 400-yard dash, the standing long jump, and the running high jump. The softball throw, volleyball, and swimming are also popular competitions.

Special Olympics events are held locally and statewide as preparation for international competition. By 1985 all 50 states and 15 other countries were involved. Today over one million athletes participate.

The events were originally sponsored by The Kennedy Foundation. But now many large corporations also subsidize the events. Famous coaches, prominent athletes, and many average citizens volunteer their time to prepare mentally retarded citizens for competition.

The Special Olympics motto, "Let me win, but if I cannot win, let me be brave in the attempt," illustrates the philosophy of the program. Participants are trained to win, but even the losers are rewarded. Every participant receives medals and ribbons.

The athletes win in other ways, too. Experts believe that the attention span of the mentally retarded is extremely short. However, when Special Olympics' athletes are motivated and interested in an activity, they often function at a very high level. In practice, coaches find that these athletes have a great deal of patience and ability to stay with a task.

Coaches teach competitors to win graciously and to lose gracefully, to play the game hard, to be loyal to teammates, to respect all people, and to be considerate of those with less ability. That makes everyone a winner!

- health clinics and other health services.
- support groups for the impaired and their families
- rehabilitative services
- general education for the public on the causes, prevention, and management of health conditions

## Legal Support

The rights of impaired people are assured by federal law. The Rehabilitation Act of 1973 prohibits discrimination against them and funds programs and research that offer benefits. In addition, public laws provide for appropriate education and assure access to vocational training.

## School Programs

Both public and private schools are committed to children with special needs. They screen children as part of a normal routine to detect vision, hearing, speech, learning, and physical problems early. If the evaluation shows an impairment, a child might be referred to a special education program. The program would provide education in the least restrictive environment for learning. Often they are mainstreamed in the regular classroom. And perhaps they receive remedial instruction as well.

Some impaired students can't attend regular schools, however. They may be taught at home by visiting teachers, or go to special schools, such as those for the deaf, the blind, or mentally retarded. Others who are severely impaired may live in institutions that provide educational experiences.

If you have classmates with impairments, be aware that they are unique individuals as you are. Like other students, they make valuable contributions to your school.

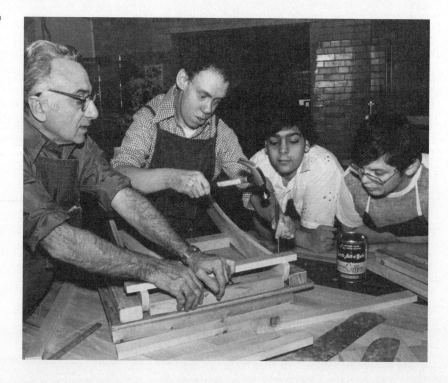

*Sheltered workshops provide job opportunities for mentally retarded people. Many businesses have their products assembled at these worksites.*

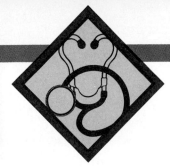

# CHAPTER CHECKUP

## Reviewing the Information

1. What are five ways the family can support an impaired family member?
2. What are five general ways an impaired person might cope with his or her own limitations?
3. Describe four conditions that might cause a person to be mobility impaired.
4. How could you alter a kitchen for someone in a wheelchair?
5. What bathroom features might be important for a person with a mobility impairment?
6. How could a mobility impaired person organize work space effectively?
7. Describe how a blind person could read a book.
8. What conditions might a health impaired person have?
9. What might cause hearing loss?
10. Describe ways a hearing impaired person can communicate with others.
11. How can impaired speech cause one's social development to suffer?
12. What are common characteristics of a mentally retarded person?
13. What does it mean to be learning disabled?
14. What are three organizations that offer support for people with special needs?
15. What are five ways organizations support people with special needs?
16. What is the Special Olympics?

## Thinking It Over

1. How might you feel if your sister lost both arms in an accident?
2. How might you help a blind friend?
3. How might you communicate with a deaf person?
4. What is the difference between being mentally retarded and emotionally disturbed?
5. How might you alter your house if a member of your family had to use crutches for a while?
6. Who would you contact to find a job for someone who was mentally retarded?
7. How does the law help protect people with impairments?

## Taking Action

1. Write a letter to an imaginary friend who is paralyzed. Ask him or her to join you for a recreational activity in which both of you could participate.
2. On paper, design your living room, kitchen, and bathroom for a blind person. Place furniture carefully.
3. Check out a book in braille at the library and feel the sensation of reading with your fingers.
4. Interview a school counselor to identify ways your school accommodates the special needs of impaired students.
5. Find out about jobs in your community for impaired people. Contact a vocational counselor or community agencies. Write a report for class.

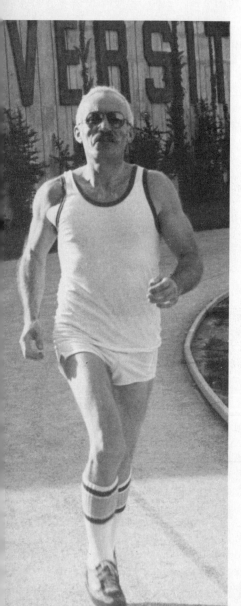

# 13 The Aging

After reading this chapter, you should be able to:

- describe the aging population.

- explain physical, social, and mental changes associated with aging.

- describe ways to meet the needs of senior citizens.

- identify common health concerns of senior citizens.

- name community resources supporting senior citizens.

## Terms to Understand

| | |
|---|---|
| disengagement | insomnia |
| extended family | senior citizen |
| fixed income | social security |
| funeral | widow |
| gerontologist | widower |

Today there are about 23 million older adults in the United States. That's about 11 percent of the total population. By the year 2030, when you will be middleaged, the elderly population is expected to reach 17 percent of the total population of our country. People live longer, often healthier, lives today because of better health care.

What is an older adult like? Many are very healthy, while the health of others has deteriorated. Older adults are people like Mr. and Mrs. Wilson, Mr. Sanchez, and Mrs. Wong.

- The Wilsons are about 70 years of age. They retired and moved near their daughter. They are active in community and volunteer work.
- Mr. Sanchez lives on his family farm. At the age of 83, he still gardens a one-acre vegetable plot.
- Mrs. Wong is 75. She lives in a nursing home. She has lost much of her memory and no longer can recognize her son.

A person who reaches the age of 65 is often referred to as a *senior citizen*. More senior citizens are women than are men. There are about three women over age 65 for every two men. Approximately half of the women are widows. A *widow* is a woman whose husband has died. Less than one-fourth of the men are widowers. A *widower* is a man whose spouse has died. Spouse is a term which can mean either husband or wife.

The senior years can span several decades, so there can be big differences between people who are 65 and those who are 95.

To help distinguish between those who have just entered their senior years from those who are much older, the terms "early retiree" and "later retiree" often are used. Early retirees are generally active, healthy, and capable of caring for themselves. On the other hand, almost half of the people in late retirement have some physical limitations.

Many older adults are vital and healthy. They look and feel far younger than their years. People might say, "She's a young 75"

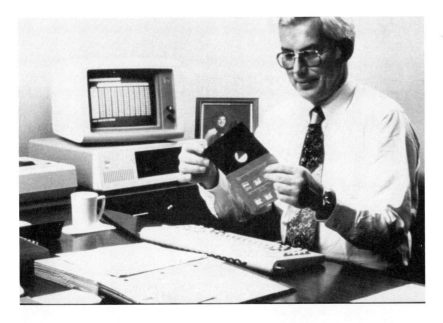

*Today more people than ever are living healthy lives after age 65. Many continue to take on new challenges.*

or "They're not old; they're just recycled teenagers!" Others who have lost their health may be immobile, confined, and lonely.

The physical, mental, and social health of an older adult affects his or her personal characteristics and lifestyles. Chronological age doesn't.

## The Aging Process

Aging is a normal part of living. People begin to age the moment they're born, and the process continues until they die. Each person can slow the aging process by following good habits of eating, exercise, and rest throughout life. But no one can prevent aging.

Three major changes are associated with the last phase of the aging process—the senior years. Most physical changes are easy to identify. Even into their senior years, people can slow the physical changes which come with age by taking care of themselves. Aging also brings dramatic social changes as a person's roles and responsibilities within the family and community change. For some seniors, these changes, in turn, bring about emotional changes.

## Physical Changes

Many early retirees feel very fit. Without the pressures of work, they feel more relaxed, and they have more time for activities such as walking, tennis, or golf. But eventually the physical signs of aging appear for all people.

A teenager once asked an elderly person, "What does it feel like to be your age?" The older woman laughed and said, "It's like having pebbles in your shoes, petroleum jelly on your glasses, cotton in your ears, a clothespin on your nose, rubber gloves on your fingers, then drinking six glasses of water and going downtown with all those

annoyances! Your body just doesn't work as it did when you were young. But people can learn to adjust!"

Your body will be at its physical peak when you're about 25 years old. After that, it slowly begins to deteriorate. By the time people reach their senior years, they usually aren't as strong physically. Their senses may be less acute. Their body responses are slower. They may have aches and pains. They often cannot endure long periods of strenuous physical activity.

Deteriorating eyesight, hearing, taste, smell, and touch make some elderly people less aware of the world around them. People who don't see as well don't notice as many things that are happening around them. Perhaps they lose the pleasures of reading and watching television. Some may have more trouble hearing conversations, doorbells, phones, community warning signals, and possible intruders. Their decreased sense of smell may prevent them from noticing smoke or gas leaks, or keep them from enjoying the appealing aromas of food, such as that of a freshly-baked apple pie. Interest in eating may be lessened further by a reduced sense of taste. On the average, young people have about 9000 tastebuds, while elderly people have only about 2700. Older people often become more aware of the stronger tastes—bitter and sour.

Some people put on weight as they grow older. Partly that's because they're less active, but their basal metabolic rate has gone down, too—two percent for every decade of adult life. Basal metabolic rate is the speed at which the body uses calories. Excess weight is a problem for many older people.

Older people commonly lose physical strength. Muscle mass decreases and is replaced by body fat. This might lead to another problem—hidden obesity. Muscle weighs more than body fat so a shift in body

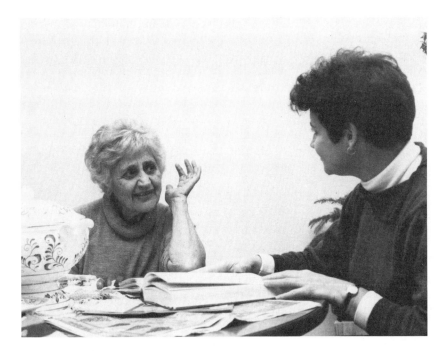

*With age, many people have a decreased sense of hearing. But they still enjoy being part of conversations.*

composition may not result in a significant change in body weight. Obesity may not be recognized by stepping on a scale.

When elderly people are sick or injured, their bodies don't heal as rapidly as your body likely does. Their bodies may have a harder time fighting infections. Injuries often occur easily; a slight fall or blow that wouldn't hurt you may seriously injure an elderly person.

Body organs and systems change. For example:

- Some older people develop digestive problems. Their stomachs get upset more easily, and they may have trouble with constipation.
- The heart must work harder to do its job if the older adult has hardened arteries or high blood pressure.
- Poor blood circulation may cause them to feel the cold much more than younger people do. An older person may feel chilly in a room you feel quite comfortable in.
- Joints tend to stiffen which may cause some pain and difficulty in movement.
- Reflexes usually become slower. If an older person is driving and an animal darts out in front of the car, it may take longer for an older person to react and hit the brakes than it would take a teenager.

## Social Changes

Almost all senior citizens experience changes in their roles, responsibilities, and relationships.

Becoming a grandparent, or even a great-grandparent, may be a new role for a senior citizen. Distance may keep ties between grandparents and grandchildren from being strong. In many families, however, grandparents live close enough to serve as baby-sitters and friends to their grandchildren.

The grandparent role is described as one of the most enjoyable in life. The husband-wife relationship may bring new pleasures with retirement. Couples may have time to do more things together and to enjoy one another more. New friendships form when retirees volunteer, join new groups for leisure activities, or travel.

More stressful role changes are caused by death or serious illness. When a spouse dies, a person must learn to function as a single person. Serious illness may change a senior citizen from a caregiver into a patient.

Successful adjustment to role changes involves accepting new responsibilities, becoming involved in new activities, and creating new relationships. For example, the new retiree substitutes meaningful activities, such as hobbies or travel, for work. People who move into their childrens' homes must learn to be a family participant rather than the family manager. People whose spouses have died find satisfaction with new friendships and perhaps remarriage. Likewise, people with physical limitations continue to live happily if they learn to compensate for lost abilities and skills.

## Mental Changes

Mental change is also part of the aging process. Signs of mental change include disengagement, lack of mental alertness, and a decrease in intellectual abilities.

When older people cease to be interested in people and activities, they are experiencing *disengagement*. They may show no interest in talking or activities. Some specialists believe disengagement is a normal part of the aging process. Others believe it results from feeling unwanted or unneeded. You can help senior citizens avoid disengagement by including them in your

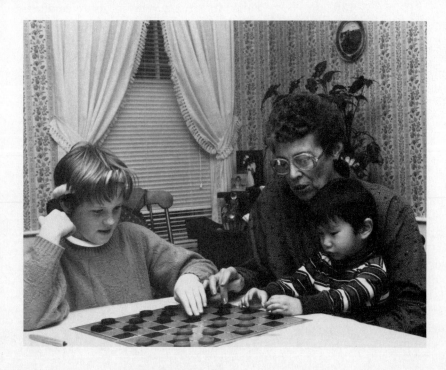

*Many older people find great satisfaction in spending time with their grandchildren.*

activities and conversations and by asking their opinions.

With aging, there may come a lack of mental alertness. For example, some older people may not be aware of danger signals that seem automatic to you. They may drive their car out in front of other cars or step onto an icy walk, not sensing the danger. When they get hurt, you may say they are "accident-prone."

Sometimes senior citizens may seem preoccupied and may not notice when others enter a room. They may not really be preoccupied at all. Instead failing eyesight or hearing may prevent them from noticing. Perhaps other older people focus their attention on a frustration that appears minor to someone your age, such as emptying the wastebasket in a room.

Many elderly people have a clear memory of the distant past but have difficulty remembering recent events. For example, they can't remember a doctor's appointment for tomorrow, but they can vividly remember their sixth birthday. They may develop habits to compensate for poor short-term memory, such as writing important dates on a calendar.

While some senior citizens lose their perception, memory, and their ability to learn, others stay "sharp as a tack." Many older adults continue to learn, particularly if they spent time studying and learning earlier in life. In fact, colleges today enroll many older adults.

## Personal Needs of the Aged

Many of a senior citizen's personal needs are like your own. Other needs are unique to their stage of life. Aging people need love and companionship, personal goals to work toward, healthful living habits, adequate income, appropriate housing, transportation, and the ability to accept death. Some senior

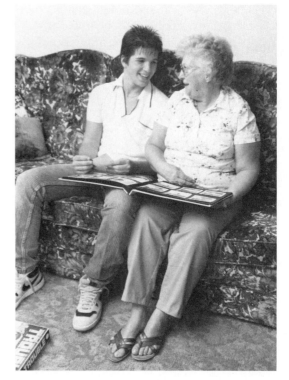

*Many older people enjoy sharing stories of their own childhood with their grandchildren. What stories of the past have you learned from an older person?*

citizens also need some form of alternative care.

## Love and Companionship

Age doesn't change a person's need for love and companionship. Yet many aging people are lonely. Living a great distance from family members contributes to loneliness and so does the death of a spouse and friends.

Older people often have more time to spend with their children and grandchildren. This offers a lot of companionship and can be a rewarding experience for everyone.

Have you seen wedding pictures where the bride and groom were senior citizens? Today remarriage among senior citizens is increasing because it provides affection and companionship. Men who remarry often live longer. In fact, for middle-aged men ages 55 to 64, research shows that the death rate is only half as high for those who remarry as for those who don't.

There are also a variety of senior citizens' organizations that provide opportunities for companionship. For example, almost every town in the United States has an organization of The American Association of Retired People (AARP). Monthly meetings and various activities offer social opportunities.

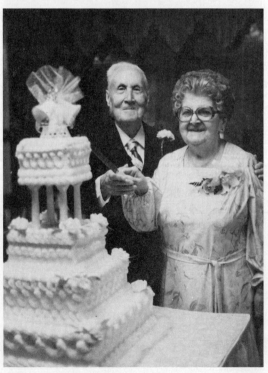

*Senior citizens often remarry to have love and companionship in their later years.*

Pets also can be great sources of affection and companionship if senior citizens are physically and financially able to care for them. Caring for a pet gives a sense of being needed and someone to talk to. People can give their affection to the pet, and the pet often returns that affection.

Some aging people complain about their relationships. They say that their families have no time for them. Or they may say that their friends are uninteresting. They may say young people don't give them respect. There are ways, however, for older people to enjoy the companionship of others and even to find new sources of friendship.

An elderly man considered the problem of companionship. He said that older people who want satisfying relationships should follow these suggestions. You might pass the ideas along to an older friend or relative:

- Keep an interest in current events. Talk to other people.
- Don't be too quick to give advice unless people ask for it.
- Be friendly. Write letters. Telephone friends and family. Arrange to be with people you like.
- Act your age. Don't impose your companionship on younger people.
- When you plan to spend some time with small children, be neat. And plan some way to relate to them. They love storytelling.

As a teenager, you may enjoy satisfying relationships with older people if you take time to get to know them. Listen to what they have to say. Write to your grandparents, or talk to them by phone. They have had years of interesting experiences to share with you.

## Personal Goals

A wise man once said, "When we cease to have goals, we begin to die!" Senior citizens need personal goals to give them a purpose, a sense of self-worth, and an interest in life itself. In retirement, some people lose self-esteem because they feel that they no longer contribute to society.

Many retirees find meaningful activity through volunteer work. Through the Retired Senior Volunteer Program (RSVP), senior citizens can volunteer for many types of helpful activities:

- Retired business executives give free business counseling to small business owners.
- Retired teachers help refugees learn English.
- Volunteers bring food to the poor.
- Volunteers help preserve the area's historic landmarks.
- Retired accountants offer free tax consulting to other retirees.
- Volunteers extend friendship to abused children and runaways.
- Retired health professionals help young former drug addicts.

The goal of many older people is to help their children. They may care for their grandchildren, help out with household tasks, or offer creative skills, such as sewing or building toys for the children. In return, they enjoy being with their families and feeling useful and needed.

Spending time on hobbies, learning new skills, and studying new subjects are goals for some people. They may travel, garden, learn to paint, or go to school. These activities provide enjoyment, spark new interests, and provide a sense of accomplishment.

## Healthful Living Habits

Wellness in the aging years depends, at least in part, on good health habits. Well-balanced diets, regular exercise, and other personal care are essential for a healthy and satisfying life.

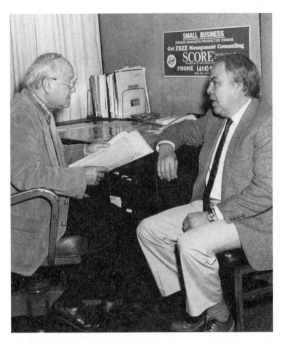

*Many senior citizens contribute to business and community organizations as volunteers.*

### NUTRITION

Older people need the same nutrients that younger people need, in about the same amounts. A balanced diet from the Daily Food Guide provides the variety of nutrients they need. However, senior citizens may need to alter their eating habits to avoid becoming overweight. Because their metabolism has slowed down and because they often are less active, they need fewer calories. In fact, after age 65, many people need 20 percent fewer calories than they needed as young adults.

Not all senior citizens eat a balanced diet, however. Emotional factors, such as loneliness or depression, may take away the pleasures of cooking and eating. Older people may not have enough money for food. Loss of teeth makes chewing difficult. Illness may cause appetite loss, digestive problems, or decreased nutrient absorption. As discussed earlier in this chapter, the senses of older people are less acute, so the flavors and aromas of food may be less appealing.

Some older people need special diets. For example, they may need a low-sodium diet if they have hypertension, a low-fat diet if they have heart disease, a soft diet if they have dental problems, a bland diet if spices give stomach trouble, or a diabetic diet.

These are guidelines a senior citizen can follow to ensure a healthful diet:

- Eat foods that are high in nutrients but low in calories to help control weight.
- Eat the main meal at noon if a heavy meal near bedtime makes it hard to sleep.
- Eat five or six small meals a day instead of three larger ones if the appetite is small. This adds interest to the day, too.
- Eat foods with high-fiber content, such as vegetables, fruit, and whole grains.

Constipation can be a problem among older adults.

- Drink plenty of fluids, especially during the heat of summer. Drinking plenty of fluids helps prevent constipation, too.
- Make mealtime pleasant when eating alone. Put a plant on the table or listen to the radio or the television.

You might offer to bring an older adult meals from time to time. If possible, find the time to stay and eat so he or she doesn't have to eat alone.

Food assistance programs are available to senior citizens on limited incomes or those with disabilities that make food preparation difficult. Home-delivered meals are prepared and brought to a person's home. Congregate meals are served at a center where people join others for food and social activities. Both of these programs receive government funding. Senior citizens eat for a very small fee. Food stamps are also available for those with limited incomes.

*Food assistance programs, such as group meals, help ensure good nutrition for older people. You might volunteer to help with these meals.*

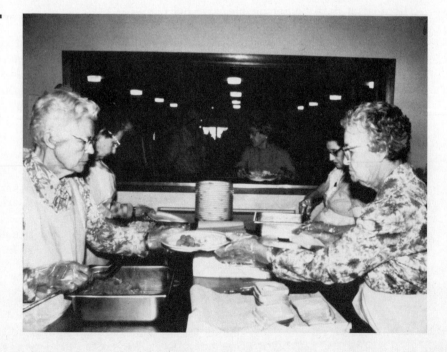

Contrary to the belief of some older people, large doses of vitamin pills will not slow the aging process. These pills cost money which many older adults can't afford.

## EXERCISE

As with people your age, or any other age, exercise contributes to a senior citizen's health. Many older adults can continue the same exercise programs they followed during middle age. Perhaps they enjoy swimming, tennis, or walking around the golf course. Recently, a 90-year-old woman reported training for another hike up a 14,000 foot mountain!

Healthy senior citizens benefit by getting moderate exercise. Moderate exercise can help them maintain muscle strength, flexibility, and coordination. It exercises the heart muscle and also improves digestion and mental outlook.

Have you seen old people walking through a shopping center at a brisk pace? Walking is good moderate exercise for many senior citizens. A shopping center is a safe, comfortable place to walk. Some senior citizens prefer walking outdoors where they can enjoy nature. If you want to know an older person better, offer to walk with him or her. You may both enjoy the experience!

People who are immobile need exercise, too. There are some exercises that can be done while standing or sitting in a chair or wheelchair. A doctor or therapist can show a person how this is done.

## OTHER PHYSICAL CARE

Besides nutrition and exercise, other physical care is important to an older adult's health and well-being:

- Since dry skin is common to aging people, a room humidifier and moisturizing creams help.
- People with dentures must clean them daily by brushing or using special cleaning products for dentures.

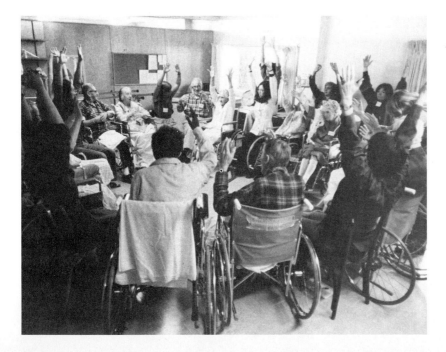

*Elderly people benefit from exercise even when they are confined to a wheelchair. What exercises might they be able to do?*

*Many older people have only a monthly social security check to pay for housing, food, transportation, and other needs.*

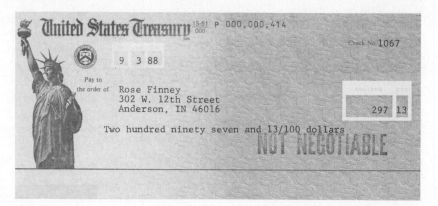

- Hygiene in the form of a daily bath, shower, or sponge bath is important. Body odors are often stronger among older people.
- People need rest as they get older but often less than they did as young adults. Sleep requirements diminish with age. Older people also have lighter sleep patterns so they awaken easily.
- Semiannual checkups are recommended unless more frequent care is needed for health problems.
- Some older people need medication. They might need help in following the physician's directions. They may need special, written instructions and a plan for taking medication. This is important for someone who has some degree of memory loss.

## Income

Senior citizens usually live on savings and fixed incomes. A *fixed income* is set at a certain sum and stays the same from one month to the next. A senior citizen's fixed income usually comes from social security or a pension. A pension is a fixed sum paid monthly to a person from a fund set up by the company from which he or she has retired. These payments come from money an employee, and perhaps an employer, put aside for retirement. *Social security* is similar, but it's handled by the federal government. The money you are required to pay for social security when you work, even as a teenager, goes toward this program.

Money worries are common among older people. Many senior citizens want to be financially independent; they don't want to burden their children. Many worry about huge medical bills and having enough savings for final expenses. For these reasons, they may not be willing to spend for daily needs.

Some senior citizens may not have enough money to meet their basic needs. They have been referred to as the "new poor." Although they lived adequately when they worked, they don't have enough for retirement years. As older people, they may have insufficient funds for basic needs, such as housing, food, heat, and medical care. This is usually true for those who must live on fixed incomes. They must pay more as the cost of living goes up, but their incomes don't go up. Many senior citizens' centers and community colleges offer financial counseling to older adults. Government programs, such as Food Stamps, Medicare, and Medicaid can help reduce financial burdens.

# Housing

Appropriate housing is important for a senior citizen's safety, emotional and social health, and perhaps medical care.

Most aging people prefer to live independently. Many continue to live safely and comfortably in the privacy of their own homes. However, those who live alone are particularly vulnerable to loneliness, stress, and being taken advantage of, or exploited, by others.

Many senior citizens choose to move near their children, perhaps in a nearby apartment. Living close allows children to check on aging parents and help them when it is necessary.

Some older people move into their children's homes. This may be for health reasons, economic necessity, convenience, or family preference. When grandparents, aunts, or uncles move in with their family, they live as an *extended family*.

Families who want to live successfully in extended families must make adjustments in their lifestyles. For example, grandparents may need to show an extra measure of patience for a teenager's music. And teens who graciously lower the volume of their music can make the home more relaxing for older adults. Everyone may need to adjust activities to provide private space for one another. The older generation is often more welcome if they avoid trying to be the major decision maker. Grandparents feel more fulfilled when grandchildren take time to be with them.

Seniors with limited incomes may choose low-cost private housing which is available in many towns. Public housing also may be available for those with limited incomes.

Retirement communities appeal to some people. They have planned activities, convenient services, and a pleasant environment. Apartments and small houses may

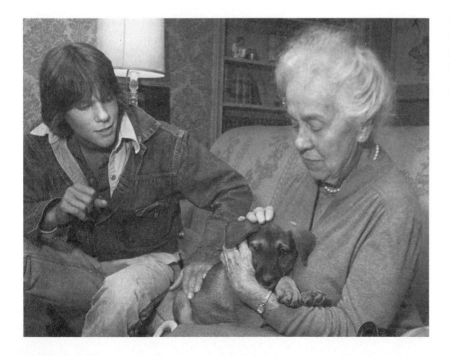

*Take time to share your recreational time with an older person. You can learn a lot from one another.*

come equipped with call buttons and grab bars in bathrooms. Many provide nursing care when needed.

Foster care is available in many communities. This is care provided by families who are paid to accommodate elderly people in their homes. Foster care has the advantage of individual care in a true home atmosphere. A disadvantage may be cost and lack of previous acquaintance with the family.

Appropriate housing for senior citizens should include these characteristics:

- adequate heat in winter.
- telephone to call for help.
- located near shopping areas, medical facilities, and community centers, or easy access to nearby public or private transportation.
- safe neighborhood with good police protection.
- neighbors who look out for each other.

## Transportation

Transportation allows independence and the opportunity to enjoy the senior years. Yet lack of transportation can be a problem for older people.

Many older people drive their own cars. But as people get older, eyesight starts to fail. Seeing at night is harder. Since reflexes aren't as fast either, a senior citizen may no longer be physically able to drive.

Others on fixed incomes may not be able to afford a car. Or perhaps they live in cities where they don't need to drive. Instead, these people need public transportation, which is convenient and low cost. Many transportation services have a lower fare for senior citizens.

Transportation needs can be met in other ways, too. Community agencies may provide free or low-cost vans to take senior citizens to stores, medical appointments, and recre-

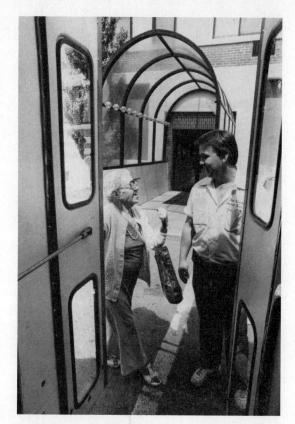

*In many communities, vans offer free or low-cost transportation to senior citizens. Perhaps you could help as a volunteer to one of these services.*

ational activities. Friends and relatives also provide transportation for older people.

## Acceptance of Death

Death is a normal part of life. It's simply the last stage of the cycle which begins at birth. Accepting death is an attitude important for everyone, especially for older people.

### DEATH OF OTHERS

Can you remember when someone in your family died? Have you ever had a friend die?

Have you experienced a life-threatening illness or injury yourself? If so, you are beginning to understand death.

Older people are more aware of death than many young and middle-aged people. Life-long friends die. A spouse dies. Not only do they miss that person, they also feel that some of their own personal history is gone. They must learn to accept the realities of death, as well as make adjustments in their daily lives.

People grieve and mourn loved ones. A grieving person may have no appetite and eat very poorly. He or she may have trouble sleeping and may tire easily. The effects of grief can take a heavy toll on older people who already may have nutritional problems and sleeping difficulties. Older people need support as they grieve so they can readjust to life.

Several activities help people mourn and accept the loss of someone close. A *funeral*, or ceremony in memory of the person who died, helps people express grief. After a funeral, grieving people need to talk to someone. For example, if your grandfather dies, your grandmother may be comforted by talking with you about him. Returning to normal routines helps relieve grief, too. This may be harder for older people who don't leave home to work. They may need new activities and interests to keep them from dwelling on their loss and perhaps to help them establish new routines.

When a spouse dies, elderly people sometimes suffer intensely. They may not think clearly. They may try to keep things exactly as they were in the past. People who have lost a spouse need to gradually make a new life for themselves. Usually it's best to wait to make major decisions until time has passed after the death, and the grieving process has diminished.

## DEATH OF SELF

Senior citizens anticipate their own death in many ways. Some are depressed or scared by the thought of dying, while others give little thought to it. Some view it as a transition. Some, who are in great pain due to disease, welcome death as a release. The way they react depends on their culture, religion, personality, and state of health.

Older people who aren't faced with immediate death have time to adjust to the idea. Time spent thinking about their past often helps to prepare for death because they see their own value over the years. Seeing old friends again and other special people helps, too. Older people should be allowed to talk about death and their concern with dying.

Many people want to put their homes and lives in order by revising their wills, getting rid of unnecessary things, and deciding how their estate should be handled. An estate includes all their money, including bank accounts and stocks, and everything they own. They may want to plan their own final arrangements, too, with a funeral director, a member of the clergy, or their family. These are important parts of accepting one's own death.

In Chapter 14, you'll learn more about dealing with the death of others and the death of one's self.

## Health Concerns of the Aging

What do your parents say to an elderly person in greeting? Many times it is, "How do you feel?" The question is a natural one because older people often have health concerns. Among their concerns are chronic health conditions, safety, fear, depression, insomnia, and memory loss.

*Older people put their estates in order. They revise their wills, which state how money and possessions will be distributed after their death.*

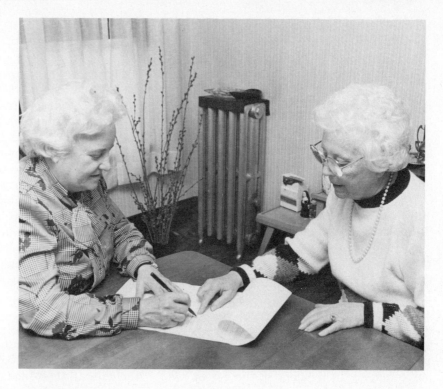

## Chronic Health Conditions

Some senior citizens learn to live with one or more chronic diseases. You know that chronic diseases are ongoing and can't be cured. Instead, many of these diseases become progressively worse as people get older. Some of the chronic conditions that are particularly worrisome to older people are:

- Cardiovascular disease. This is the leading cause of death in the United States. Cardiovascular disease also can be disabling. High blood pressure can damage the kidneys and cause a stroke. Strokes vary in severity. They can cause partial or complete paralysis, speech problems, and memory loss.
- Osteoporosis. Also called brittle bone disease, this disease can cause curvature of the spine and bone fractures to happen easily.
- Diabetes. This chronic condition can cause loss of eyesight and incurable infections requiring amputations.
- Arthritis. This condition causes pain, stiffness, and crippling in the joints.
- Cataracts and glaucoma. These eye conditions are more common among older people and can lead to blindness. A cataract, a clouding of the eye's lens, often can be surgically removed. Glaucoma, an increased pressure in the eye, can be treated with medication if it's detected early enough.

## Safety

The greatest fear of many elderly people is having a serious accident. They fear the

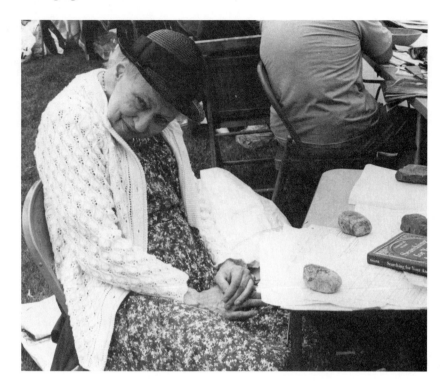

*Bone loss is a natural part of aging. Severe bone loss from osteoporosis can cause a hump.*

resulting loss of independence and the need to be cared for by someone else in a place other than their own home. They may also be afraid that their bodies will never heal completely.

A safe environment for older adults is much like a safe environment for the mobility impaired. Call buttons, non-slip floors, and grab rails in bathrooms help provide safety. In Chapter 12, you learned how a home can be adapted for people with physical limitations. The following offers other safety tips that can help protect the aged:

- Smoke alarms help provide security in case of fire. These are important safety devices in any home. They are especially important for the elderly whose decreased sense of smell may prevent them from being alerted to a fire.

- Handrails on steps help prevent falls.
- Canes and walkers make moving around easier and safer for people who are unsteady on their feet. Slippery-soled shoes should be avoided.
- For a person with failing eyesight, bright lights are important.
- Hot-water thermostats set no higher than 110° F help prevent burns.

Practicing safety habits helps prevent accidents and helps keep an older person from injury. Safety guidelines listed in Chapter 4 are important to follow, too.

## Fear

Some senior citizens fear the uncertainties of old age: illness, injury, and the unknown. They also may fear the loss of independence and loss of financial security.

Others are afraid of being the victims of personal assault. Some fear death.

As people get older, they can change their environment and lifestyle so they feel more secure. For example, they might move into a home with no steps, little maintenance, and fewer costs. Family, friends, and community organizations can help relieve their fears and make them feel more secure by having someone check on them regularly. Telephone reassurance is a program handled by community organizations, such as churches. Calls are made each day to check on the well-being of older people and offer friendly conversation. Friendly visitation is another program for senior citizens who live alone. Volunteers visit regularly to see if the elderly are safe and well, and they offer friendly conversation.

Fear for personal security is very legitimate. Senior citizens are easy prey to assault because they often can't protect themselves. Some may remain indoors because they're afraid to go out. They may become lonely and depressed because they miss people and outside activities. In the summer, some may suffer heat exhaustion because they won't open windows. Security features on doors and windows help reduce fear of assault. Daily telephone calls, transportation so older people don't have to go out alone, and planned activities provide the security of being with others. Protective services are also provided by government agencies to ensure that the elderly aren't abused. Reports of abuse are checked. If necessary, older people are helped to find other housing.

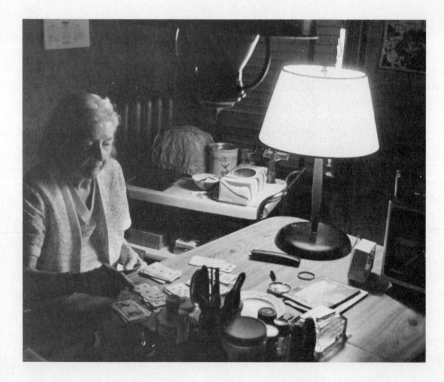

*Fear often keeps elderly people from enjoying pleasures outside their homes.*

Many reduce the fear of death by practicing their religion or by simply turning attention away from thoughts of death. Developing interests in life is a very effective way to reduce the fear of death!

## Depression

Depression may occur more frequently later in life. In fact, some authorities view depression as the leading problem among the very old.

Depression may have a physical cause. If so, doctors can treat it. However, depression often has emotional or social causes. Older people may feel depressed when they can't do many of the things they once enjoyed, when friends die or move away, and when they think their families don't have time for them. Forgetting things may embarrass and depress them. Being inactive may cause a listless feeling. Loss of body functions can be humiliating. People who can't get around easily might feel trapped.

Depression is relieved by changing habits, finding new relationships, and being as mentally and physically active as possible. Families and friends can help relieve a loved one's feelings of depression, spending time with him or her, and showing respect. This promotes self-esteem, which in turn, greatly reduces depression.

## Insomnia

*Insomnia*, the prolonged inability to get adequate sleep, plagues some older people at times. That may seem strange if you have seen them go to sleep in movies, church, or other places during the day. But they may be sleepy during the day because of interrupted sleep at night.

Insomnia is caused by many things. Older people need less sleep. Yet they may try to keep the same sleep schedule they followed during middle age so they spend a lot of time lying in bed awake. Insomnia may result from indigestion, pain, over-excitement, worry, fear, or depression. Coffee and other stimulants also interfere with sleep.

Insomnia may be relieved with good sleep habits. Dark, quiet rooms with good ventilation help promote sleep. Warm milk has properties which help induce sleep. Avoiding caffeine-containing beverages, such as coffee, tea, and colas, helps, too. Establishing regular sleep habits by going to bed at the same time each day is beneficial. Or an older person might wait until he or she is sleepy before going to bed.

## Memory Loss

Memory loss is common among older people. Yet memory loss is often offset with increased wisdom, reasoning, and understanding from years of living. Memory loss isn't an inevitable part of growing older. Many people in their 80's and 90's still have excellent memories.

*Gerontologists*, specialists in the aging process, disagree on the subject of memory loss. Some believe older people are better at long-term memory than younger people. You may say that your grandfather is very forgetful because he forgets what he did last week. Yet he can still tell stories about his childhood. Some gerontologists say that elderly individuals remember only those things that are important to them. Others attribute poor memory to a general decrease in awareness.

Memory loss can be caused by certain health conditions. Alzheimer's Disease causes severe memory loss, disorientation, and eventually death. Although middle-aged people may also get this disease, many victims are elderly. Small strokes and atherosclerosis can cause memory loss, too.

Refer to Chapter 7 for more information about these diseases. Other causes of memory loss, such as severe pain, infections, and lack of B vitamins, can be treated by a physician.

Some older people have developed practices which they think help them remember better. They write down important things. They have a special place for each belonging. They do only one thing at a time. Sometimes they take notes when they read. They also live by set routines. People with severe memory loss need the help of a family member or other caregiver.

## Alternative Care for the Aging

When older people become unable to take care of themselves, alternative care is required. Various types are available.

Nursing homes are one alternative to independent care. Actually only five percent of older people live in nursing homes. Other forms of care are day care and home care.

### Nursing Homes

Nursing homes are appropriate for some senior citizens. The type of home chosen depends on a person's health. There are four types:

- Residential care is group living for people who need help with various everyday activities, such as cooking, bathing, dressing, eating, and grocery shopping. They don't need medical or nursing services.
- Intermediate care includes nursing care for various medical treatments such as blood pressure readings.
- Skilled nursing care has 24-hour special nursing services, such as physical therapy, medicine, and changing bandages.

- Extended care is like long-term hospital care with 24-hour nursing and medical help.

Laws help ensure that nursing home living provides pleasant and comfortable surroundings, as well as good health care. The chart on this page may help you select a satisfactory nursing home for someone in your family.

## How to Choose a Nursing Home

1. Get a list of nursing homes in the community from the Department of Public Health. Or ask a doctor and friends to recommend several homes.
2. Call the nursing homes and ask if they have vacancies. Inquire about their services and their fees.
3. Visit the homes that seem to meet the needs of the person needing care. During the visits, observe the staff, the food, the activity program, and the ways patients are treated. If possible, have the person requiring care also visit and help make the choice.
4. Choose a home that has these qualities:
   - good care for residents
   - location convenient to family and friends
   - friendly, competent, caring staff
   - well-prepared food, attractively-served and in adequate amounts
   - clean building, free of unpleasant odors
   - interesting activity program
   - doctor on call 24 hours a day
   - licensed by a state or local agency
   - safety equipment, such as fire and smoke alarms, good lighting, grab bars, and call bells
   - ample grounds for outside activities, if the person is able to enjoy the outdoors.

## Day Care

Day care centers for elderly people are increasing in this country because they fulfill many daytime needs. Many older people don't want to move away from home, but they can't cook or handle personal chores any more. Others live with children who work and cannot give care 24 hours a day.

Day care facilities offer many services. Transportation is available to and from home if needed. During the day, food, activities, and simple medical care are provided. Personal care, exercise, and outside entertainment are part of most programs. Because day care is a group program, there are opportunities for senior citizens to socialize with others near their own age, too.

## Home Care

In-home care is an increasingly popular form of care. It appeals to those who want to remain in their own homes but who lack ability to totally care for themselves.

A home-care provider comes to the home at regular intervals depending on the need. Or the caregiver might live in and provide 24-hour assistance. This might be especially important for someone in a wheelchair, for example. The home-care provider cooks, cleans, bathes, shops, and does other necessary chores. Sometimes a trained nurse provides in-home medical treatment.

## Community Support Systems

A greater percentage of Americans are over 65 today than ever before, and that percentage is rising. As a result, many more services are available for senior citizens.

Four major government agencies serve the elderly. They are The Department of Human Services, The Department of Health, the Mental Health and Mental Retardation

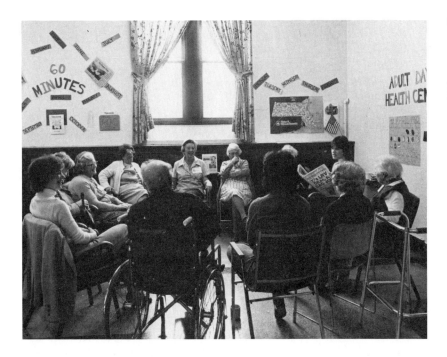

*Many senior citizens, who live at home with others, need day care. Activities there provide physical, social, and emotional care.*

# SPOTLIGHT ON SENIOR CITIZENS

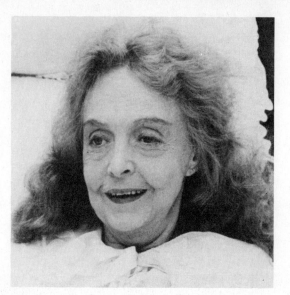

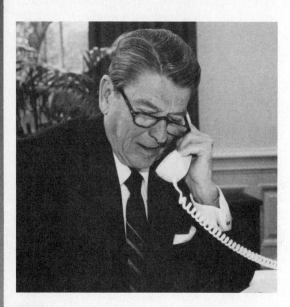

**M**r. **Ronald Reagan**, the 40th President of the United States, has been admired and respected all over the world. In fact, he has been judged one of the most popular presidents we've ever had!

Mr. Reagan is the oldest person to have served as president in the country's history. He was born in 1911, making him 69 years old when he was first elected. He has governed with health and vigor.

Once he was debating with a younger presidential candidate and someone tried to introduce Mr. Reagan's age as an issue. Mr. Reagan replied with a quip that the audience loved. He said, "I am not going to exploit for political purposes my opponent's youth and inexperience."

**M**iss **Lillian Gish** is an outstanding actress. After 75 years of continuous acting success, she has been honored, after most people her age have retired, with the Life Achievement Award from the American Film Institute. Born in 1898, she began making movies in 1912. During the days of silent movies, she was known as the "first lady" of motion pictures. She is probably best known for her work in the theater, for her popular roles in *Hamlet* and *Life with Father*. In the mid 1980's, she continued appearing in movies, such as *Sweet Liberty*, where she acted with Alan Alda.

**M**iss **Clementine Hunter**, a famous artist from The Cane River in Louisiana, continues to paint in the golden years of her life. She's over 100 years old! Her primitive-style oil paintings have been exhibited in many art galleries all over the country, including The Smithsonian Institution in Washington, D.C., The Museum of Folk Art in New York City, and The New Orleans Museum of Art.

Miss Hunter paints scenes of the Old South. She focuses on activities in rural areas, particularly on life in the black community. Her most loved paintings feature families picking cotton, children playing, people doing laundry, and pecan gathering.

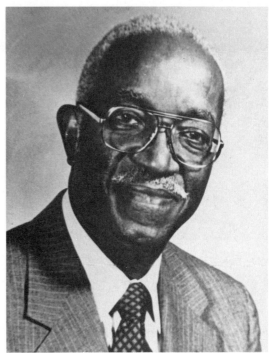

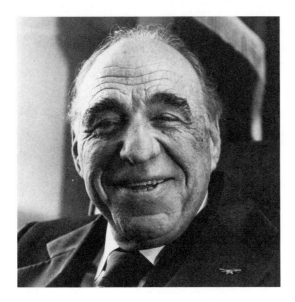

**M**r. **Henry Gonzales** from Texas is the first American with Mexican ancestry in the United States House of Representatives. Mr. Gonzales was born in 1916 and continues to serve his state and nation as a political leader and decision maker.

Educated as a lawyer, he has worked as a juvenile probation officer. During his years as a representative, he has worked to eliminate segregation.

Over 70 years old, Mr. Gonzales continues to enjoy a rich home life. He and his wife have eight children. He still enjoys swimming, biking, and baseball.

**D**r. **John Hope Franklin**, the James B. Duke Professor Emeritus of History at the Duke University School of Law, is over 70 years old. He not only teaches law, but he continues to publish books as well. Recently he published a biography of a famous black historian.

Dr. Franklin is an able spokesman for black people in America. He has worked in the civil rights movement for 35 years. And he doesn't let his age stop his work! More than 60 honorary degrees have been given to this man who continues to work toward new goals.

At his North Carolina home, Dr. Franklin enjoys his hobby—a greenhouse filled with orchids. He has more than 800 red and white flowers called the John Hope Franklin orchid.

## Services for Senior Citizens

| For All Senior Citizens | For Homebound Senior Citizens | For Senior Citizens with Special Needs |
| --- | --- | --- |
| Congregate meals | Housekeeping | Day care centers |
| Legal services | Home-delivered meals | Protective services |
| Transportation | Telephone reassurance | Health care |
| Recreational activities | Information | |
| Counseling | Health aides | |
| Information | Shopping assistance | |
| Housing | Friendly visitation | |

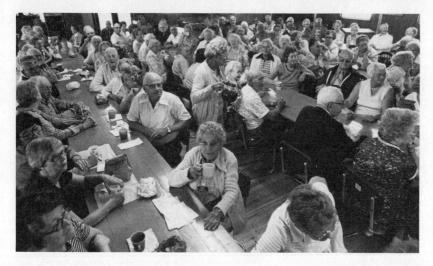

*Congregate meals are one of many social services provided to senior citizens.*

Organization, and Area Agencies on Aging. These agencies provide both in-home and outside-the-home services. The chart above lists major community services.

Numerous social organizations exist for older men and women. The largest of these organizations is The American Association of Retired Persons (AARP). You learned earlier how the AARP acts as a source of companionship for senior citizens. It also provides travel services, adult education, temporary employment, volunteer programs, and a monthly magazine.

Community organizations, such as colleges, churches, and the YMCA, have organized senior citizens' programs and centers. These organizations also offer field trips, classes, meals, and other services depending on need and interest.

Even business recognizes the benefit of serving older adults. Senior citizens' discounts at movies, in restaurants, and on public transportation help people on fixed incomes. Banks may offer free financial counseling. Travel agencies often plan trips to match the pace of older people.

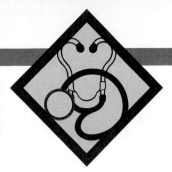

# CHAPTER CHECKUP

## Reviewing the Information

1. What percent of the U.S. population is over 65 years of age?
2. List five physical signs of aging among senior citizens.
3. What are three social changes common among older people?
4. How might senior citizens successfully adjust to new roles after retirement?
5. Describe disengagement.
6. What are four sources of companionship for senior citizens?
7. What are three reasons an elderly person might not eat balanced meals?
8. What are two benefits of exercise for senior citizens?
9. What are five characteristics of appropriate housing for senior citizens?
10. Describe these programs—congregate meals, telephone reassurance, friendly visitation, and home-delivered meals.
11. Describe five chronic health conditions common among senior citizens.
12. What are three safety tips aging people may follow to avoid injuries?
13. What are three common fears of senior citizens, and how might these fears be relieved?
14. How can depression be relieved?
15. Describe ways to combat insomnia.
16. What are the reasons for day care for the elderly?
17. List three agencies which provide services for the aging.

## Thinking It Over

1. How might you describe the aging population?
2. How might you offer companionship to an older adult?
3. What exercises might a senior citizen do while seated in a wheelchair?
4. Why is a fixed income a problem for retired people?
5. What is the difference between social security and a pension?
6. How might a senior citizen with a physical disability get groceries?
7. How might a bathroom be made safe for an aging person?
8. Describe a senior citizen you know who lives an active, productive life.

## Taking Action

1. Read magazines and newspapers to learn about three productive senior citizens. Write a brief description of their activities.

2. Find out more about social security benefits from the government office. Determine how much money a person would receive in monthly social security income if he or she had been making $24,000 annually before retirement.
3. Interview an older person to learn about his or her retirement plans.
4. Make a "Senior Citizen's Yellow Pages" in class. Find out about community services for the aging in your town.

# 14 Care of the Terminally Ill

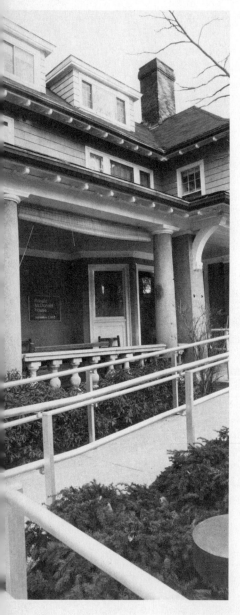

After reading this chapter, you should be able to:

- describe how dying people and their families respond to terminal illness.

- name sources of community care that meet the special needs of the dying.

- identify how to help the person who has a terminal illness.

## Terms to Understand

| | |
|---|---|
| autopsy | denial |
| bargaining | grief |
| casket | hospice |
| cremation | mourning |
| deceased | terminal illness |

With the great advances in medical science, people are living longer and healthier lives than ever before. Just as the stages of birth, growth, and adulthood are part of life, so is the final stage—death. It is the time of separation from the people, places, and things in life.

Death can occur at any age. It may be a sudden, accidental death or a prolonged process of dying from a chronic illness. No one escapes death. Certainly, death will come to your family, your friends, and eventually to you. How people respond is an entirely individual experience.

People who experience the death of someone they care about must cope with the loss of companionship and many emotions. Understanding the process of death and dying makes it easier to handle the changes that occur. It helps caregivers better support the dying family member or friend.

*Terminal illnesses* are diseases without cures that eventually result in death. AIDS, severe heart disease, Alzheimer's disease, and some types of cancer are terminal illnesses. You learned about these diseases in Chapter 7. The length of time a person lives with a terminal illness varies from person to person. It may be months or even years. Prolonged dying can be physically and emotionally painful.

Regardless of the amount of time they may have left, the remaining lifetime of terminally ill people is very important. Dying people experience the same emotions in varying degrees as healthy people. They still respond to touch, humor and the news. They want quality of life in their remaining days. They want to enjoy what time they have left

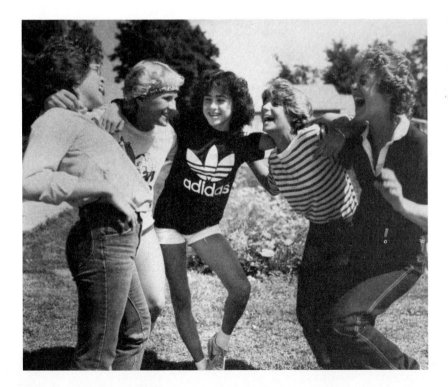

*Take time to enjoy others. Life can end at any time—without warning.*

with people they love, activities they enjoy, and without pain.

## The Individual's Response to Impending Death

Death isn't easy to understand or accept. The way people respond to the fact that they are dying depends on their age, personality, philosophy of life, the support of family and friends, and how well they can communicate their feelings. For many people, it's a hard struggle. But, in general, mature people, who have close family ties and who can share their feelings openly, do better at accepting their own death.

Being diagnosed with a terminal illness causes many different emotions in a person—denial, anger, fear, guilt, and sadness, among others. Working through these feelings is the way people come to accept their impending death. Responses to death don't occur in any typical order, and emotions may switch back and forth. Not everyone responds in the same way or experiences the same feelings.

People who are trying to accept that they are dying often shift their behavior and mood suddenly. This is a normal part of the coping process. Sometimes it's hard for others to understand erratic behavior and mood changes. One day the person will be outgoing and unable to stop talking. The next day he or she will be sad and withdrawn. A dying person may snap at a best friend or close family member. These responses are normal and should never be taken personally.

When family members and friends recognize and understand emotions related to death, they can deal more effectively with the dying person and with their own feelings.

## Denial

Denial means not believing or accepting something. In the case of those with terminal illness, *denial* means that people refuse to believe or accept that their own death is near. The person thinks, "It can't be true," "This isn't really happening to me," or "There must be some mistake." People who deny death often can't talk or even think about it. Some go to many different doctors expecting to find one who says that their illness can be cured. Others prefer to be alone or spend time with someone who doesn't know they are terminally ill.

Terminally ill people may deny their illness to protect themselves. Denial keeps them from having to suddenly face a situation too horrible to comprehend all at once. Denial gives them time to become more emotionally ready to accept death.

Some people continue to deny that they are dying until the very end. They talk about their future plans and what they'll do when they're better. Family and friends may think people experiencing denial are being brave. Really, they're often afraid. Often people will deny that they are dying in order to protect those close to them.

The best way to help people through the denial response to terminal illness is to be available when they need you. Display the attitude, "When you're ready to talk, I'm here." Listening is considered a strong form of communication.

## Anger

Anger is another way people respond to terminal illness. The person's behavior might say, "Why me?" or "What did I do to deserve this?" Sometimes anger is directed at specific people, perhaps the doctor. Anger may be directed at you for no reason at all.

Being with someone who responds to

death with anger is difficult, especially when you care about them. Your first reaction may be to lash back with angry remarks. But this only magnifies the anger. Try not to take angry remarks personally.

Deal with the anger within dying people by allowing them to express their emotions. Be a sounding board for complaints. Without being overly attentive, agree so they're encouraged to talk. Let them know that being angry is normal.

Help a dying person find a physical outlet for anger. A younger person might throw darts or use a punching bag. Or perhaps you could take a brisk walk together or even have a pillow fight.

## Fear

Facing death may be more fearful than anything else in life. There are many fears that come with death:

- death itself
- the dying process
- pain
- loss of control over body functions
- risks of medical treatments
- the unknown—after death
- being left alone, especially at the time of death
- uncertainty of the future

People show fear in different ways. Many people can't admit outright that they're afraid. Instead, some have physical symptoms such as muscle tension, talking fast, fidgeting, or whining. Others show fear through crying and nervousness. Some may try to hide fear by joking.

People who fear death should be encouraged to talk about it. Sharing apprehension lessens fear. Just sitting with a dying person brings comfort and eases fear. You don't need to offer suggestions or advice. Like reducing anger, physical exercise can also be an outlet for fear.

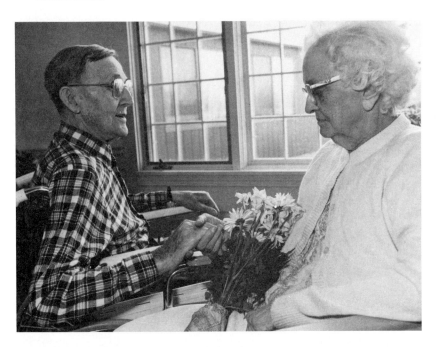

*Just being with others who care helps relieve the fear of death.*

## Guilt

You might wonder how anyone could feel guilty about dying. After all, it's no one's fault, certainly not the fault of the sick individual. But some people feel guilty anyway.

People with a family may feel guilty that they are abandoning them. If they're the wage earner or have no insurance, they feel guilty about no longer providing financial support. They feel guilty about the trouble their illness is causing family and friends. Or they feel guilty about money spent on medical care, and perhaps leaving behind huge medical bills.

Reassure the terminally ill person that they've done all they can for their family and friends. If the person has been a good, devoted family member or friend, say so and give examples.

## Bargaining

Have you ever wished that something just weren't so? You'd give anything you could to change it. That's *bargaining*. The dying person may want so much to live that he or she tries to bargain in an attempt to postpone death. For example, "I've led a good life. Just let me live until I graduate." Or, "Just let me keep going until my kids get through school."

Most bargains are made silently with no one else knowing, except perhaps a member of the clergy. Usually bargaining is a helpful response because it gives the person hope, even if it lasts for only a little while.

## Sadness

In time, most terminally ill people come face-to-face with their imminent death. Knowing that they are losing everything

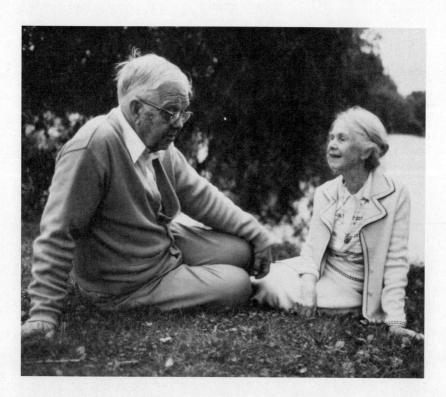

*When a person finally accepts the reality of death, he or she can often find peace and meaning in life.*

and everyone they love makes them very sad. The thought of separation becomes a great burden. Many people show sadness in a quiet manner. Maybe they'll cry a little.

At this point, avoid trying to cheer up the terminally ill person. Instead, you can be helpful by sharing your time. There is little need for words. You can express your feelings with a touch of the hand or just sitting beside them.

Some people think back on their lives during this time. They recall a lifetime of events, trying to see some value. Be there to listen.

## Acceptance

After dying people work through their other emotions, they usually accept death. This is a peaceful response, but not a happy or sad one. Acceptance comes as a relief after the struggle of screaming through anger or crying through sadness.

Acceptance is usually a quiet time for a dying person. Often the person is tired, weak, and sleeps a lot. Don't mistake the withdrawal and distance for lack of love.

As a caregiver, eliminate irritations, such as the sound of television. Avoid a lot of visitors. Make your own visits brief. Short visits can be special. What you say is not important. You may not need to say anything. Just be there.

## The Family's and Friends' Response to Impending Death

Grief and mourning are common responses to the impending death of a loved one. Many factors influence the response of family and friends. Often it's hardest to accept the death of a young person.

## Grief

*Grief* includes the emotions felt by family and friends when someone special is dying

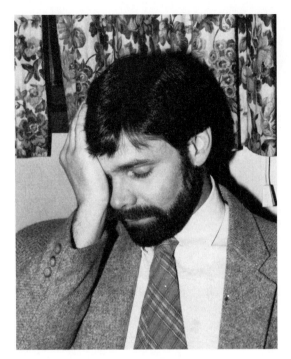

*Grief is a normal reaction to the death of someone you love. It's okay to cry.*

or dies. Grief often starts when people first hear that someone they care about is terminally ill and often lasts long after death occurs. The extent of grief usually is determined by how closely people have lived each day with the dying person.

The finality of death is often a shock to family and friends, even when they've prepared themselves. The first reaction to death is often disbelief or a time when they may feel nothing at all. Death leaves an emptiness. It often takes time for the reality and the finality of death to sink in.

Sadness is a normal reaction when people realize that the person they care about will never be with them again. Initially people cry, sometimes hard. They may need a few days away from normal routines of work, school, or friends to collect their thoughts. As time goes on, they often need quiet time alone or with family and friends, just to talk. It's important not to withdraw from others since support is part of the healing process.

Sometimes the emotional trauma of having someone close to you die or become terminally ill causes physical problems. Feeling nauseous, perspiring heavily, feeling tenseness in the throat, and sleeplessness are symptoms that last for short periods. As time goes on, they usually happen less often as the person learns to cope with the death or terminal illness of someone very close to them.

Sometimes the knowledge of impending death or death itself causes anger for a family member or friend. "How dare this happen!" expresses anger at fate. "If the nurses had given better care, my mother would be alive today," shows anger at medical personnel. "How can he die and leave me alone?" is an example of anger toward the dead person. Anger is a normal reaction, and getting the anger out is part of the coping process.

Some people suffer from guilt because they feel helpless in the face of death. They feel that somewhere, somehow they may have done something to prevent it. They can't answer the question, "Why that person? Why not me?" Terminal illness doesn't come to people because of the kind of person they are or because of anything anyone else did or didn't do. So there's nothing to feel guilty about.

Grief is part of accepting death and dying. But it shouldn't consume someone's life. A sick person doesn't need to be visited everyday. Caregivers, friends, and family shouldn't feel guilty about giving themselves a break to do other things or enjoy themselves. Nor should they feel guilty after the person dies because they didn't spend enough time with the dying person or show enough love. Seeing a movie, riding a bike, attending a dance, or picking a bouquet of flowers are good therapies for the grieving process and they help relieve depression.

Even though family and friends grieve, death may be welcome when terminal illness lasts a long time. There may be a sense of relief that the person's suffering is over.

## Mourning

*Mourning* is the process of separating from the deceased. The *deceased* refers to the person who has just died. This doesn't mean forgetting the person. Memories are comforting. But people need to rebuild their own lives and maybe live a little differently. Living without a parent, a best friend, or a brother or sister is a big adjustment.

Mourning is a process that takes time. For most people, it lasts about four to 12 weeks. By then life resumes, and people adjust their lifestyles.

While mourning, people often daydream, thinking about the deceased and things they did together. They may want to visit the person's private spaces, touch his or her belongings, and look at pictures of him or her. This lets them hold on for a little while until they're ready to let go.

Some people want quiet time alone to get in touch with their feelings. Or they want time to express their feelings to others. When people can't work through their emotions or put feelings into words, the feelings come out in other ways. Restless sleep or loss of appetite are common.

In time, people resume normal living patterns. They are no longer sad when they think of the dead person. Instead, they talk easily about happy memories. This is an indication that they have confronted and resolved—not forgotten—their loss. They're able to pack away the deceased's belongings because they've accepted the finality of

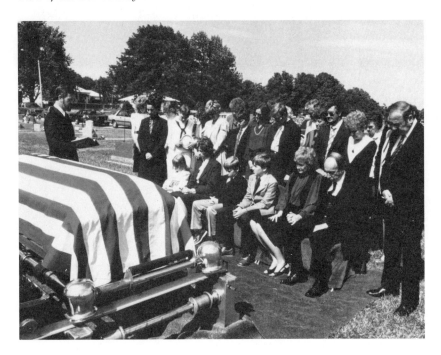

*Among certain ethnic and religious groups, certain customs, such as wearing dark clothing, are part of the time for mourning.*

death. They can again enjoy socializing. In other words, they've mourned and resumed living.

## Death—At What Age?

Terminal illness can strike people of any age. Age affects how people handle their own death and how others respond.

The death of a child often seems the most tragic. A young child dies with unfilled hopes and unrealized opportunities. But children often accept their own death more easily than adults do. They have less fear of dying. They haven't been conditioned to death, and very young children might not even understand it.

Instead, children fear separation from their parents, the hospital, medical treatments, the dark, and pain. Family members need to stay with the dying child almost all the time. This puts a burden on the family, especially if there are other children.

Terminal illness is hard to accept among adolescents, too. Teenagers are often confused and angry when they must face death. Their confusion is directed toward a body which won't respond and heal the way they want it to. Anger and resentment is often directed at parents who have always been able to nurture them back to health. They may feel their parents have let them down. There is sadness at life suddenly being withdrawn as they move into the time of their greatest potential. These emotions, along with the normal emotions of the teenage years, make it especially hard for a teenager to deal with his or her own impending death.

The adolescent years are normally the most active stage of life. Even during the dying process, teens should be helped to stay as active as possible. They should be encouraged to maintain their normal routines of school, dating, and recreation if their illness permits.

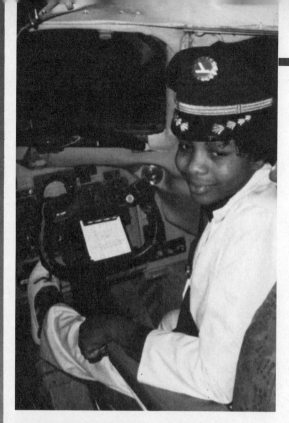

They've provided pets, computers, and bikes. They've arranged meetings for children with Mickey Mouse, sports celebrities, movie stars, and even the President.

Why do they do this? They know that dreams are important to children. And yet, some children will never have simple dreams fulfilled because their hope and time are running out. These children, whose primary dream is to regain health, also have little dreams that have special meaning. These little dreams may be just the inspiration that keeps their spirits high and motivates them "to hang in there" when things get tough.

Sometimes making a dream come true brings tears. Sometimes the joy is translated into a gleam in the eye or a shy smile. Sometimes it miraculously helps bring improved health, if only for a short time.

The Dream Factory exists for three reasons:
- to put smiles on the faces of seriously ill children
- to promote a better family atmosphere during a time of suffering
- to involve entire communities in the pleasure of granting wishes to children in need

Volunteers who support the Dream Factory are active in many ways. They seek out seriously ill children and ensure that their dreams are fulfilled. Through special projects, they raise funds necessary to make dreams come true. Never do they want to refuse any child.

# WHEN YOU WISH UPON A STAR . . . YOUR DREAMS COME TRUE

If you suddenly faced a serious illness, what would you wish for? A trip to Disneyland? A racer bike? A meeting with Brooke Shields? A horseback ride in the Colorado mountains?

For the Dream Factory, the wish of a seriously ill youngster is their command. Since 1980, this organization has been making dreams come true for many children, aged three to 13. The Dream Factory has sent children to camp, on cruises, and to a Dallas Cowboys' football game.

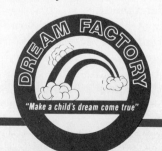

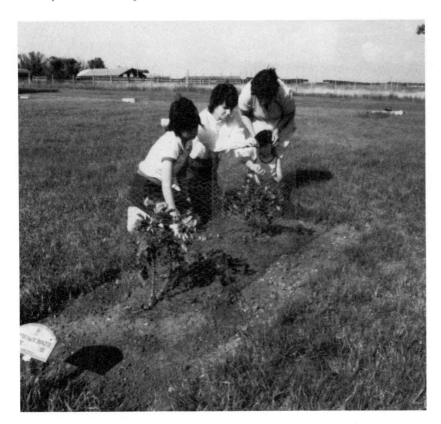

*Death leaves a void that affects many people.*

The midlife years are the time of greatest life achievement and responsibility. Loss of life then may be viewed as deserting a family and a career where the person plays a big part. Death of a parent, a family wage earner, a volunteer community leader, or a company manager leaves a big void that affects many people.

The death of older adults is easier to accept because it's more expected. They've lived long lives, and many are ready to die. Perhaps they've lost their spouse already, or maybe they've been chronically ill for many years. Many have prepared for death by writing a will and by lessening others' dependence on them. Older adults, unlike those much younger, die knowing they are leaving behind many accomplishments and memories.

Regardless of age, a terminally ill person needs adequate and appropriate medical and personal care to help ensure the highest quality of life during his or her remaining days.

## Sources of Care for the Dying

People have a right to die with dignity and respect. If possible, they should be allowed to choose where they will spend their last days.

Many dying people require special medical care or a great deal of personal care. Skilled medical care in a hospital or nursing home may be necessary. In other circumstances, a sensitive friend or relative can provide quality of life for a terminally ill person at home.

# Home

If possible, many people prefer to die at home. They like being in familiar surroundings, close to people they love. Dying at home gives them the freedom to make their own choices, perhaps about mealtime or bedtime. But dying at home may also commit them to a much bigger decision—not to use life-sustaining equipment available in hospitals. This might include the use of a respirator, a machine that breathes for the person.

Many terminally ill people return home after treatment in a hospital. Perhaps the hospital can do nothing more for the patient. Psychologically, that's often hard for the dying person and the family to accept. At home, caregivers may not be able to prolong life either, but they often can add to the quality of life with love and special attention. Before the illness progresses too far, the dying person may be able to do many things for himself or herself, as well.

Some families choose home care because dying at home is less costly. Health insurance may not pay for maintenance care in a hospital or nursing home. The sick person or a family member should check the insurance policy before the decision to stay in a hospital or return home is made. Financial assistance for terminal illness is often available from a local public health department, the Social Security Administration, and the Veterans' Administration.

Caring for a dying person is like caring for someone with a chronic illness. In Chapter 11 you learned how to care for a sick person in the home. Physical, emotional, and social needs must be attended to. This takes time, energy, and patience. Care includes providing for comfortable surroundings, nutritious meals, relief from pain, personal hygiene, medical treatment, emotional support, and social opportunities.

Keeping family life normal is often a challenge during a terminal illness, and sometimes it's impossible. Some families must adjust to many changes. A husband might have to fix dinner, clean the house, and care for his sick wife in addition to going to work everyday. A teenage daughter might need to get a part-time job to help the family finances because her dying mother can no longer work. Living with someone who is gradually dying is stressful for all other family members at home. But it's usually accepted as part of family life and not considered a burden.

# Hospital or Nursing Home

Many terminally ill people choose to stay in the hospital or a nursing home until their death. This may be the best solution for the patient and the family. Some terminally ill people require around-the-clock medical care. A hospital or nursing home can also relieve loneliness for those who live alone or whose families need to be away. Hospital or nursing home care also offers security and protection and provides for basic daily needs. Some terminally ill people prefer to stay in a nursing home because they don't want to burden their family with added responsibility.

While hospitals and nursing homes provide excellent care, many people don't like to give up the control they had at home. These are typical rules the patient and family must accept at the hospital:
- set visiting hours
- no young children allowed
- set schedules for meals, activities, and therapy
- few personal items in the room
- lights out at a certain time

Nursing homes are often the best solution as long as the home matches the person's physical needs. The surroundings are much more homelike; sometimes personal possessions are allowed. Rules are more flexible. And for those who are able, there are many social activities. There are four basic types of nursing facilities: extended care, skilled care, intermediate care, and residential care. Extended care is most like a hospital, while residential care is for people who don't need medical services. Nursing homes are described more fully in Chapter 13.

## Hospice

Many of the people who die of terminal illnesses every year participate in the hospice program. Started in Europe many years ago, it was introduced in the United States in 1974. *Hospice* is a program designed to help people die with as much comfort and dignity as possible. The program also provides psychological support for the families.

Hospice is a type of care, not a place. In most cases, this total care is part of outpatient programs, although many hospitals and nursing homes have hospice care. The dying person remains at home as long as possible. Hospice services provide assistance for a person's last days.

The dying person's wishes are respected as much as possible. He or she is involved in making decisions about personal and medical care with suggestions from the doctor and family.

In this program, symptoms such as pain are controlled and treated. Nobody pretends the disease can be cured.

Medical care is handled in a team approach with doctors, nurses, social workers, volunteers, counselors, and others. Together, they help the patient and family.

With hospice, the needs of both the patient and family are provided for. If the patient's spouse or child needs counseling, a trained professional is available to talk. Patients and their families are accepted into hospice

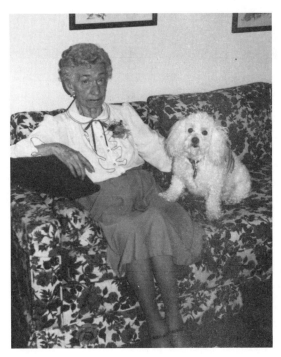

*A hospice program is planned to be as homelike as possible. Pets may continue to provide companionship. They also help a dying person feel needed.*

programs based on need, not their ability to pay the bills.

## Community Organizations

In the last ten years, people have started talking openly about dying. The public has become aware of what dying people need. Both national and local organizations help meet the needs of terminally ill people.

### AMERICAN CANCER SOCIETY

The American Cancer Society (ACS) is a national organization with local chapters in many cities across the country. The ACS sponsors special programs for people with cancer, as well as their families.

**CanSurmount** is a mutual support program. It brings together the patient, family, a CanSurmount volunteer, and health professionals. On a physician's referral, a trained CanSurmount volunteer, who is also a cancer patient, meets with the patient and family. The goal of the program is to provide mutual help and understanding. The program includes education and support.

**I Can Cope** addresses the learning and psychological needs of people with cancer and their families. It's a series of eight classes covering: learning about the disease, learning to cope with daily health problems, learning to express feelings, learning to live with limitations, and learning about local resources. Through lectures, group discussions, and study assignments, the course helps people with cancer regain a sense of self-control over their lives.

### MAKE TODAY COUNT

**Make Today Count** is a national support group for people with life-threatening illnesses, their families, and any interested people. It was started by an incurable cancer patient who saw a need to meet and talk openly with other cancer patients and their families. By sharing what they're going through, members help each other live more meaningful lives.

### CANDLELIGHTERS

**Candlelighters** is a support group of parents whose children have died. They meet regularly to share experiences, concerns, and feelings. They give each other strength to get over the loss of their children and to offer hope for the future.

## Support of the Dying

Diagnosis of an incurable disease hits people as a tremendous shock. One dying person describes the experience as being "hit by a locomotive, but I was still alive." When the shock wears off, the reality of dying sets in. This burden is often too great for the dying person to bear alone.

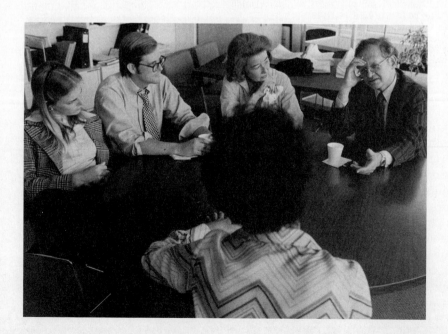

*Groups, such as I Can Cope, meet regularly to learn how to deal with the process of death. A psychologist might talk about the fear of dying.*

Family and friends can play a big part in sharing the burden of death by meeting the dying person's needs and helping whenever possible.

## What the Dying Person Needs

People who are terminally ill have many needs—physical, psychological, and social. And those needs change from day to day. Some needs are related to the dying process. Others are personal needs that anyone has from day to day. Regardless, a dying person's needs can be met with the help of sensitive caregivers.

### PHYSICAL NEEDS

Staying active as long as possible helps maintain self-esteem. If possible, encourage a person with impending death to work, go to school, do the dishes, or whatever is the usual routine. Being able to get up everyday and do something says, "I have value. I can still contribute."

For those whose illness is advanced, encourage them to be as active as the disease allows. In some cases this may only mean getting out of bed and sitting in a chair. If possible, allow them to get up on their own. Respect their age, and don't treat adults in a child-like way even if you must do a great deal for them.

In the final days of a terminal illness, people are usually very ill, and they require a great deal of physical care. They often have severe problems with pain and body odor. Their appetite might be gone, and they tend to be very inactive.

The terminally ill, especially cancer victims, often suffer unbearable pain. At the least, pain is irritating. At its worst, pain can cause people to be so preoccupied that they can't think of anything else. Medicines and treatments can relieve the pain. But there are some simple things the caregiver can do to make the dying person comfort-able. Refer to Chapter 11 for ways to relieve pain. Other therapies include:

- Deep breathing. Very slowly, have the person take in air through the nose, then slowly release the air through the mouth. Take eight to 10 seconds for each full breath. This relieves tension which eases pain.
- Guided imagery. Have the person lie back with eyes closed. Describe in detail the person's favorite place—seashore, garden, snow-covered mountain. Help the person feel as though they're a part of the scene you're describing. This distracts from pain.
- Thick mattress padding or a sheepskin on top of the bed sheet or chair. This is especially helpful for very thin people.
- Positioning in the bed or chair. Find out what positions are most comfortable, and help him or her change positions every couple of hours. Pillows add comfort.
- Soft mellow music. Playing music with string instruments is relaxing.

As the body deteriorates, it often develops odors. There are odors from wounds that won't heal, bad breath, and possibly from accidents with urine and stool. To minimize the odors:

- Bathe the person every day. Offer mouth care every few hours.
- Change the bed linens everyday, or more often if needed. Sprinkle oil of wintergreen on the sheets for a fresh smell.
- Keep the room well ventilated. If you can, open a window.
- Use room deodorizers or an air freshening machine.

Sick people need nourishing food, but they often lose their appetite or even feel nauseous. Refer to Chapter 11 for ways to make mealtime pleasant and appealing. To relieve nausea, have the person sip on gingerale or eat a bit of dry popcorn or crackers.

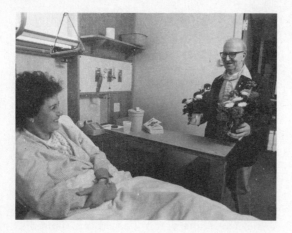

### PSYCHOLOGICAL NEEDS

Sharing feelings is the best way to meet the emotional needs and deal with the trauma of dying. But sharing is a two-way communication. Provide a "safe" environment where the dying person can talk about his or her feelings in privacy and confidence. Don't judge the comments, but be an active listener. Be prepared to share your feelings, too. Are you sad? Are you angry and hurt? Are you afraid? If you are, then say so. The dying person will appreciate your honesty, and your openness will encourage his or her openness, too.

As you support a dying person's emotions, don't feel like you have to say anything, especially "the right thing." Just your presence meets the dying person's greatest need—reassurance that he or she is loved.

To gain the courage to face death, many people use religious beliefs as a source of strength. Members of the clergy are trained to offer solace, provide hope, and help ease family crises for the dying.

### SOCIAL NEEDS

People need to be with other people whether they're healthy or whether they're dying. The support of family and friends helps people cope with their own imminent death. As a caregiver, look for ways to involve others in the dying person's life. The chart, "Give a Hand," on page **339** gives some ideas.

## How to Help

Most people want to help and be with someone who's dying. But they may feel uncomfortable, perhaps afraid. They ask, "What should I say? What should I do? How can anything I do or say help someone who's dying?"

The way to help someone who's dying is to be there, and be yourself. Be the same caring friend or family member you've always been. At first, this may feel awkward, but soon most people begin to feel natural and their words and actions come without thinking.

Consider the special needs of the dying person. Offer to help and then do what you've offered.

## Death

Caring for a dying person may last a long time. During those weeks or months, caregivers prepare mentally and emotionally for the moment of death. Physical signs usually suggest that death is near. Caregivers must also prepare for certain responsibilities just after death occurs.

## Signs of Imminent Death

Many family members and friends want to support the person emotionally during the last hours of life. The caregiver should be

## Give a Hand

When someone you know is facing a terminal illness, you may feel helpless. You want to help, but what do you do or say? You can help and feel good yourself at the same time.

- Cry together and laugh together. Both are natural and okay.
- Take your friend for a ride. Sightseeing provides distraction and something to talk about.
- Always call before you visit. But do visit. It relieves loneliness.
- Visit often. If you like, bring something homemade, such as a card, taped music, or wall poster.
- Celebrate holidays by decorating the hospital room or home.
- Call for your friend's shopping list for food, toiletries, reading materials, and other things. Then deliver them at a convenient time.
- Bring reminders of happy times to share, such as photos.
- Listen to the person's reminiscences. It feels good to remember happy times.
- Call just to say "hello." Send a friendly card. But don't let calls and cards replace visits.
- Bring a game that the sick person can play in bed. Mental stimulation is important.
- What's new? Magazines, newspapers, and other news keeps the person from feeling the world is passing by.
- Talk about the illness and death if the sick person initiates it. Or ask, "Do you feel like talking about it?" Probably all you'll have to do is listen.
- Don't always feel you have to talk. You can sit silently together.
- Help the person feel good about his or her appearance. Compliment the person on looking good, as appropriate. Don't make phony compliments. They'll make you seem insincere. Offer to provide a shampoo or shave.
- Talk about the future—tomorrow and next year. The person can feel part of the future now.
- Ask the person to do something for you. This promotes feelings of usefulness.
- Don't forget the family. Offer to stay with the sick person to give them time away. Or invite the person out.
- Help with housework. During an illness, the family still faces dirty dishes and other chores.
- Babysit or take the children out of the house. That gives everyone a break.

alert to these common signs of imminent death so others can be contacted. Just before death, perhaps within a few days, the body systems and senses gradually deteriorate. The patient may or may not be awake.

Muscles lose their tone. Eventually the person needs help just to sit up. It may be difficult to swallow. It may even be hard to keep the eyelids open.

Blood circulation slows down. The arms and legs may look blue and feel cold. The underside of the body may appear darker because the blood pools there. The person's pulse may feel very weak.

Mental confusion often occurs. The dying person may not be able to keep track of the day, time, or even who you are. Reassure them by telling them the day, time, and your name. Hallucination is not uncommon. Don't be surprised to hear the person call out to someone who has already died or to talk about his or her life earlier as if it were today.

Breathing becomes difficult, shallow, raspy, and irregular. Sometimes the person may stop breathing for 10 to 30 seconds. Every breath seems like the last.

Senses may not be as sharp. Vision becomes blurred. Sometimes the person's eyes become more sensitive to light. Hearing is the last sense to go. So even if the person doesn't answer, go ahead and talk. He or she may still hear you.

Being with the person during the last few days can be difficult for family and friends. It's time for everyone to start letting go. If the dying person is conscious, it's important to assure him or her that family and friends will be all right.

Some family members and friends want to be present at the time of the person's death. They want to be able to touch or talk to the dying person. If you're in this situation, choose what's right for you. There's nothing wrong with leaving the room. It's hard to see someone you love die.

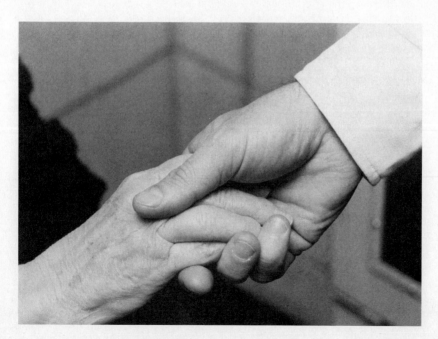

*Touch is an important and meaningful way to communicate your care and concern for a dying friend or relative.*

*A flat electro-encephalogram test, which shows no brain waves, is one indicator of brain death.*

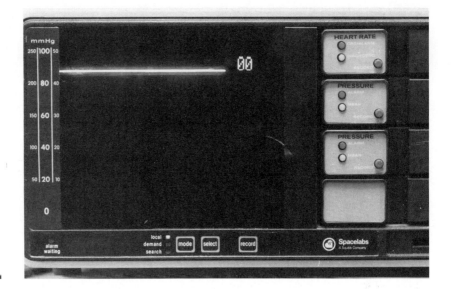

## Death—A Definition

The actual moment of death is very brief. It's the time when breathing and heart beat stop.

According to laws in some states, a person may be considered legally dead before actual death occurs. This is true when the brain has stopped functioning, even if sophisticated equipment can keep the heart and lungs going. Death is defined by most laws and health professionals as when the body meets four conditions:

- no reflexes
- permanent coma, or a very deep state of unconsciousness
- no brain waves, or flat electroencephalogram test
- no breathing or movement without a mechanical respirator

## Immediate Care after Death

After death occurs, family and friends need to deal with their own emotions. Children may need special help understanding the loss of a parent or other very close relative. These are some healthful ways you might cope when you learn that someone close has died:

- hug or be hugged by someone you care about
- cry
- breathe deeply
- go somewhere to be alone
- stay with the dead person for a few moments
- hold hands with a friend
- think about your happiest memory of the deceased
- take a walk in the sunshine
- do something helpful like inform others of the death

The next of kin must make an immediate decision about an autopsy. An *autopsy* is a medical exam of the body organs to learn the cause of death. This may be important health history for a family to know. For most terminally ill people an autopsy isn't necessary.

## Final Arrangements

Following death, there are many final arrangements that must be made immediately. Terminally ill people often choose to pre-plan these arrangements themselves, knowing that decisions are hard when the family is emotionally upset. If not, surviving family members or friends make the arrangements. The major decision is for the disposal of the body through organ donation, cremation, or burial.

Some body organs or an entire body may be donated to science or to an organ transplant program. These agreements usually are made far in advance of death, unless death is caused by an accident. In most cases, the family knows about the agreement. Some states put an organ donor agreement on the back of the driver's license. A signature on a license isn't legally binding, but it indicates the deceased's wish to contribute to life after death.

*Cremation* is reducing the body to ashes using heat. The ashes may be buried, scattered, or kept in a container. The process of cremation isn't costly for the family.

Burial is a common arrangement. The body is put in a *casket*, or box-type container used for burial. The casket is lowered into the ground and covered, or placed in a vault for above-ground burial.

Following death, a funeral director or cleric usually handles the body and carries out the family's or friends' wishes. An obituary, or death notice in the newspaper, is prepared. As you know, a funeral is a ceremony to honor the deceased. It is the time for survivors and friends to say goodbye, to grieve, to get support from others, and to deal with the finality of death.

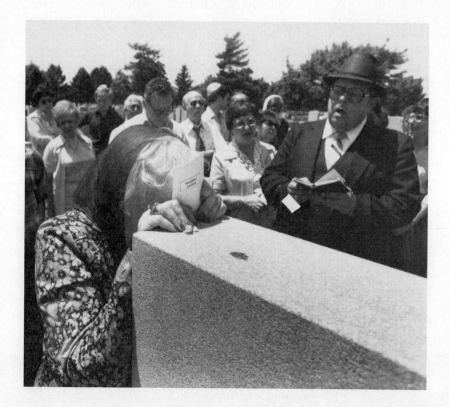

*Many families have a ceremony at the gravesite as a time to honor the deceased and to say their personal goodbyes.*

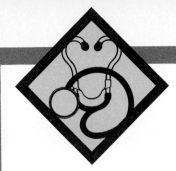

# CHAPTER CHECKUP

## Reviewing the Information

1. What is a terminal illness?
2. Describe the common responses a person may have to his or her own death.
3. Describe the ways family and friends might grieve for the deceased.
4. What is mourning?
5. How might a teenager feel when faced with his or her own terminal illness?
6. What are the advantages and disadvantages of caring for the terminally ill at home?
7. What care can be provided by a nursing home or hospital that can't be provided at home?
8. What is hospice care?
9. Describe three community programs for people with incurable diseases.
10. How might you help a terminally ill person relieve pain?
11. Why is it helpful to keep a dying person active for as long as possible?
12. What kind of psychological support might you give a dying person?
13. Describe the signs of imminent death.
14. What is an autopsy, and why might it be done?
15. How might people let their family and doctor know if they desire to donate their body organs when they die?
16. Why is a funeral important to many families?
17. What is the Dream Factory?

## Thinking It Over

1. Imagine for a moment that you have an incurable disease. How would you feel?
2. Describe how you might help a friend who is dying of leukemia.
3. Where might you go for community support if you were caring for a grandparent with cancer?
4. Would you consider donating your body to science? Discuss the pros and cons.
5. How would you feel about caring for a terminally ill relative in your home?
6. How might family members deal with the death of a loved one immediately after the time of death?

## Taking Action

1. If you were to die today, how would you be remembered? Write your obituary for your local newspaper.

2. Read the obituaries in your local newspaper for a week. Compile the ages of the deceased. Are you surprised at the ages?
3. Write or call the American Cancer Society to learn about their programs for the terminally ill.
4. If there is a hospice program in your community, volunteer to help.
5. Discuss with your parents or grandparents the final arrangements they want for themselves.
6. Practice guided imagery with a friend.

# 15

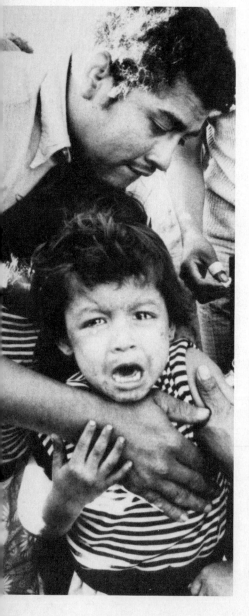

# Community, National, and World Health

After reading this chapter, you should be able to:

• identify ways the community controls infectious disease.

• discuss how pollution, natural disasters, overpopulation, and community violence affect public health.

• identify how citizens can contribute to public health.

## Terms to Understand

| | |
|---|---|
| acid rain | pollution |
| decibel | quarantine |
| epidemic | radiation |
| famine | sewage |
| ozone | smog |
| pollutants | |

Individuals, families, and communities depend on each other for good health and well-being. Health concerns don't stop at community, or even national, boundaries, however. The health concerns of the world's citizens are closely linked to each other.

Today the world is described as a global village. A disease such as AIDS, which was first seen in Africa, has quickly spread to people in the United States, perhaps carried by travelers. Insects common in one part of the world are spread through food shipped elsewhere, affecting crops or spreading disease. Poisonous gases released by industry in one country are carried by air currents to another. Hunger in Africa, disease in Malaysia, or disaster in Mexico City are shown by satellite on television, and citizens around the world contribute to relief efforts.

National and community policies and activities affect your family's health, too. Controlling infectious disease, environmental hazards, and community violence, as well as responding to the problems of overpopulation and natural disasters, are important to public health. The private, government, and international agencies you learned about in Chapter 4 are dedicated to public health. It is also your responsibility to help promote public health.

## Infectious Diseases

Americans are healthier today than ever before. During the past century, progress has been made in reducing and, in some cases, wiping out many infectious diseases that threatened lives for decades. This is one reason why people in the United States live longer today than they did 100 years ago.

Less than 100 years ago, diseases such as smallpox, diphtheria, measles, scarlet fever, influenza, and tuberculosis were the leading causes of death. These communicable diseases moved very quickly through the population. The rapid spread of many diseases rose to epidemic levels. An *epidemic* occurs when a communicable disease affects large numbers of people. *Quarantine,* or isolating and restricting a person or family with disease, was a common way to prevent the contagious disease from spreading. In those days, communities didn't have the knowledge or technology to control these diseases.

Today many infectious diseases that once were killers can be controlled. Improvements in sanitation practices, nutrition and eating patterns, and housing standards help control disease. Scientists also have a greater understanding of the body's ability to defend itself against disease.

Most infectious diseases have been brought under control. But the pathogens that cause them are still in the environment, and people still are susceptible to infectious disease. People must know how to protect themselves from getting sick. Good health practices, such as good nutrition and rest, help maintain physical immunity. Personal hygiene, as well as sanitary practices

| Changes in Life Expectancy in the United States | |
|---|---|
| Birth Year | Life Expectancy at Birth |
| 1900 | 49.2 years |
| 1910 | 51.5 years |
| 1920 | 56.4 years |
| 1930 | 59.2 years |
| 1940 | 63.6 years |
| 1950 | 68.1 years |
| 1960 | 69.9 years |
| 1970 | 70.8 years |
| 1980 | 73.7 years |

*Source: National Center for Health Statistics*

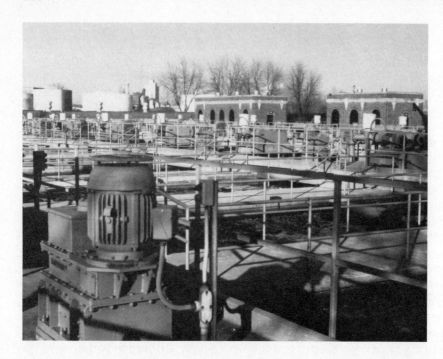

*A sewage treatment facility helps ensure the safety of the community water supply.*

within the home, help control disease. In Chapters 7 and 11, you learned how to control the spread of disease at home.

Many people are immunized regularly to help build immunity. An immunization schedule is given on page **242.** Infectious diseases within the community are controlled largely through the activities of local and state public health departments. These are some, but not all, of their activities:

- Maintaining water purification facilities to ensure that water used at home and in public places is safe for drinking and cooking.
- Maintaining sewage treatment facilities to remove, treat, and dispose safely of waste materials from the home and public areas. *Sewage* is formed from human waste, food, detergents, and other substances.
- Ensuring the safe and correct removal and disposal of garbage from private and public places. Food and other organic material decays and promotes the spread of disease.
- Spraying certain areas with pesticides to kill insects that might spread disease.
- Seeing that restrooms in public areas, such as parks, are kept clean.
- Picking up stray animals that might become or already may be infected with rabies.
- Inspecting the cleanliness of public eating places and food manufacturing plants. This includes making sure that certain food industry employees are regularly checked for contagious diseases, such as hepatitis and tuberculosis.
- Maintaining health clinics for people who can't afford their own physicians.
- Collecting data on diseases from doctors and hospitals, then analyzing the data so they can warn the public about disease outbreaks.

- In some states, requiring the testing for sexually-transmitted diseases before issuing marriage licenses.
- Coordinating immunization programs.
- Educating the public about public health practices.

## Environmental Hazards

What is a "quality" environment? Some people would say that it's a small town or perhaps a farm. Others would describe a quality environment as a modern city. A few would say that it's a natural wilderness or a mountainside resort.

A quality environment is not a place. It's the surroundings that promote good physical, emotional, and social health. Clean air, pure water, and safe food sources are among the things that many people expect.

Some of the most serious issues facing Americans deal with the environment. People have been creative in controlling or conquering the land. The accomplishments have changed the environment, often at a great price. Forests have been cut to clear land for farmers. Rivers, rich with fish, have been used to carry industrial wastes away from factories. Mountains and valleys have been changed to make room for highways. Coastlines have become a place for high-rise hotels, rather than waterfowl. People now know that land and natural resources have limits. This affects the health and well-being of present and future generations.

Hazards in the environment that cause air, water, and soil to become contaminated can cause health problems. Medical discoveries and improved health practices have increased the life span for the average person. Yet, Americans haven't been able to control or remove many environmental hazards that shorten lives and cause disease.

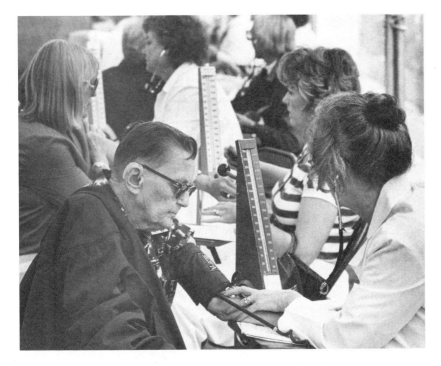

*The public health department may work with other organizations to sponsor a community health fair. Citizens are screened for various medical conditions at the health fair.*

Pollution from man-made industries and activities is a major environmental hazard. *Pollution* is the harmful change in the environment that occurs when unclean or dangerous substances are present. These substances are called *pollutants*. Pollutants are harmful to people and other forms of life. Exhaust fumes, aerosol sprays, industrial waste products, loud noises, and radioactive substances are all pollutants. With more and more technology, the amount of pollution also increases.

## Air Pollution

Air pollution is the contamination of air with harmful gases and particles. It is unhealthy for human beings, as well as animal and plant life.

Almost no place is completely free of air pollution. The amount of air pollution depends on the geographic location, the number of people that live in the area, the type of industry present, and the weather conditions.

### CAUSES OF AIR POLLUTION

Chemical substances in the air are one end result of manufacturing and burning fuel for energy. The air outside your home is polluted by exhaust from vehicles, industry, and other sources.

One major air pollutant is carbon monoxide. Carbon monoxide is a gas released in the exhaust of cars, trucks, buses, and other vehicles. Two other pollutants, nitrogen oxide and hydrocarbons, are also given off. With more vehicles on the road than ever before, the risk to clean air is greater. In the past, lead in gasoline put too much lead into the air. This is changing now that many cars run on unleaded gas.

Industry is the second major cause of air pollution. Fuels used in industry may produce toxic, or poisonous, gases, such as sul-

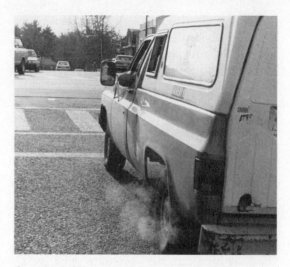

*Cars have been one of the major air polluters. How might you help control air pollution if you are a driver?*

fur dioxide and nitrogen dioxide, and harmful particles that float in the air. These substances are released into the atmosphere through factory smokestacks.

Besides vehicles and industry, air pollution comes from many other sources. As you read, you will realize that not just outdoor air is polluted. Even the air within homes and public buildings can be polluted.

- Insecticides and fertilizers applied to crops are released into the air. Insecticides are chemicals that kill insects, and fertilizers provide the nutrients plants need to grow. Without these chemicals, there may not be enough food for people to eat so the benefits outweigh the risks.
- Asbestos is a mineral fiber once commonly used as a building material. Because it has been found to cause severe lung problems and some forms of cancer, it is being removed from old structures. Now asbestos is used safely in insulated form in items such as potholders and protective clothing.

- Burning leaves can pollute and affect breathing. That's why many communities don't allow people to burn leaves or trash.
- Smoke from cigarettes, cigars, and pipes can pollute the air in your home and other buildings.
- Some household chemicals, such as spot removers and paint thinners, can produce harmful fumes.
- Formaldehyde is a chemical that is used on some fabrics, carpeting, and certain types of insulation. This chemical can give off unhealthful vapors.
- Fluorocarbons are gases used in aerosol spray cans to force the contents from the can. Fluorocarbons help destroy the protective ozone layer in the atmosphere. *Ozone* is a gas that helps shield the earth from the sun's harmful ultraviolet rays. Without the protective ozone layer we would be exposed to more harmful rays, and the world's climate would become warmer.

## WEATHER AND AIR POLLUTION

Does it surprise you that weather and air pollution are interrelated? Weather affects the spread of air pollution, while air pollution can affect climate and cause rain, snow, and sleet to be polluted. When the air is dry, air currents move pollutants away from industrial areas. But then the pollutants travel with the wind to places thousands of miles away and can affect other people and places. Air pollution can affect the quality of air around the globe.

Moist or humid conditions, clouds, and fog keep pollutants in place. Do you live in a city with a smog problem? If so, you probably have heard a daily smog report with the weather report. *Smog* is a yellowish-brown combination of smoke, chemical fumes, and fog. If the air currents can't move

the pollution away, the air becomes even more polluted, causing poor visibility and difficult breathing.

*Acid rain* is a combination of pollutants with rain, snow, or sleet. When fossil fuels, such as oil and coal, are burned by industry for energy, sulfuric and nitric oxides are formed. Rain combines with these oxides in the air, and they return to Earth as acid rain. Acid rain inhibits the growth of crops and forests. It pollutes the water supply, affecting fish and other animals. It also corrodes buildings and other structures.

The world's temperature is heating up. Some scientists believe this is caused by air pollution damaging the protective ozone layer in the earth's atmosphere. Even a two-degree temperature change in the earth's atmosphere could seriously influence conditions that affect health, such as agricultural production of food.

## HEALTH RISKS OF AIR POLLUTION

Air pollution affects people's health in many ways. Breathing problems are common. Air passages become clogged with tiny particles so some people have more difficulty getting the oxygen they need. As air pollution has increased, more people suffer from respiratory diseases such as allergies, asthma, pneumonia, and emphysema. Lung cancer is more common where levels of air pollution are high. Itching or burning eyes, frequent coughing, headaches, skin rash, or a feeling of nausea may be caused by air pollution.

During heavy smog, when oxygen levels are especially low, individuals are encouraged to take health precautions. People with respiratory problems are advised to reduce physical activity, so they avoid shortness of breath and chest pains. Everyone may experience eye discomfort, so it's better to stay inside. Driving should be reduced since more

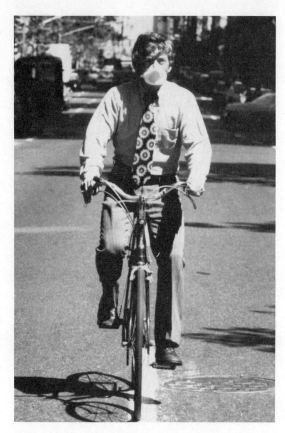

*Pollution is a threat to personal health.*

## ACTIONS AGAINST AIR POLLUTION

Industry, government, and citizens are all working to reduce air pollution. The amount of pollution partly depends on the kind of fuel industry uses. Industries are trying to use fuels that emit fewer harmful pollutants into the air and that are also available and not too expensive. Natural gas, a "clean" fuel, doesn't cause much pollution, but it's in short supply and expensive. Coal and shale oil, on the other hand, are reasonably priced and abundant, but they produce more air pollution. Factory managers need to consider profit, of course, but they still need to be responsible for air quality.

State and federal governments have set standards for air quality. The Environmental Protection Agency (EPA) is a federal agency that sees that these standards are followed. They enforce standards to protect the environment. They regulate the kinds of fuel and the amount of pollutants that industry can emit into the air. For example, the federal government set standards that required automobile manufacturers to make engines that gave off fewer pollutants in their exhaust. It is the EPA's job to make sure these standards are adhered to. The United States also works closely with some other countries to protect the world's air.

You can make an important effort to reduce air pollution. For example, you might work with an environmental action group that talks to legislators and industry leaders about clean air laws. You can also reduce air pollution by the way you use your car. Using public transportation and sharing rides with others puts fewer cars on the road. You can keep your car's engine and exhaust system in good working order so it emits fewer pollutants. And you can use non-aerosol consumer products. Being a nonsmoker and discouraging others from smoking also helps reduce air pollution.

vehicles add more carbon monoxide and other pollutants to the air. Smoking should also be curtailed because it adds to the already heavily polluted air. Alcohol consumption during a smog alert can cause an even greater health risk than usual. This is because the combination of drinking alcohol while breathing air low in oxygen can even further affect one's thinking and judgment than drinking alcohol alone.

High levels of air pollution can also keep agricultural crops from reaching their full growth. This can affect the abundance of nutritious foods available.

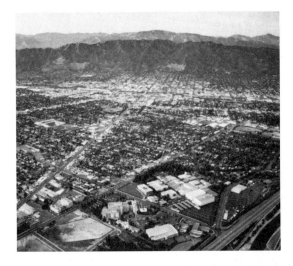

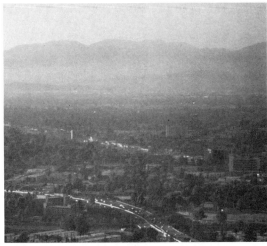

*Many government, industry, and consumer efforts are helping to improve the quality of air.*

# Water Pollution

The world is very dependent upon water resources for drinking, for food, and for recreation. Yet, for years, waterways have been used to dispose of waste materials. The result is water pollution in many places. Some water sources can't be used for drinking.

Others are unfit for fish. A few can't even be used for swimming or other kinds of water sports and recreation.

Two sources of water must be protected from pollution—surface water and groundwater. Surface water includes streams, rivers, and lakes. Groundwater consists of underground streams that supply wells and springs. Clean water from both sources is essential to the well-being of human beings and to the earth's total environment.

## CAUSES OF WATER POLLUTION

Water is polluted by sewage, industrial waste, and agricultural drainage. Waterways first became polluted when individual and community sewage systems dumped untreated sewage into nearby rivers or streams. Today most cities have sewage treatment and water purification systems that help ensure clean water. Many rural areas use septic tanks to treat sewage. But in some places sewage still gets into the water supply because there is no adequate sanitation system.

Industrial wastes make their way into the water supply in these ways:

- Acid rain carries industrial wastes in the air back to Earth where they become a part of both surface and groundwater sources.
- Toxic chemicals that are by-products of manufacturing are often sealed in metal drums and stored underground. If the drums leak, chemical wastes may seep into the groundwater. It's difficult to predict how or where chemical wastes will affect the millions of streams in the underground water system and contaminate the water supply.
- Sometimes unscrupulous manufacturers try to cut costs by illegally dumping toxic chemicals and other wastes directly into rivers and streams.

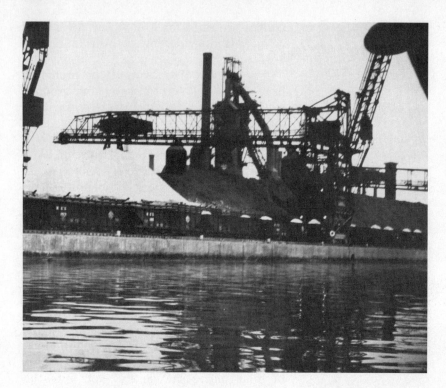

*Industrial pollution is a worldwide problem. As countries industrialize, rivers and lakes are more likely to become polluted. In the U.S., the Environmental Protection Agency has established rules for chemical waste disposal. Even so, some chemicals pollute water and soil, thus affecting food sources.*

• Hot water from factories or electric power plants pollutes even though it's free of contaminants. A change in water temperature can kill or injure fish and plants that grow in water.

The purity of water is also threatened by agricultural chemicals. Chemicals that have been sprayed on crops, such as pesticides or fertilizers, may wash back into rivers, lakes, and oceans or seep into the groundwater. Although most of these chemicals break down into harmless substances, others may affect water life. If a toxic or poisonous chemical reaches the groundwater, it may pass into the underground water system.

## HEALTH RISKS FROM WATER POLLUTION

How does polluted water cause disease? Pathogens and chemicals pose health risks.

Pathogens in the water supply can spread diseases through a community. Hepatitis and typhoid are two of the diseases spread by pathogens in unclean water. This is often a problem when natural disasters such as floods hit, causing sewage to get into the water supply. Places with poor sewage treatment also have this problem.

Many chemicals in water threaten human health and wildlife. Some chemicals are carcinogenic, or cancer-causing. Most water purification systems can't remove all chemical pollutants in water.

Water pollution affects the delicate balance of nature. Plants and fish die, so the food supply is affected. Eating fish or shellfish contaminated by polluted water is an unseen hazard. They may not appear diseased, but eating them can cause you to become very ill.

## PROTECTION FROM WATER POLLUTION

Once water becomes polluted, it takes a long time before the water source returns to a healthful condition. For example, when an oil tanker spills oil into the ocean and onto the beaches, the ocean needs 30 years to clean its coastline. In the meantime, plants, birds, fish, and humans are affected.

The Environmental Protection Agency monitors the water supply as well as the air. Laws control the kind of materials that can be dumped into water supplies.

Thanks to public pressure and federal and state laws, many polluted lakes and rivers are gradually being cleaned up. Lake Erie, one of the Great Lakes, once was so polluted that few forms of life could live in the waters. Many industrial cities dumped their wastes there until it became a "dead" lake. The combined efforts of citizens, industry, and governmental agencies have restored Lake Erie to a much healthier condition.

You can contact your community health department to learn about the purity of your water. Never drink contaminated water or use it for ice cubes, food preparation, or even to brush your teeth. If your water comes from your own well, be careful to keep it pure. If you're unsure of your drinking water's safety, purify it to kill any harmful germs. Chapter 5 gives you instructions for water purification. These methods cannot get rid of chemical pollutants, however. Avoid eating fish, shellfish, or seafood caught in polluted water, and refrain from bathing or swimming there.

## Landfills and Waste Disposal

As the number of people on Earth increases, more people who use more products must live in the same amount of space. With a larger population, there are more waste products to dispose of and less space to dis-

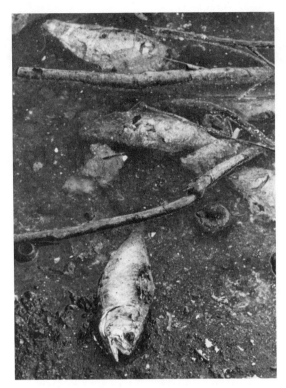

*A single oil spill can pollute the coastline for many years. This makes the water and beach unsafe for swimming and endangers plant and animal life.*

pose of them. Garbage from households and public places as well as industrial wastes—by-products or leftovers of manufacturing—must be disposed of properly. Every year people and industry discard tons of garbage and other wastes that are hauled to landfills. There it is supposed to be handled in a safe, sanitary way to protect the environment and public health. However, many landfills, both industrial and public, don't meet minimal safety and health standards.

Even while toxic industrial wastes are being hauled to a dump site, they pose potential health hazards. If the vehicle transporting the wastes has an accident and the

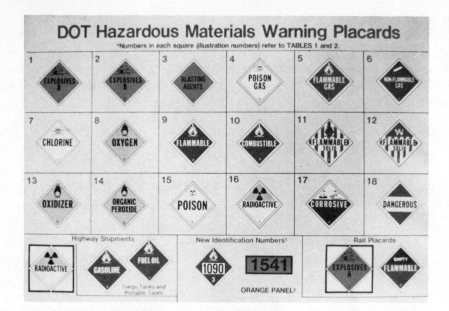

## DOT Hazardous Materials Warning Placards
*Numbers in each square (illustration numbers) refer to TABLES 1 and 2.

*Hazardous materials are hauled by trucks to safe disposal sites. A caution on the truck warns drivers of the truck's load.*

wastes are spilled, then toxic fumes can fill the air, and toxic chemicals can contaminate the ground as well as nearby water.

Industries and consumers are taking a serious look at ways to handle both nontoxic and toxic waste. Besides carefully managed garbage disposal, nontoxic garbage can be handled in responsible ways. Garbage has been used to create an energy supply for electricity. Many Americans are recycling glass, metals, and paper. They take these waste products to recycling centers so resources can be used again and again, and so there is less waste to be disposed of.

Toxic wastes pose a far greater problem. They are often expensive to dispose of safely and effectively. These materials can be sealed in drums, carefully transported, and buried in toxic landfills or waste sites. However, accidents can occur during transportation. Drums can occasionally leak and contaminate the ground and groundwater.

Industries around the nation and world need to take responsibility for the toxic chemicals they produce. In the United States, the EPA watches over the production, use, transportation, and disposal of chemicals for public well-being. Internationally, the World Health Association is also concerned about hazardous materials.

## Noise Pollution

Does it surprise you that noise can be another form of pollution? The environment is filled with noise of all kinds. But in recent years, the noise level in some cities has increased. Now environmental noise is considered a kind of pollution.

### CAUSES OF NOISE POLLUTION

Noise is actually excessive sound. It becomes a pollutant when it's disturbing, damages hearing, or both. The intensity of a sound, its frequency, and its length all determine if a sound is really noise pollution.

A *decibel* is a measurement to show how loud sounds really are. It tells the amount

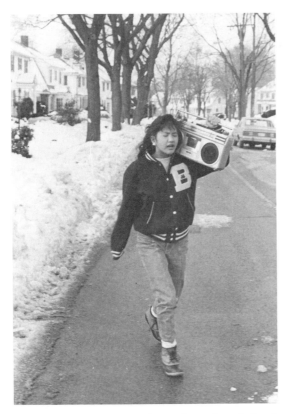

*Listening to loud music for prolonged periods of time causes permanent ear damage. Loud music may also annoy other people who are nearby.*

of pressure being put on the ear by various noises. The normal ear can hear sounds that range from one decibel to over 150 decibels.

Noise levels above 85 decibels, for long periods of time, cause permanent hearing loss. Compare the average decibels in these sounds to learn how loud 85 decibels is:

- Leaves rustling                    20 decibels
- Normal conversation         60 decibels
- Sound of a vacuum           70 decibels
  cleaner
- Music of a live rock band   125 decibels
- Jet engine at take-off          130 decibels

## HEALTH RISKS FROM NOISE POLLUTION

Environmental noise contributes to a variety of health problems. Loss of hearing is the most obvious damage. One in every 10 Americans is exposed, on a regular basis, to noises loud enough to cause a hearing loss. One-third of all college freshmen suffer from a hearing loss. Why? Some say it's because teenagers listen to very loud music so often.

Ask yourself: are you regularly exposed to sounds at high-decibel levels? If so, what causes the loud sounds? Is it necessary to be near those high-decibel sounds?

After going to a rock concert, you might experience temporary hearing loss that comes back in a few hours. Permanent damage to the ears may be caused as well, meaning that hearing cannot be restored or corrected to the original levels. Loud sounds destroy the sensory hair cells inside the inner ear. Sensory hairs transmit sounds of both high- and low-decibel levels.

Noise pollution affects rest and relaxation. Over time, it may cause emotional stress that can lead to physical health problems. For example, headaches, irritability, high blood pressure, ulcers, and nervous system disorders may be related to environmental noise.

The body treats loud noise as a warning signal of danger. Although most sounds aren't related to danger, your body still reacts as if you've been threatened. When you hear a jackhammer, siren, or other loud sound, your blood pressure and breathing and heart rates may increase. Your muscles become tense. Hormones, which are body chemicals, may be released into your bloodstream, causing you to perspire.

Some people say that loud noises don't bother them. However, studies show that even people who are asleep in a high noise area have higher heart and breathing rates

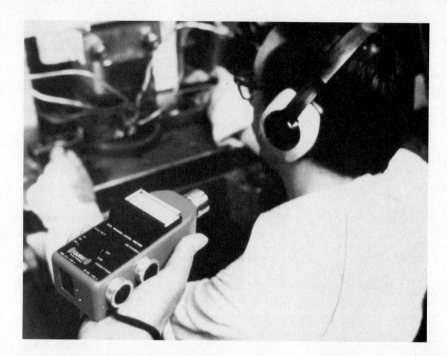

*An industrial hygienist measures the noise level in a manufacturing plant with electronic equipment called a sound-level meter. Checking and helping control other types of pollution caused by manufacturing are also part of the job.*

than they do when they sleep in a quiet place. People living in neighborhoods with high noise levels make more visits to the doctor than those living in quieter neighborhoods. And a noisy learning environment can interfere with learning and with mental development.

### PROTECTION FROM NOISE POLLUTION

Noise pollution is usually easy for individuals to control. You can protect yourself from noise with some simple precautions:

- Turn down the volume on your stereo or television.
- Limit the length of time you listen to loud noises.
- Use earplugs if you must be near loud noises.
- Help deaden noise in a room by using drapes, rugs, and upholstered furniture.
- Plant trees and shrubs outside to reduce loud noises around your house.

- Find out about the noise standards in your community, and see if anything can be done to control noisy conditions.

Noise is a problem in many workplaces. Industries are required to meet governmental regulations that control noise on the job. If you work in a place with too much loud noise, talk to your boss about it or to the labor union, if you belong to one. If the noise isn't controlled, workers can also contact the Occupational Safety and Health Administration (OSHA). OSHA is a federal agency responsible for setting workplace safety standards and enforcing them. The EPA also sets standards that limit the noise of newly-built trucks, motorcycles, and construction equipment.

## Radiation Pollution

*Radiation* is a form of energy. Light rays, heat radiation, radio waves, X-rays, and cosmic rays are types of radiation.

## SOURCES OF RADIATION

Radiation comes from four main sources: nature, medical treatment, consumer products, and nuclear energy.

Natural radiation has been present in the water, sun, soil, and air since the formation of the galaxy. When you feel the warmth of sunshine, you are enjoying a form of natural radiation. The ultraviolet light of sunlight damages skin over time, but it's not considered a pollutant. Two natural materials are radioactive—uranium and radium. Most people don't come in daily contact with these materials.

Using radiation for medical diagnosis and treatment purposes is a positive use of radiation. X-rays permit early diagnosis of diseases and injuries. In small amounts, radiation treatments and radioactive drugs are successful in fighting cancer.

Some consumer products, such as microwave ovens, color televisions, and smoke detectors may give off very small amounts of radiation. When they work properly, their radiation level is very low. Microwave ovens do **not** put radiation into food.

Nuclear energy is a highly efficient power source produced from radiation. When nuclear energy is produced, radioactive waste is a by-product. Disposing of this radioactive waste presents a problem that scientists around the world are trying to solve. A major fear is that radioactive materials will leak into the water supply. Because wastes from a nuclear reactor or weapons plant remain radioactive for as long as 250 centuries, the problem is complex.

## HEALTH RISKS OF RADIATION

How much radiation is good, and how much may be harmful? In small amounts, radiation isn't harmful. However, scientists know that prolonged exposure, over time, can cause cancer and damage genes, causing birth defects. They don't know how much radiation the body can tolerate. They don't know how much actually causes cancer or how much can harm a developing fetus. Scientists are, however, continuing to work to find answers.

Nuclear power production is heavily regulated by laws and government agencies so that radiation is contained. Even with regulation, human error and machinery failure are possible, and radiation can be leaked into the air, water, and land. Nuclear power plants at Three Mile Island, Pennsylvania (1979) and in Chernobyl, Russia (1986) had failures that caused radiation leaks and threatened human life and health. With these incidents, scientists learned more about the potential dangers and ways to avoid future problems. And, each time, people had to judge the risks and benefits of using nuclear energy.

## PROTECTION FROM RADIATION

Protection from radiation is an individual, national, and international responsibility.

Because medical and dental X-rays give off radiation, be cautious about the number of X-rays you receive. Except for a medical emergency, pregnant women should avoid X-rays, especially during the first three months of pregnancy, to protect the developing fetus from radiation. Medical technicians who work near X-ray machines should wear a lead "apron" or operate the machine from behind a protective lead wall. Lead is an excellent radiation barrier.

National and international efforts are at work to protect citizens from harmful radiation. Two agencies of the U.S. Government are responsible for the safety of nuclear energy. The Department of Energy is responsible for new energy sources, for energy conservation, and for establishing energy policies. The Nuclear Regulatory Agency

*Federal laws heavily regulate the production of nuclear power in order to control the amount of radiation that escapes into the atmosphere. However, there is still public concern over the use of nuclear energy.*

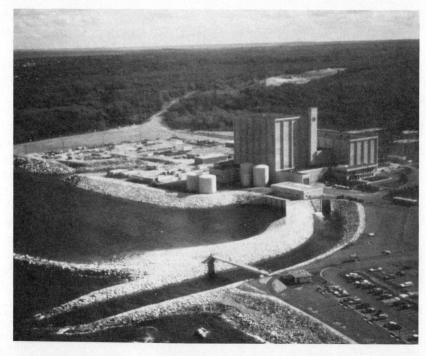

*Solar energy, or heat energy from sunlight, is safe and nonpolluting. Many homes and buildings use solar energy for heating and cooling.*

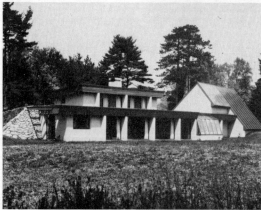

approves and regulates nuclear power plants and their operations.

Many people are concerned about the benefits and risks of nuclear power. Probably the most effective action you can take to avoid radiation pollution is to study and learn more about it. Then you can better understand the benefits, risks, alternatives, and safety precautions. Only then will you be prepared to urge decision makers in industry and government to take actions in the best interest of the public.

## Natural Disasters

People can control many parts of their lives. However, natural disasters continue to be out of their control and threaten their well-being. Disasters, such as floods, tornados, hurricanes, and earthquakes, strike both the rich and the poor, the young and the old. They strike in the center of cities just as easily as in the middle of fields. Anyone could be the victim of a disaster.

Natural disasters affect the health and safety of individuals, families, and communities in many ways:

• The disaster itself causes many kinds of injury, as well as death.
• Water supplies get contaminated, so communicable diseases and infections spread.

- People have no way to refrigerate food, so it spoils. Food poisoning will result if they eat spoiled food.
- Many lose their homes and possessions. They need clothing and shelter for personal protection.
- A disaster is stressful for its victims. People may experience physical, emotional, and social problems as they face their loss and try to rebuild their lives.
- Medical staff and supplies are often scarce in relation to the increased need.

The United States is well equipped to handle many natural disasters. Emergency relief plans and modern technology make it possible to provide quick and efficient help for most disasters.

Some organizations respond to the immediate needs of individuals and communities during disasters. The American Red Cross, the Department of Civil Defense, The Salvation Army, and the United States National Guard provide disaster relief. The feature on pages **360** and **361** shows how a Red Cross nurse helps in a community after a disaster.

Natural disasters threaten cities and villages all over the world. Some disasters have been known to wipe out entire communities and kill thousands of people.

Many parts of the world, particularly remote, impoverished, or overpopulated areas, aren't able to efficiently handle the results of a disaster. They have inadequate medical and emergency equipment, few health professionals, and unsophisticated communications systems. Clothing, food, water, and medicine may be needed in staggering amounts which they don't have.

In times of disaster, members of the world population often work to help the victims. Together many nations and their citizens share the responsibility of meeting human needs without regard for a country's politics. For example, quantities of food, water, medicine, and clothing, along with medical staff, are quickly airlifted around the globe. Being a citizen of the world is important to global health and human survival.

## Overpopulation and Hunger

Do you ever feel that there are too many people around you? Overpopulation is a concern to cities and countries around the globe. During the last 100 years, the population of the world has increased by 300 percent. This means that more and more people are sharing natural resources, such as food, water, land, and fuel. Some worry that there may be too many "passengers" aboard Planet Earth.

### Public Health Is Your Responsibility!

You, your family, and your friends can respond in many different ways to health concerns in the community, the nation, and the world.

- Be informed about the causes of public health problems, and learn ways that you can help prevent disease.
- Be a good citizen, and practice habits that promote the public's health and well-being.
- Contribute food, supplies, or money to disaster victims.
- Volunteer your time to help disaster victims, perhaps by distributing clothing or preparing and serving food.
- Join a volunteer organization that helps people in need.
- Participate in fund-raising efforts for volunteer agencies whose goals include protecting or providing for the health and well-being of others.
- Be alert to legislation on issues that affect public health and the environment. Communicate your beliefs with letters to decision makers in government.

# DISASTER RELIEF

The American Red Cross has over a 100-year history of caring for victims of disaster, providing emergency food, clothing, shelter, and health care. In 1985 alone, the Red Cross spent over 50 million dollars of the American public's voluntary contributions to help victims of hurricanes, fires, mudslides, airplane crashes, and many other disasters.

A nurse is an important part of the Red Cross disaster team. In May, 1986, a tornado, with winds exceeding 250 miles per hour, devastated two towns in Missouri. Two people were killed and many more were injured. A total of 632 families were affected by the tornado. Margaret Wichard, R.N., a Red Cross disaster nurse, was on the scene to help the victims.

Margaret visited disaster victims to evaluate their homes for health problems, such as contaminated food and water. She advised them on safe ways to handle their food supply and on how to purify water.

Following a disaster, many homes don't have functioning kitchens. Often extensive damage makes the homes unlivable. Until families can arrange alternative ways to prepare food, the services of the Red Cross feeding van are available to them. It makes rounds of the disaster areas to provide three meals per day. Hot items, such as beef stew, vegetable soup, sloppy joes, and coffee, are served. Supplemental foods such as fruit, boiled eggs, wheat crackers, and oatmeal cookies are distributed also.

Disaster nurses staff temporary shelters where victims stay until they can return to their homes. They are usually located in school gyms, or other buildings. In shelters, nurses take care of all kinds of physical and psychological health problems.

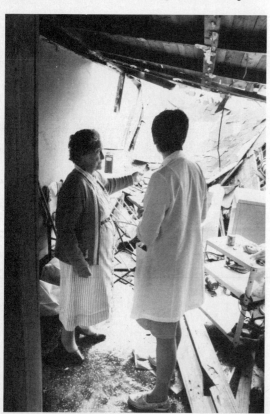

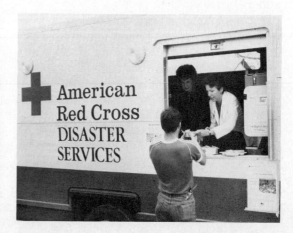

They must be especially careful about the spread of communicable diseases because many people live in very close quarters. Red Cross service centers help disaster victims with their losses. Interviewers assess the damages each home sustained and provide funds for food and clothing.

Talking about and facing such major losses is emotionally stressful. Reactions might include insomnia, periods of crying, or depression. A nurse, such as Margaret, helps parents and their children cope with their emotional reactions. She also replaces lost medicines, finds ways to pay medical bills, and screens for flareups of chronic diseases, such as high blood pressure.

A tornado strews a good deal of debris about a community. When victims begin to clean up, many step on nails or broken glass. To prevent health problems, the Red Cross works with local public health officials as they immunize local citizens.

Other Red Cross nursing functions at the site of a disaster include staffing morgues, contacting hospitals about victims they've treated, and referring victims to local resources. A morgue is a place where the dead are kept until they have been identified.

The American Red Cross has a commitment to care for victims of manmade and natural disasters. Nurses such as Margaret, who provide vital health services, are an important part of the relief effort.

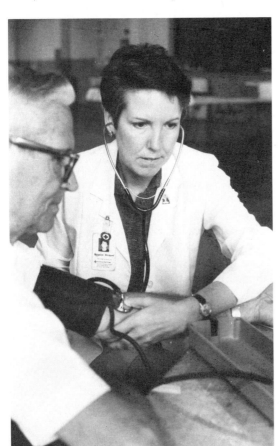

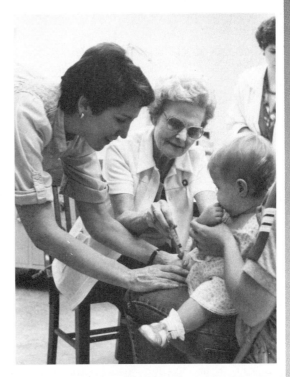

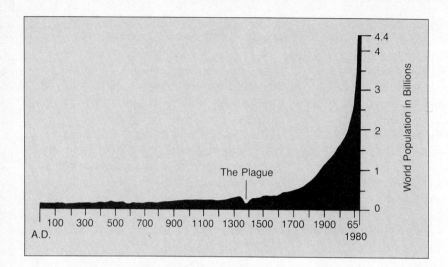

The Plague

World Population in Billions

4.4
4
3
2
1
0

100  300  500  700  900  1100  1300  1500  1700  1900  65
A.D.                                                      1980

*The world population has increased dramatically over the past 100 years, in large part due to better health care. How will continued population growth affect health?*

In 1900, there were about one-and-a-half billion people on Earth. Today there are almost five billion people. And by the year 2025 the world population is expected to be over eight billion! There are two reasons why the world population has grown rapidly in recent years. First, more babies are being born who survive infancy. Second, improved medical care has made it possible for people all over the world to live longer.

Overpopulation affects public health in many ways. When large numbers of people live close together, disease can spread more quickly. Sanitation problems increase when facilities and housing are inadequate for serving large numbers of people. With more people, a larger supply of nutritious food and safe water is needed. Less space is available for recreation. Traffic increases, causing congestion and more pollution. And, as many persons move from rural villages to cities, finding employment becomes a real concern. Unemployment leads to poverty which makes it difficult to afford housing, food, and medical care.

Concerns about world hunger and malnutrition are closely linked to concerns about the size of the world population. Malnutrition means that people don't get all the nutrients their bodies need. Approximately one in five people around the world is malnourished. Even in the United States where grocery shelves are full, people at poverty level are malnourished. In some countries, the population is growing faster than food can be produced. When these countries experience agricultural problems, such as crops being destroyed by flooding, drought, or insects, famine results. *Famine* is an extreme scarcity of food and usually leads to starvation and death.

Malnutrition seriously affects health, physical energy, and growth. When their bodies aren't properly nourished, people are subject to disease and extreme lack of energy. Emotional and social needs are difficult to meet when physical needs for food, even water, aren't fully met. Severe malnutrition can affect brain development and may cause death. Children and the elderly suffer most when food supplies are short.

World population growth will be a major international issue for the rest of this century and into the next. Many nations rec-

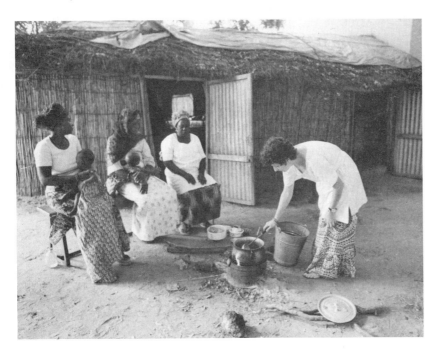

*Nutritionists in many parts of the world work to fight hunger and malnutrition. A Peace Corps volunteer gives a nutrition lesson using traditional cooking methods and foods recently introduced as a local crop.*

ognize that food resources for survival and health must be shared among nations around the globe.

## Community Violence

Violence has a serious effect on the health of a community. Physical injury, emotional stress, social alienation, even death are among its results.

Fortunately, most people aren't victims of personal violence. However, an increasing number are rightfully concerned about safety in their home, their workplace, or their community. Even the fear of violence may be harmful. Experiencing real or needless fear over long periods of time is stressful and can affect a person's emotional and physical health.

Many factors contribute to violence. Drug and alcohol abuse, which you learned about in Chapter 3, are closely linked to physical assault, rape, and other acts of violence. Overcrowding, poverty, unjust conditions, inability to communicate, greed, lack of self-esteem, and other emotional and social problems contribute to violence as well.

Every day you are exposed to real or imagined violence on television and in movies, and in newspapers and advertisements. Many mental health professionals believe that seeing frequent violence actually may contribute to a person's violent behavior. A person may copy violent behavior as a way to handle conflicts or extreme stress.

The problems that lead to acts of violence are complex and must be addressed by community and national efforts. As a citizen, you can support citizens-against-violence programs or help remove conditions that lead to violence. You can also help and support the victims of violence.

To protect yourself and others from personal abuse, refer to the guidelines found in Chapter 5.

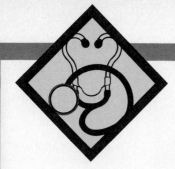

# CHAPTER CHECKUP

## Reviewing the Information

1. Describe four ways the public health department helps control the spread of communicable disease.
2. What is a quality environment?
3. What are five pollutants?
4. What are four causes of air pollution?
5. How might smog affect health?
6. How are weather and air pollution interrelated?
7. Where does acid rain come from, and what does it do?
8. How does water get polluted?
9. How does water pollution affect health?
10. What could you do to check the safety of your water supply?
11. What are the hazards of toxic wastes?
12. Why is noise called a pollutant?
13. What are the health effects of noise pollution?
14. What are some hazards of too much radiation?
15. What are two government agencies that help protect people from pollution?
16. How do natural disasters affect public health?
17. How do countries respond to global disasters?
18. How does overpopulation affect health?
19. What factors contribute to community violence?
20. Besides injury, how does violence affect personal health?

## Thinking It Over

1. Why is the world often called a global village?
2. Why have environmental health hazards increased in recent years?
3. As a citizen, how might you help control air pollution? Water pollution?
4. What are ways you can protect yourself from noise pollution?
5. Why is flooding a public health hazard?
6. Why are natural disasters often worse in many places outside the United States?
7. Why are overpopulation and hunger so closely linked?
8. How might you act as a private citizen to promote public health?

## Taking Action

 1. Use the library to research how water purification plants or landfills work. Write a report.

 2. Find out about a natural disaster that could affect your community. Write how you and your family might protect against personal injury and disease from that disaster.

 3. Follow a local environmental issue. Summarize your findings, then write your opinion.

4. Contact the local public health department to learn how the agency controls communicable diseases.

5. Research or interview to learn about a local, national, or international program that provides food to the needy.

# Careers in the Health Field

16

After reading this chapter, you should be able to:

- describe personal qualities appropriate for a successful career in the health field.

- describe how to obtain a job.

- explain the value of volunteer, part-time, and summer jobs.

- identify entry-level and professional jobs in the health field.

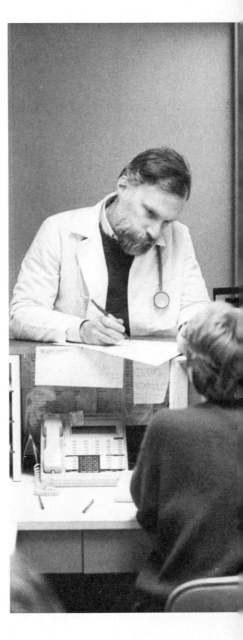

## Terms to Understand

| | |
|---|---|
| career | licensed practical nurse |
| career ladder | references |
| dietitian | registered nurse |
| entrepreneur | resume |
| entry-level job | surgical technician |

Are you committed to a healthful life style? Do you enjoy helping people feel comfortable and healthy? Do you like to learn how the body functions? If you answered "yes" to these questions, you may want a career in the health field.

The need for health care workers in the United States is growing rapidly. In its report on jobs, the U.S. Bureau of Labor indicated that the need for health workers is expected to increase by 50 percent or more by 1995. In fact, health care is one of the fastest growing professions in the United States today! Some experts feel that health occupations are developing faster than workers can be trained.

A career in health care has a wide range of job possibilities for people with many talents, interests, and levels of education. These include nutritionists, dental hygienists, nurse's aides, physicians, laboratory

## Start Now to Think About a Career

1. Take time to know yourself:
   - Your values and attitudes
   - Your personal qualities
   - Your interests
   - Your skills and abilities
   - Your goals
2. Look closely at occupations that interest you:
   - Talk with your parents, relatives, and friends' parents.
   - Talk with your teachers.
   - Talk with school counselors.
   - Talk with people who hire employees.
   - Read job descriptions in help wanted ads and career brochures.
3. Take advantage of opportunities:
   - Related courses in school
   - Work-study programs
   - Volunteer programs
   - Part-time and summer jobs
   - School and community clubs

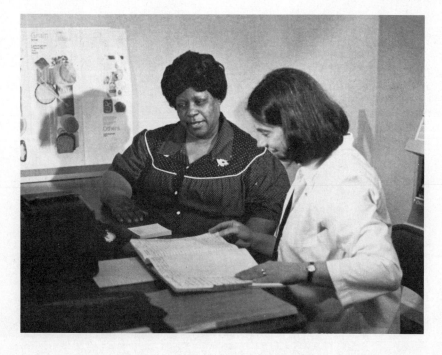

*The "Help Wanted" advertisements in local newspapers list a variety of jobs in health care and promotion.*

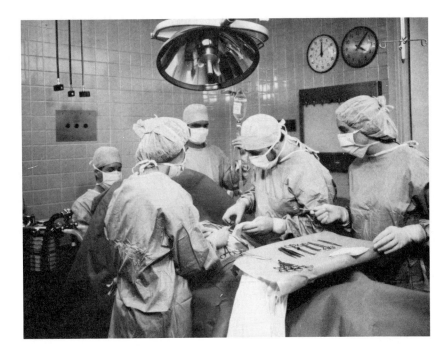

*People on a surgical team have many years of specialized training.*

technicians, and medical scientists. Many new health care opportunities are also emerging for people with specialized interests such as sports, computers, communications, and art.

If you are interested in knowing more about working in health promotion or care, investigate factors that help ensure success. Take a variety of volunteer, part-time, and summer jobs in the health field to learn more about this career field. Then look closely at health-related careers. One might be right for you!

## Success in the Workplace

Your own health, as well as your attitudes and skills, are keys to success in the workplace. Many personal qualities needed in the health field are common for employees in any job. Others are unique for people to work successfully in health care and promotion.

## Personal Health and the Job

Health and safety are important factors in successful job hunting and work itself. Throughout this book, you've learned that your lifestyle and daily decisions affect your total well-being—how you look, feel, and act. These same qualities influence your success on the job. In fact, they may even determine if you get a job!

When you're healthy, you feel good. Good health shows all over! It helps make you a happy, pleasant worker. In turn, you're likely to be more energetic and productive.

Personal habits affect your health and ultimately your value as an employee. A balanced, nutritious diet contributes to good health. Adequate rest and a balance of work and leisure contribute to physical and mental wellness. Exercise makes your body physically fit.

Safety habits are good work habits. Work-related accidents commonly occur when employees lack knowledge and job skills. Many workers think that accidents only happen to others. This attitude may cause carelessness. Then accidents occur.

People who don't follow safety rules established for their job are likely to get hurt. For example, an employee in a hospital kitchen can easily get cut if knives are handled carelessly. Or laboratory workers may infect themselves with disease if they aren't careful with the materials they're testing. OSHA, which you learned about in Chapter 5, has regulations for safety in many jobs.

Fatigue and illness cause workers to decrease their productivity. On the other hand, healthy, rested employees are aware of dangers and can give attention to safety. They have less absenteeism, fewer doctor visits which require time off, and better attitudes toward work.

Alcohol or drug abuse interferes with normal patterns and affects people's judgment and behavior. Use of alcohol or drugs also increases accidents at work. Experts estimate that 40 percent of all work-related accidents involve drinking. After a late party with heavy drinking or drugs, a worker may not get to work on time and may be sluggish, irritable, and careless on the job. Drug or alcohol use on the job or during lunch hours is dangerous, particularly for people working with equipment or when the user must care for patients who need very specific, well-monitored care. Thus, people who drink heavily or use drugs often lose their jobs.

## Attitudes at Work

Attitudes are the way people feel and think. For example, if you believe school is important, if you enjoy being there, and if you think your teachers are fair, you have a good attitude toward school. On the other hand, a person who hates school, who thinks teachers are unfair, and who feels education is not important has a poor attitude toward school. You know that attitudes affect success in school. Attitudes are equally important for success at work.

Supervisors and managers who have observed workers for a long time have identified attitudes important in all types of work. A good employee is:

- friendly. Cheerful workers and friendly smiles make other workers feel good. Customers or patients want to return to businesses, offices, and hospitals where workers are friendly.
- positive. Productive workers are people who respond to problems and challenges with an "I can do it" approach and who are willing to try.
- energetic. Employees who are willing to do extra work and give extra time to their jobs impress their supervisors as mature, responsible people.
- adaptable. Change is part of the world of work. Workers who are successful are those who learn to adapt to new procedures and to new and different management styles.
- helpful. Successful workers help each other. They are generous with their time, their knowledge, and their praise.
- reliable. Individuals who work just as well when the supervisor is absent as when he or she is present are reliable. A reliable employee is also on time and honest.
- responsible. Responsible employees understand that businesses and other organizations must make a profit or provide a service. They do their part to reach the goals of the organization. They take responsibility for their own actions. They do not try to blame others for their own mistakes.
- willing to learn. Few people have all the skills needed for a job. But if they're

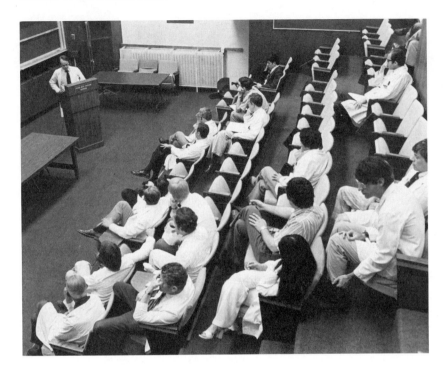

*Health professionals continue to learn about advances in health care and promotion. In this way, they provide the best service to their patients or clients.*

willing to learn, they can gain skills for many jobs. Employees also must be willing to learn new skills for the jobs they already have.

- loyal. Valuable employees show loyalty by their comments and by their service. If a person can no longer be loyal, he or she should leave the organization.

Workers with negative attitudes, on the other hand, are often less productive and more likely to make mistakes. Their bad attitudes also may rub off on others. Employers often avoid hiring employees who:

- criticize others
- are close-minded
- are not reliable
- are selfish
- feel no responsibility to the organization, other employees, or their clients.
- complain frequently
- are not friendly

All the elements of a good attitude just discussed are important qualities in a health care worker. In addition, other characteristics contribute to success. Specifically, health care workers should be caring people, concerned about the welfare of others. They need to be patient, understanding, and accepting of people who may think and act differently from themselves. They must be careful with details of care. Someone's health, even life, might depend on it. For example, a person who prepares food trays must serve the right food prescribed by the doctor. The wrong food could interfere with the person's health.

## Skills in the Health Field

A career in health promotion or care requires certain skills. Some skills apply to many fields of employment. Others are especially important to health careers.

These general skills are important for jobs in the health field:

- good work habits. Effective workers begin to work as soon as they arrive at work. They take care of equipment. They keep a clean and neat work area. They're well organized and they follow the rules of the job, including work habits that help control the spread of disease and keep the area safe for patients, consumers, and employees.

- communication skills. Good health care employees must be able to communicate information to others and must be able to listen well to what others are saying so they get all necessary information. Many times a health care worker must also be able to teach patients and consumers how to care for themselves. They may need writing skills for filling out reports and forms accurately and clearly. Perhaps they need good counseling skills so they can speak and listen well.

- interpersonal skills. Most health care jobs involve person-to-person contact. So a successful worker must get along with patients, consumers, supervisors, and co-workers.

- emotional control. Emotional control is especially important in the health care field. Patients need a quiet, stress-free environment for recovery. Nurses, technicians, and doctors realize that strong emotional responses often interfere with their abilities to give quality patient care.

- accuracy. When dealing with a person's health, there's little room for error. For example, medication must be given in exactly the correct amounts. One unit of medicine may help the healing process, whereas a double unit may be a dangerous overdose.

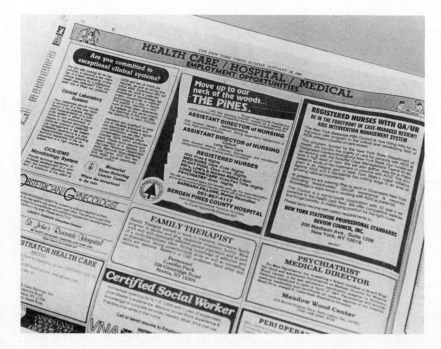

*Because the health field provides services to the public, good interpersonal skills, such as counseling, are important.*

- documentation skills. A health professional must be able to record vital signs, signs and symptoms of illness, care prescribed, and care given. For example, a medical technician who documents the exact readings of test results makes it possible for a doctor to diagnose illnesses correctly.
- ability to think and act quickly. Often this skill is critical to life. For example, the emergency team of an ambulance service must decide immediately what care to give in order to keep a person living while they are on the way to a hospital.
- math skills. Many new machines used in health promotion and medical care require math skills. Calculating nutrients in diets, preparing medication, and handling insurance claims are some tasks requiring math ability. Some knowledge of computers is often helpful.

For each job, very specific knowledge and skills are also required. In some cases, on-the-job training is sufficient. Other jobs may require technical training in a vocational program. Still, others require a college degree and perhaps medical school.

## Health Care Opportunities for Teens

If you are like most people your age, you are not ready to choose a career. But there are many ways you can learn more about a health profession and, at the same time, earn money and develop job skills. For example, if you need a summer job and you're also thinking about a medical career, you might work as an aide in a hospital for the summer. Part-time and summer jobs and volunteer work help many teens decide whether or not they are interested in a certain job area.

## Volunteering

Volunteer teens handle many responsibilities in health promotion and health care organizations. They carry mail, run errands, visit with patients, serve trays, and transport patients. They may work in emergency rooms, in offices, in pharmacies, in nursing homes, in private homes, in laboratories, or even on a hospital floor in patient care.

Junior volunteers represent the most popular volunteer program for teens in health care. Hospitals, nursing homes, and many other health-related institutions have volunteer programs for students. Recently teens have begun to volunteer in health care programs such as shelters for the homeless. Helping operate adult transportation services for the aged is satisfying for many teens.

Some high school clubs volunteer their services. For example, Future Homemakers of America members often work in nursing homes to entertain patients and make their mealtime more pleasant. The Health Occupations Student Organization may volunteer as a group in community centers that provide physical therapy.

If you want to offer your help, contact the volunteer officer of a hospital, therapy center, or other health care organization. Or ask your high school guidance counselor.

## Part-time and Summer Jobs

Part-time and summer jobs offer opportunities to learn about careers in health care and health promotion. Part-time workers may work at a wide variety of jobs such as a housekeeper's aide, maintenance worker, technician's helper, cook, clerk, or nurse's aide.

As a part-time or summer employee, you can observe and work with employees who have chosen health care and promotion as a profession. You'll observe patients or clients.

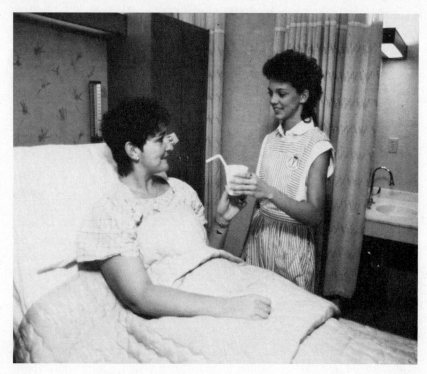

*Volunteer work helps teenagers gain valuable insights and experience in the health field.*

Clients are people who use or buy services or things. You'll learn about the working environment and schedules. All these observations can help you decide about health care or promotion as a career.

If you're interested in a job, contact the personnel officer at your local hospital, nursing home, or other health promotion or health care organization. Or perhaps a local doctor's or dentist's office has an opening.

When you apply for a job, try to get an interview, and then present yourself in a mature manner. Dress neatly. Plan ahead how you can present yourself favorably!

Before you go for the interview, practice filling out an application form, such as the one on page **373**. When you go for the interview, take names and addresses of people for references. *References* are people an employer can contact to find out about your character and abilities. Bring your social se-

curity number, too. If you don't have one, apply for a social security number before you start job hunting. Read the feature "Getting a Job" on pages **374–375** to learn how to prepare for and conduct yourself during an interview.

## Careers in Health Service

A *career* is work you do for many years in a specific field. For example, your teacher has a career in education. The police chief has a career in law enforcement. Your doctor has a career in medicine. Within a career a person might have many different jobs.

When a person enters a career, the first position he or she gets is usually called an *entry-level job*. As people become experienced and more skilled, they usually move into new positions. As they move to more responsible positions, we say they are moving up the *career ladder*. If they acquire

# Job Application

**THE CHILDREN'S HOSPITAL**
300 Longwood Avenue, Boston, Massachusetts 02115
An Equal Opportunity Employer

EMPLOYMENT APPLICATION

## PERSONAL DATA

NAME | last | first | middle | SOCIAL SECURITY NO.

PRESENT ADDRESS | street & no. | city/town | state | zip | TELEPHONE NO.

PERMANENT ADDRESS | street & no. | city/town | state | zip | TELEPHONE NO.

ARE YOU A U.S. CITIZEN? ☐ YES ☐ NO
ARE YOU A PERMANENT RESIDENT OF THE U.S.? ☐ YES ☐ NO
ARE YOU AUTHORIZED TO WORK IN THE U.S. ☐ YES ☐ NO
VISA TYPE

HAVE YOU EVER BEEN EMPLOYED BY THE HOSPITAL? ☐ YES ☐ NO
WHEN?
WHAT DEPARTMENT?
IF YOU ARE UNDER 18 WHAT IS YOUR BIRTHDATE?

IN CASE OF EMERGENCY WHOM SHOULD WE CONTACT? NAME: | last | first | middle init. | relationship

ADDRESS | street & no. | city/town | state | zip | TELEPHONE NO.

## EDUCATION

CIRCLE HIGHEST GRADE COMPLETED

| | GRAMMAR | HIGH | COLLEGE | GRADUATE |
|---|---|---|---|---|
| | 1 2 3 4 5 6 7 8 | 9 10 11 12 | 1 2 3 4 | 1 2 3 4 |

| SCHOOL | NAME | CITY | STATE | DATES ATTENDED | Did you Graduate? | Grade Average | MAJOR | DEGREE |
|---|---|---|---|---|---|---|---|---|
| HIGH SCHOOL | | | | TO | | | | |
| COLLEGE | | | | TO | | | | |
| COLLEGE | | | | TO | | | | |
| SCHOOL OF NURSING | | | | TO | | | | |

ACTIVITIES

## INTERESTS & SKILLS

TYPE OF WORK PREFERRED | FIELD OF INTEREST | DATE AVAILABLE | SALARY EXPECTED

WHAT HOURS ARE YOU AVAILABLE FOR WORK (EXCLUDING ANY NEED TO BE ABSENT FOR RELIGIOUS REASONS)
☐ DAYS ☐ EVENINGS ☐ NIGHTS ☐ WEEKENDS
☐ FULL TIME ☐ PART TIME
☐ REGULAR ☐ TEMPORARY

SUPPORT STAFF SKILLS | TYPING SPEED | TEST RESULTS | TRANSCRIPTION | MEDICAL TERMS | FOREIGN LANGUAGE (Indicate)

SPECIAL INTERESTS

## PLEASE DO NOT WRITE BELOW THIS LINE

JOB TITLE | JOB CODE | GRADE

SALARY ALLOCATION

| | COST CENTER | PERCENT | ANNUAL DOLLARS |
|---|---|---|---|

EMPLOYMENT DATE | EMPLOYEE REPLACED | TELEPHONE EXT. WHERE EMPLOYEE CAN BE REACHED

WEEKLY SALARY (Base Salary Only)
$ _____ Per Hour
$ _____ Per Week
MONTHLY SALARY
$ _____ Per Month
$ _____ Per Year
SHIFT PREMIUM
☐ EVENING/NIGHT
☐ WEEKEND
☐ FULL TIME
☐ PART TIME
☐ TEMP. F.T.
☐ TEMP. P.T.
☐ COOP STUDENT
☐ OTHER

TIME SHEET | TOTAL

HOURS PER WEEK | HOURS PER MONTH | OTHER PREMIUMS INCLUDED IN GROSS PAY $ _____

| M.C. | S. | VC | CO. |
|---|---|---|---|

DEPARTMENT | LOCATION | EXT.

AUTHORIZED SIGNATURE | DATE

03392 6M 6/86

# GETTING A JOB

Getting a job involves selling yourself to an employer. Remember that you are the best salesperson for you! By presenting yourself in a mature, professional manner, you're more likely to be hired. The following paragraphs offer some tips for getting a job.

First, find a job opening that interests you. Look in newspapers. Ask your friends. Talk to your parents. Watch for "Help Wanted" signs. Or perhaps send a letter of inquiry to find openings.

Plan your first contact carefully. If it's by letter, be sure the letter is brief (one page only), neatly typed, and free of errors. Let someone check it for you. The letter should include a realistic statement of your goal—describe the kind of job you are looking for and why you are interested. Be sure to include your address and phone number. You might include a resume, too. A *resume* is a short outline describing your experiences and skills. Look at the example of a job letter and resume on pages **374** and **375**.

Prepare carefully for an interview or first contact. Dress neatly. Groom your hair, face, and nails carefully.

Plan what you will say. Think of past experiences that might make you a good choice for the job. Identify those qualities and skills you already have that will be helpful in carrying out this job. For example, if the job is delivering trays in a nursing home and you enjoy working with people, be prepared to say so. If you've helped care for an older relative in your home, tell about that, too.

| Sample Resume | |
| --- | --- |
| **Jennifer Ann Smith** | |
| Permanent Address: | 110 Main Street Miller City, Texas 77001 |
| Telephone Number: 409-821-1100 | |
| Age: 16 | |
| Height: 5'4"    Weight: 110    Health: Excellent | |
| Education: | Junior, Miller City High School G.P.A.—84.6 |
| Work Experience: | Teens for Health, Miller City, volunteer health aide Mrs. Jan Morales, babysitter Mr. Craig Benden, babysitter |
| School Activities: | Junior Class, secretary History Club, committee chairperson Student Council, member Varsity Tennis Team, member |
| References: | Mrs. Helen Wright, English Teacher Miller City High School Miller City, Texas 77001 |
| | Mr. John Harris, History Teacher Miller City High School Miller City, Texas 77001 |
| | Dr. Thomas Russell, Coordinator Teens for Health P.O. Box 300 Miller City, Texas 77001 |

The first interview usually determines whether or not you will get the job. Arrive on time, or early. But never arrive late. Do not smoke, chew gum, or wear dark glasses.

When you meet the interviewer, shake hands with a firm grip. Look at the person directly in the eye. Be seated only when asked to sit. Use good posture.

Be prepared to talk about yourself, your skills, and your attitudes. You may be

- documentation skills. A health professional must be able to record vital signs, signs and symptoms of illness, care prescribed, and care given. For example, a medical technician who documents the exact readings of test results makes it possible for a doctor to diagnose illnesses correctly.
- ability to think and act quickly. Often this skill is critical to life. For example, the emergency team of an ambulance service must decide immediately what care to give in order to keep a person living while they are on the way to a hospital.
- math skills. Many new machines used in health promotion and medical care require math skills. Calculating nutrients in diets, preparing medication, and handling insurance claims are some tasks requiring math ability. Some knowledge of computers is often helpful.

For each job, very specific knowledge and skills are also required. In some cases, on-the-job training is sufficient. Other jobs may require technical training in a vocational program. Still, others require a college degree and perhaps medical school.

## Health Care Opportunities for Teens

If you are like most people your age, you are not ready to choose a career. But there are many ways you can learn more about a health profession and, at the same time, earn money and develop job skills. For example, if you need a summer job and you're also thinking about a medical career, you might work as an aide in a hospital for the summer. Part-time and summer jobs and volunteer work help many teens decide whether or not they are interested in a certain job area.

## Volunteering

Volunteer teens handle many responsibilities in health promotion and health care organizations. They carry mail, run errands, visit with patients, serve trays, and transport patients. They may work in emergency rooms, in offices, in pharmacies, in nursing homes, in private homes, in laboratories, or even on a hospital floor in patient care.

Junior volunteers represent the most popular volunteer program for teens in health care. Hospitals, nursing homes, and many other health-related institutions have volunteer programs for students. Recently teens have begun to volunteer in health care programs such as shelters for the homeless. Helping operate adult transportation services for the aged is satisfying for many teens.

Some high school clubs volunteer their services. For example, Future Homemakers of America members often work in nursing homes to entertain patients and make their mealtime more pleasant. The Health Occupations Student Organization may volunteer as a group in community centers that provide physical therapy.

If you want to offer your help, contact the volunteer officer of a hospital, therapy center, or other health care organization. Or ask your high school guidance counselor.

### Part-time and Summer Jobs

Part-time and summer jobs offer opportunities to learn about careers in health care and health promotion. Part-time workers may work at a wide variety of jobs such as a housekeeper's aide, maintenance worker, technician's helper, cook, clerk, or nurse's aide.

As a part-time or summer employee, you can observe and work with employees who have chosen health care and promotion as a profession. You'll observe patients or clients.

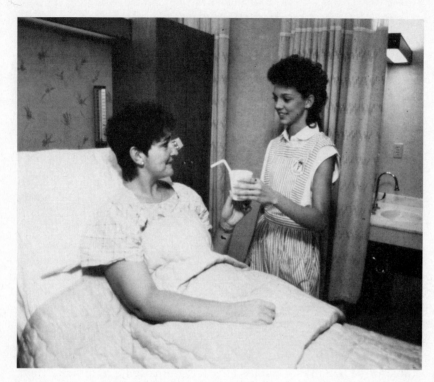

*Volunteer work helps teenagers gain valuable insights and experience in the health field.*

Clients are people who use or buy services or things. You'll learn about the working environment and schedules. All these observations can help you decide about health care or promotion as a career.

If you're interested in a job, contact the personnel officer at your local hospital, nursing home, or other health promotion or health care organization. Or perhaps a local doctor's or dentist's office has an opening.

When you apply for a job, try to get an interview, and then present yourself in a mature manner. Dress neatly. Plan ahead how you can present yourself favorably!

Before you go for the interview, practice filling out an application form, such as the one on page **373**. When you go for the interview, take names and addresses of people for references. *References* are people an employer can contact to find out about your character and abilities. Bring your social se-

curity number, too. If you don't have one, apply for a social security number before you start job hunting. Read the feature "Getting a Job" on pages **374–375** to learn how to prepare for and conduct yourself during an interview.

## Careers in Health Service

A *career* is work you do for many years in a specific field. For example, your teacher has a career in education. The police chief has a career in law enforcement. Your doctor has a career in medicine. Within a career a person might have many different jobs.

When a person enters a career, the first position he or she gets is usually called an *entry-level job.* As people become experienced and more skilled, they usually move into new positions. As they move to more responsible positions, we say they are moving up the *career ladder.* If they acquire

# Job Application

**THE CHILDREN'S HOSPITAL**
300 Longwood Avenue, Boston, Massachusetts 02115
An Equal Opportunity Employer

EMPLOYMENT APPLICATION

## PERSONAL DATA

| NAME | last | first | middle | SOCIAL SECURITY NO. |
|------|------|-------|--------|---------------------|

| PRESENT ADDRESS | street & no. | city/town | state | zip | TELEPHONE NO. |
|---|---|---|---|---|---|

| PERMANENT ADDRESS | street & no. | city/town | state | zip | TELEPHONE NO. |
|---|---|---|---|---|---|

ARE YOU A U.S. CITIZEN? ☐ YES ☐ NO    ARE YOU A PERMANENT RESIDENT OF THE U.S.? ☐ YES ☐ NO    ARE YOU AUTHORIZED TO WORK IN THE U.S. ☐ YES ☐ NO    VISA TYPE _____

HAVE YOU EVER BEEN EMPLOYED BY THE HOSPITAL? ☐ YES ☐ NO    WHEN? _____  WHAT DEPARTMENT? _____   IF YOU ARE UNDER 18 WHAT IS YOUR BIRTHDATE?

IN CASE OF EMERGENCY WHOM SHOULD WE CONTACT?  NAME: ___ last ___ first ___ middle init. ___ relationship

| ADDRESS | street & no. | city/town | state | zip | TELEPHONE NO. |
|---|---|---|---|---|---|

## EDUCATION

CIRCLE HIGHEST GRADE COMPLETED

GRAMMAR **1 2 3 4 5 6 7 8**    HIGH **9 10 11 12**    COLLEGE **1 2 3 4**    GRADUATE **1 2 3 4**

| SCHOOL | NAME | CITY | STATE | DATES ATTENDED | Did you Graduate? | Grade Average | MAJOR | DEGREE |
|--------|------|------|-------|----------------|-------------------|---------------|-------|--------|
| HIGH SCHOOL | | | | TO | | | | |
| COLLEGE | | | | TO | | | | |
| COLLEGE | | | | TO | | | | |
| SCHOOL OF NURSING | | | | TO | | | | |
| ACTIVITIES | | | | | | | | |

## INTERESTS & SKILLS

| TYPE OF WORK PREFERRED | FIELD OF INTEREST | DATE AVAILABLE | SALARY EXPECTED |
|---|---|---|---|

WHAT HOURS ARE YOU AVAILABLE FOR WORK (EXCLUDING ANY NEED TO BE ABSENT FOR RELIGIOUS REASONS)
☐ DAYS  ☐ EVENINGS  ☐ NIGHTS  ☐ WEEKENDS    ☐ FULL TIME  ☐ PART TIME    ☐ REGULAR  ☐ TEMPORARY

| SUPPORT STAFF SKILLS | TYPING SPEED | TEST RESULTS | TRANSCRIPTION | MEDICAL TERMS | FOREIGN LANGUAGE (Indicate) |
|---|---|---|---|---|---|

SPECIAL INTERESTS

---

**PLEASE DO NOT WRITE BELOW THIS LINE**

| JOB TITLE | JOB CODE | GRADE |
|---|---|---|

**SALARY ALLOCATION**

| COST CENTER | PERCENT | ANNUAL DOLLARS |
|---|---|---|

EMPLOYMENT DATE    EMPLOYEE REPLACED    TELEPHONE EXT. WHERE EMPLOYEE CAN BE REACHED

WEEKLY SALARY (Base Salary Only)  $____ Per Hour  $____ Per Week    MONTHLY SALARY  $____ Per Month  $____ Per Year    SHIFT PREMIUM  ☐ EVENING/NIGHT  ☐ WEEKEND    ☐ FULL TIME  ☐ PART TIME  ☐ TEMP. F.T.  ☐ TEMP. P.T.  ☐ COOP STUDENT  ☐ OTHER

TIME SHEET          TOTAL

| HOURS PER WEEK | HOURS PER MONTH | OTHER PREMIUMS INCLUDED IN GROSS PAY  $____ |
|---|---|---|

| M.C. | S. | VC | CO. |
|---|---|---|---|

DEPARTMENT ___ LOCATION ___ EXT. ___

AUTHORIZED SIGNATURE ___ DATE ___

03392 6M 6/86

# GETTING A JOB

Getting a job involves selling yourself to an employer. Remember that you are the best salesperson for you! By presenting yourself in a mature, professional manner, you're more likely to be hired. The following paragraphs offer some tips for getting a job.

First, find a job opening that interests you. Look in newspapers. Ask your friends. Talk to your parents. Watch for "Help Wanted" signs. Or perhaps send a letter of inquiry to find openings.

Plan your first contact carefully. If it's by letter, be sure the letter is brief (one page only), neatly typed, and free of errors. Let someone check it for you. The letter should include a realistic statement of your goal—describe the kind of job you are looking for and why you are interested. Be sure to include your address and phone number. You might include a resume, too. A *resume* is a short outline describing your experiences and skills. Look at the example of a job letter and resume on pages **374** and **375**.

Prepare carefully for an interview or first contact. Dress neatly. Groom your hair, face, and nails carefully.

Plan what you will say. Think of past experiences that might make you a good choice for the job. Identify those qualities and skills you already have that will be helpful in carrying out this job. For example, if the job is delivering trays in a nursing home and you enjoy working with people, be prepared to say so. If you've helped care for an older relative in your home, tell about that, too.

## Sample Resume

**Jennifer Ann Smith**

| | |
|---|---|
| Permanent Address: | 110 Main Street Miller City, Texas 77001 |

Telephone Number: 409-821-1100

Age: 16

Height: 5'4"  Weight: 110  Health: Excellent

| | |
|---|---|
| Education: | Junior, Miller City High School G.P.A.—84.6 |
| Work Experience: | Teens for Health, Miller City, volunteer health aide Mrs. Jan Morales, babysitter Mr. Craig Benden, babysitter |
| School Activities: | Junior Class, secretary History Club, committee chairperson Student Council, member Varsity Tennis Team, member |
| References: | Mrs. Helen Wright, English Teacher Miller City High School Miller City, Texas 77001 |
| | Mr. John Harris, History Teacher Miller City High School Miller City, Texas 77001 |
| | Dr. Thomas Russell, Coordinator Teens for Health P.O. Box 300 Miller City, Texas 77001 |

The first interview usually determines whether or not you will get the job. Arrive on time, or early. But never arrive late. Do not smoke, chew gum, or wear dark glasses.

When you meet the interviewer, shake hands with a firm grip. Look at the person directly in the eye. Be seated only when asked to sit. Use good posture.

Be prepared to talk about yourself, your skills, and your attitudes. You may be

## Sample Letter of Introduction

110 Main Street
Miller City, Texas 77001
April 2, 1988

Dr. Barbara Jones
Dentistry Clinic
220 Main Street
Miller City, Texas 77001

Dear Dr. Jones:

My high school counselor, Miss Pat Smith, told me that you have a summer and part-time job open for a clerk in your dental office. I am interested in applying for the position and believe that I can work successfully in an office such as yours. Working in a dental office would also give me a chance to learn more about the health field as a possible career.

In high school, I have had several responsible positions. I am secretary of the junior class and serve on the student council. My overall grade average is 84.6. I also work as a community volunteer in the Teens for Health program and babysit frequently. I enjoy working with people.

In May I will finish my junior year at Miller City High School. I will be available for employment on June 1. During my senior year, my schedule enables me to work from 3 to 5 p.m. after school.

Enclosed is my resume with more information about my background. References are included.

I would like to schedule an interview to learn more about the job in your dental office and to tell you about my abilities.

Sincerely,

*Jennifer Ann Smith*

Jennifer Ann Smith

---

asked about previous work, about school, extra-curricular activities, hobbies, and personal interests. Tell about past work and volunteer experiences you have had— even if they were just helping your parents with house or yard work. School and club activities also tell a lot about you.

Speak of your past work with confidence. For example, you might say, "This will be my first paid work, but I have had responsibilities for work at home for several years. I regularly shovel snow for our family in the winter and mow the grass in the summer. I also babysit my sister after school while my parents work."

Employers will also be impressed by work with community groups. For example, talk about your work as a scout.

When you tell about past employment, explain what work you did and what skills you acquired. Never complain about your previous boss or position. Be positive!

When the interview is over, shake hands and thank the person for talking with you. If you are interested in the position, say that you will look forward to hearing about the job in a few days.

Leave your telephone number with the interviewer. Then arrange to be near the telephone for calls. Or have someone available to take a message for you so that you don't miss a call.

The persistent, well-prepared person often gets a job. You will be that person if you work to find a job and if you present yourself well to employers.

You can succeed! Good luck!

more education, they have more opportunities. See the charts on pages **377** and **379** to see the variety of levels of training needed in three different occupational areas.

Because there are so many different occupations in health care, the U.S. Office of Education has arranged them into clusters. A career cluster is a group of jobs that are similar to each other. For example, a farmer, a rancher, and an animal breeder are grouped together in a cluster because they all work in agriculture.

In health care there are three major career clusters. The first is made up of physicians. The second includes nursing, pharmacy, therapy, and dietetics. The third group is made up of medical technologists and technicians.

Many other people work in health care services, but their jobs don't fit neatly into a single cluster. Assistants, such as therapy assistants, nursing assistants, and dietetic assistants perform a combination of clerical and patient care tasks. They assist health care professionals such as dentists, physicians, therapists, nurses, and dietitians. Training for these positions varies considerably but most require only on-the-job training.

Still others work in new fields which are emerging in health care.

## Medicine

Physicians are general practitioners or specialists in the field of medicine. They may be doctors of medicine (M.D.) or doctors of osteopathy (D.O.). Seven out of 10 physicians are specialists. They concentrate their study and practice in one particular field of medicine. Common specialties are surgery, dermatology, pediatrics, obstetrics, gynecology, urology, radiology, and pathology. Chapter 4 gives more information about many specialities.

## Health Care Workers with Post-High School Training

| Worker | Responsibilities |
| --- | --- |
| Dental hygienist | Cleans teeth, develops X-rays |
| Dietetic technician | Takes diet records, calculates nutrients in menus and patient food choices |
| Electrocardiograph technician | Operates machines that check heartbeat |
| Emergency medical technician | Drives emergency vehicles and gives emergency care |
| Licensed practical nurse | Gives patient care |
| Medical laboratory worker | Takes blood tests, urine tests, and other medical tests |
| Medical records technician | Develops and maintains records |
| Radiology technician | Takes X-rays |
| Surgical technician | Prepares equipment for surgery |

A physician's training includes a college degree, a medical degree, and a period of supervised, on-the-job training including a one-year internship and a one- to three-year residency. Usually these programs require 10 to 12 years of study after high school.

A career as a physician might be right for you if:

- you have a strong desire to promote health and treat illness
- you are a good student, especially strong in science
- you are willing to go to school for many years
- you won't mind being "on call" 24 hours a day for emergencies

Recently physician's assistants have begun to work closely with doctors. They interview patients, take medical histories, order tests, and, in general, assist a physician. A physician's assistant must work under the supervision of a licensed physician. Licensing means that a doctor or other professional has passed the requirements to provide specific kinds of health care in the state he or she works in.

Generally the training for a physician's assistant consists of a four-year program following high school. Training programs are located in medical schools, in teaching hospitals, and in community colleges.

## Nursing

Careers in nursing include registered nurses (R.N.), nurse practitioners, licensed practical nurses (L.P.N.), and nurse's aides.

*Registered nurses* are licensed to practice professional nursing. They are graduates of state-approved schools of nursing, which are often four-year college programs, and have passed a state board examination.

Nurse practitioners are registered nurses who have a master's degree. A master's degree is a two-year graduate degree earned

| Occupations in Emergency Medical Care | |
|---|---|
| Education | Occupation |
| Medical School & Residency | Physician |
| College | Nurse Practitioner |
| | Registered Nurse |
| Post Secondary | Medical Technologist |
| | Licensed Practical Nurse |
| Short-Term Training | Laboratory Assistant |
| | Emergency Medical Technician |
| High School | Secretary |
| On-the-Job Training | Admitting Clerk |

after receiving a bachelor's degree. They may work in hospitals, clinics, schools, industries, or private homes. Often they have supervisory positions. They usually practice with physicians, assist in surgery, and treat routine diseases. Some nurse practitioners operate community health programs, conduct research, or teach. A licensed midwife is a nurse practitioner who specializes in pregnancy and childbirth.

*Licensed practical nurses* provide patient care under the direction of physicians and registered nurses. They do not have as much nursing education as an R.N., and they do more routine, less complex tasks. To qualify as an L.P.N., a person completes a state-approved practical nursing course, which usually requires two years of training after high school, and passes a written examination. In Texas and California, a licensed

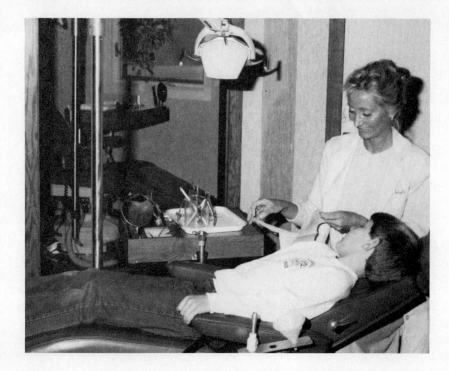

*In a pediatric dental office, the staff work carefully to make their young patients feel comfortable.*

practical nurse is called a licensed vocational nurse (L.V.N.).

A nurse's aide gives patients care which requires limited skill. Nurse's aides are in increasing demand as care for the elderly increases. Many work in nursing homes. They are trained either on-the-job or in training programs lasting three to six months. There are training programs for nurse's aides in hospitals, community colleges, and technical schools.

## Dentistry

Dentists specialize in the care of teeth and gums. They examine teeth and diagnose disease and dental abnormalities. Their work includes filling cavities, extracting teeth, treating gum diseases, making dentures, straightening teeth, and other services.

A dentist must complete a four-year college degree and four more years in dental school. State licensing is also required.

Some dentists specialize in one area of dentistry. They might become orthodontists who straighten teeth, periodontists who care for gums, pediatric dentists who only work with children, or oral surgeons. A specialty requires additional years of study.

Dentists employ other professionals for the dental care team. Dental hygienists clean teeth and provide other patient care under the direction of the dentist. Dentist assistants do office work and aid the dentist during examinations and treatment. A hygienist receives at least one year of training after high school, and an assistant can often learn on the job.

## Pharmacy

Pharmacists specialize in medication. They generally work in hospitals or drugstores where they prepare and dispense medicines prescribed by doctors and dentists. They need a license to practice. To get

## Occupations in Nutrition and Food Service

| Education | Occupation |
|---|---|
| University | Registered Dietitian |
| Post Secondary | Dietetic Technician |
| | Dietary Manager |
| | Executive Chef |
| High School | Secretary |
| | Clerk |
| | Cashier |
| On the Job Training | Cook |
| | Assistant Cook |
| | Dishwasher |

a license they must complete about five years of specialized training beyond high school and pass a special examination. These professionals attend a college of pharmacy and then gain supervised practical experience, called an internship, under the direction of a licensed pharmacist within a hospital or drugstore pharmacy. Licensed pharmacists display a state certificate in the places where they work.

Some pharmacists own businesses related to their profession. They may operate a drugstore. Or they may buy and sell a wide range of medical supplies.

## Dietetics

Dietetics is the health profession that specializes in nutrition. *Dietitians* provide nutrition counseling to individuals and to groups. They set up and supervise food service for a variety of institutions, including hospitals. These professionals also promote good eating habits through education and research.

Approximately five years of education and training beyond high school are required to be a dietitian. A bachelor's degree, with a major in foods and nutrition or institutional management, is the basis for a dietitian's training. To be a registered dietitian (R.D.), The American Dietetic Association requires an internship or an optional coordinated program handled through a university as well as passing a registration examination. In some states, dietitians are also licensed through another examination.

A dietetic technician has a two-year associate's degree. A diet manager has one year of training. Both work under a registered dietitian.

## Therapy

Therapists work with people who have physical or occupational injuries or limitations. Physical therapists provide treatment and exercises to help people restore muscle use. Occupational therapists work with people to restore abilities to live independently and to earn an income. Speech pathologists work with children and adults who have speech, language, or voice disorders. Their work includes evaluation and diagnosis as well as treatment.

## Occupations in Physical Therapy

| Education | Occupation |
|---|---|
| University | Licensed Physical Therapist |
| Post Secondary | Licensed Therapist Assistant |
| High School | Secretary |
| | Clerk |
| On-the-Job Training | Therapist Aide |

A bachelor's degree in a specialized field of therapy is required, and many continue for a master's degree. Licensing requirements vary from state to state.

## Psychology

Psychiatrists, psychologists, psychiatric nurses, and clinical social workers are health professionals who work with mental, emotional, and social problems. A psychiatrist primarily tests for severe mental disorders, prescribes medicine, and treats patients in hospitals. A clinical psychologist administers tests for emotional health, makes diagnoses, and treats emotional disorders. A clinical social worker does work similar to a clinical psychologist but also specializes in one-on-one therapy and group counseling. A psychiatric nurse provides care for mentally ill patients under the direction of a psychiatrist in a mental institution.

A psychiatrist is a doctor with specialty training. A psychologist needs a college degree and three to four years of graduate work for licensing. A clinical social worker has a college degree, with training in helping families with social problems. A psychiatric nurse is one with on-the-job experience in psychiatry.

These professionals work in hospitals, clinics, mental health centers, rehabilitation centers, and nursing homes.

## Technology

Health technologists and technicians work in laboratories that are necessary for diagnosing and treating patients. Many owe their jobs to new technology in medical procedures and equipment.

Biomedical equipment involves the use of sophisticated machines to monitor the body's functions and conditions. For example, computerized tomographic machines link equipment with a computer to make X-rays of the brain. Mammographic machines use X-rays to examine the breasts for irregularities. Diagnostic medical sonographic machines produce images from sound waves to examine body organs. Computerized scanners are used to take pictures of the inside of the body.

Scientists in medical technology design and test biomedical equipment. They have college degrees in science, engineering, and related fields. Many also have master's and doctoral degrees.

Technologists and technicians operate these machines. And as a rule, they are trained right in the health care facility where they work. However, some receive one or two years of training at community colleges or vocational schools. A technologist performs more skilled work than a technician, and thus, needs more education and training.

There are many types of health technologists and technicians:

- Dental hygienists clean teeth and perform other services in a dental office.
- Electrocardiograph technicians run tests that monitor heart function.
- Emergency medical technicians work in teams to care for the injured.
- Technicians work in critical health care areas. For example, setting up surgical instruments and operating machines is the responsibility of the *surgical technician.*
- Other technicians work in radiology (X-rays), blood banks, and operating rooms. A blood bank is a place where blood donations are taken, stored, and dispensed.

## Health-Related Occupations

Many other workers are necessary to keep hospitals and health facilities operating. Doctor's offices need clerical workers and

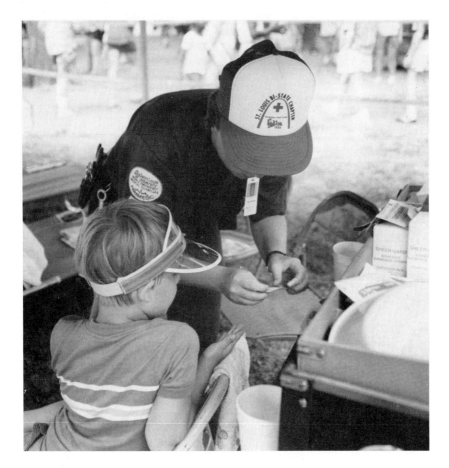

*Health technicians help provide many services, such as providing first aid at a county fair.*

secretaries. Accountants, clerks, and insurance officers are needed in hospitals. Medical librarians organize journals and other references for medical staff. Public relations professionals write health newsletters and organize seminars from the hospital or clinic for the community. The hospital laundry, hospital maintenance, and hospital housekeeping departments also provide career opportunities. Pharmaceutical companies and medical supply companies provide careers and training in medical sales.

If you enjoy working in a helping profession but do not want training in medical or nursing care, you may want to investigate one of these important jobs.

# New Opportunities in Health Care

The world of health care is growing, expanding, and changing. New technology, new procedures, and increasing government commitment to health care has given rise to many new careers.

## Worksite Health Programs

Today many large companies employ health care workers for health promotion and medical care at the worksite. For example, a company may have a clinic where workers can get dental work done and where they may be treated for simple illnesses.

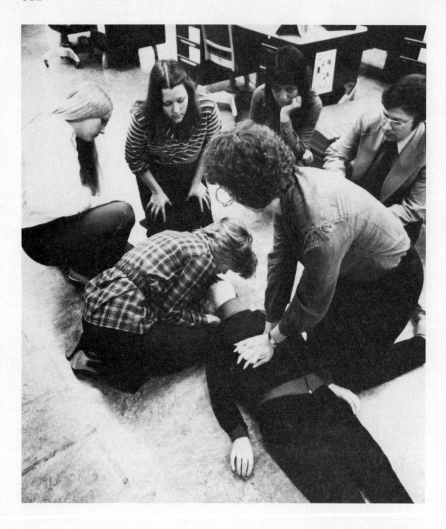

*Worksite wellness programs, a new trend in health promotion, will provide more and more jobs for health professionals in the future.*

Health care workers often check employees for health risks, such as high blood pressure. Many companies have worksite wellness programs, which may include seminars on CPR, smoking cessation (programs to stop smoking), stress reduction, and back injury prevention. Others offer company-wide weight control programs, exercise classes, and workout facilities. The cafeteria menu might even be labeled as low-calorie, low-sodium, and low-fat/low-cholesterol foods.

## Health Media

Writing about wellness, illness, the treatment of disease and injury, and new medical advances is a challenging occupation. Today many health reporters for newspapers, television, and radio are health care professionals such as doctors, nurses, and dietitians. If you like the field of communications, as well as the field of health care, you may want to investigate health care careers within the media.

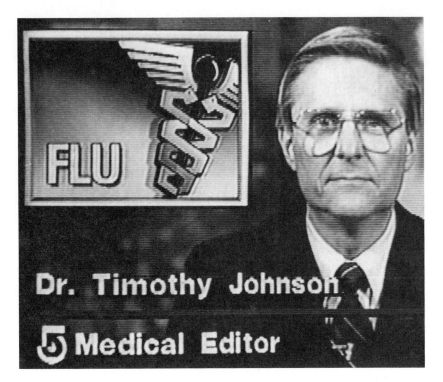

*Today many health professionals appear on TV or radio to update the public on health issues.*

If you are a skilled artist, you might explore the field of medical illustration. Medical books, for both consumers and health professionals, need artists who also understand physiology.

## Sports Medicine

Five professions combine their training in health and physiology to work with the athlete. Physicians, athletic trainers, physical therapists, exercise physiologists, and dietitians have established careers in a new area of health practice called sports medicine.

You have read about the work of physicians, physical therapists, and dietitians, so you know what they do and how they're trained. Athletic trainers and exercise physiologists complete a special college curriculum. Trainers work with athletes as they train for specific sports, and trainers work to prevent and treat sports injuries. Exercise physiologists teach athletes and coaches about ways the body responds to various athletic activities.

## Computer Science

Computer use in health care is increasing daily. For example, medical pictures taken by X-ray machines, ultrasound scanners, and other imaging, or picture, devices use computers to make internal outlines of the body clearer and to make body features stand out. In addition, miniature computers combined with electrical equipment greatly expand independence for the impaired. For instance, people who are paralyzed from the neck down may operate a wheelchair using a computer device attached to a wheelchair headrest.

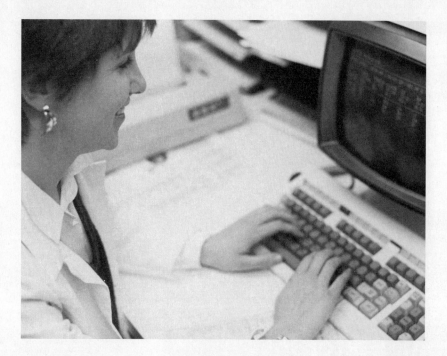

*Dietitians and dietetic technicians use computers to plan menus for patients who must follow special diets.*

## Research

Exciting things are happening in medical research. If you enjoy science, health care, and laboratory work, you may want to consider research. Today there are many new life-giving discoveries in all areas of the health field.

Medical research is done in universities, hospitals, and medical industries. Medical scientists have advanced degrees from universities. Laboratory technicians may be trained to work with them on the job.

## Entrepreneurship

*Entrepreneurs* are people who have their own businesses. They assume the risks and the management of the business. An entrepreneur needs business management skills, as well as skills related to a product or a service.

Some health care providers choose to work independently and not in a hospital, clinic, or doctor's office. These entrepreneurs offer services to businesses and individuals. Health care entrepreneurs include:

- home-health aides, who go into private homes for a few hours of general patient care daily. This may include homemaking duties.
- live-in caregivers, who give daily care and live with the elderly or other people who are not physically independent. This may include simple nursing, homemaking, and transportation.
- consulting dietitians, who have their own offices and work with people who need special diets. Their clients might include diabetics, obese people, athletes, and people with anorexia or bulimia.
- nurse practitioners who have their own businesses. They provide private care under the supervision of a physician.
- occupational therapists, physical therapists, and speech therapists, who have

their own offices or clinics or who go into the home to give therapy.

- private-duty nurses, who work in homes or for individuals who want additional nursing while they are hospitalized.
- visiting dentists, who take equipment to homes or to remote community centers, to perform dental work for patients who cannot get to a regular dental office.

## Environmental Health

A sanitarian works to enforce laws regarding sanitary standards for community water, food, and sewage. Sanitary engineers protect water and air and control contamination. Environmental technicians and aides work to assist in the protection of food, water, and air. All these workers represent careers in environmental health care. These are emerging occupational opportunities that may interest people who like the out-of-doors and are interested in caring for people.

## Career Information

If you want to know more about careers in health promotion and care, consult these resources:

- the vocational or career counselor in your school
- health professionals in your community
- the publication, "200 Ways to a Health Career," available from the National Health Council, 1740 Broadway, New York, NY 10019
- the publication, "Health Careers Guidebook," available from the Department of Health and Human Services, U.S. Government Printing Office, Washington, DC 20402

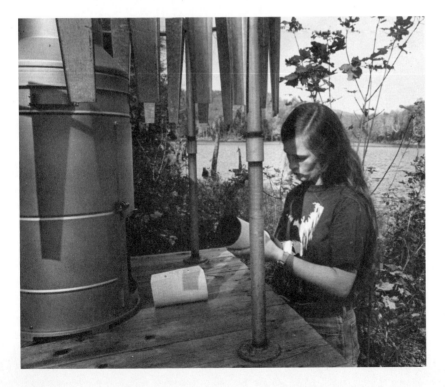

*An environmental technician tests the safety of water downstream from industries which may cause pollution.*

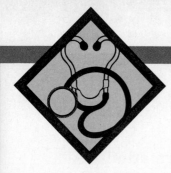

# CHAPTER CHECKUP

## Reviewing the Information

1. How might a person's health affect his or her job?
2. Name five attitudes that are important for success in any kind of job.
3. Name three personal attitudes that are important for someone who works in a health-related occupation.
4. Describe five skills important for an employee in the health field.
5. What volunteer jobs might help you learn about the health field?
6. Explain how a part-time job may help a person choose a health career.
7. Where might someone look for a job in the health field?
8. What tips could you give someone who was going for an interview?
9. What are the differences between a registered nurse and a licensed practical nurse?
10. Name three health occupations that require only a high school diploma.
11. Name three health occupations requiring one to three years of training after high school.
12. Name three health occupations that require four years of college or more and a special examination.
13. Name three new career opportunities in the health field.
14. Where could you find information on health careers?

## Thinking It Over

1. Explain why you think a person might choose to become a physician.
2. Evaluate your own health. How might your health and health habits make you a productive employee in the health field?
3. Suppose you are going for a job interview. What personal qualities, skills, and experiences would you tell a potential employer about?
4. How might references help get a job?
5. Describe a job in the health field that might interest you.
6. Name a health organization, such as a hospital, and list as many jobs as you can in that organization.

## Taking Action

 1. Write a brief paper describing jobs in the three health career clusters.

 2. Visit the library and research a medical specialty. Prepare a description for the class.

 3. Write to your state hospital association and ask for brochures on health careers in your state.

 4. Write a personal plan for getting a volunteer or part-time job in the health field.

5. Interview the school nurse to learn about nursing education and jobs. Write a brief report.
6. Find out about vocational or college programs nearby that prepare people for careers in health.

# Glossary

**abrasion** (uh-BRAY-zhun). A skin scrape, such as when one falls off a bicycle and scrapes a knee.

**acid rain.** A combination of pollutants and rain, snow, or sleet.

**acne** (AK-nee). Pimples and blackheads resulting from clogged skin pores.

**Acquired Immune Deficiency Syndrome.** See AIDS.

**addictive.** Habit-forming. People who use addictive substances over a period of time develop a physical and psychological need for that substance.

**adrenalin** (uh-DREN-uh-lin). Body chemical that helps prepare the body for action by increasing heartbeat rate, while suppressing digestion.

**aerobic** (uh-ROE-bik) **exercise.** Vigorous, sustained exercise, such as running, bicycling, swimming, or jumping rope.

**afterbirth.** The placenta and other membranes discharged from the uterus a few minutes after birth of a baby.

**AIDS** (Acquired Immune Deficiency Syndrome). Viral disease spread by intimate contact or through blood transfusions. It destroys the body's ability to fight off disease and infection.

**alcoholism.** Illness characterized by physical and psychological addiction to alcohol.

**alienation** (ay-lee-uh-NAY-shun). Feeling left out or cut off from others. Some people deliberately alienate, or set themselves apart, from others.

**allergy.** A sensitivity to a substance which may have no effect on other people. When people with an allergy to a substance come in contact with that substance, they may develop any of these symptoms: sneezing, coughing, runny eyes or nose, rash, swelling, headache, or digestive upsets.

**Alzheimer's** (ALZ-hime-urz) **Disease.** Chronic disease in which physical changes within the brain cause a person to gradually and steadily deteriorate mentally, physically, and socially.

**ambulatory** (AM-byoo-lah-tore-ee) **surgery.** Surgery that does not require an overnight stay in the hospital.

**amino** (uh-MEE-no) **acids.** Chemical compounds, contained in proteins, that are used to build and repair the body.

**amniocentesis** (am-nee-oh-sen-TEE-sis). A sample of the fluid surrounding the fetus in the uterus is withdrawn and analyzed for a variety of possible defects or disorders in the fetus.

**amputation.** Surgical removal of an arm, leg, finger, hand, or foot.

**anorexia nervosa** (an-uh-REX-ee-uh nur-VO-suh). Eating disorder in which a person who has an intense fear of becoming fat resorts to self-imposed starvation.

**antibiotics** (an-tee-by-AH-tiks). Medicines used to combat bacterial infections.

**antidote** (AN-tih-dote). A substance used to counteract the effects of a poison.

**antihistamines** (an-tih-HISS-tuh-meens). Medicines used to relieve a stuffy or runny nose resulting from an allergy or cold.

**arteries.** The body's largest blood vessels; they carry oxygen-rich blood from the heart to the rest of the body.

**arthritis** (are-THIE-tis). Chronic disease marked by painful, swollen, and inflamed joints, especially the joints of the fingers, wrists, arms, legs, hips, and feet. Over a long period of time the joints can become weakened and bone tissue can be destroyed.

**asbestos** (as-BESS-tuhs). A mineral fiber once used as a building material and in fireproof clothing because it is a good insulator and is fireproof. It is now known to cause serious lung diseases.

**asphyxiation** (as-FIX-ee-AY-shun). Occurs when something interferes with a person's breathing so much that the lack of oxygen causes unconsciousness or even death.

**assault.** A violent physical attack on one person by another person.

**asthma** (AZ-muh). Condition in which the bronchial tubes that lead from the windpipe to the lungs become partially obstructed, resulting in difficult breathing, wheezing, and coughing.

**atherosclerosis** (ath-ur-oh-skle-ROH-sis). Disease resulting from buildup of fatty deposits on the lining of the arteries. This causes the passageway to narrow and interferes with blood flow.

**autopsy** (AW-top-see). Medical exam of a body after death to determine the cause of death.

**avulsion** (uh-VUL-shun). Type of wound received when a piece of skin or a body part is torn or cut from the body, such as when a finger is cut off by a saw.

**bacteria.** Tiny one-celled organisms that can cause disease and infection.

**bargaining.** Behavior often exhibited by those with terminal illness in which they try to trade or bargain in an attempt to postpone death.

**basal metabolic** (BAY-sul meh-tuh-BOL-ik) **rate.** Speed at which the body uses calories.

**bassinet.** Small, basketlike infant bed.

**bedpan.** A shallow container for a bedridden woman to use for urination, or a bedridden man or woman to use for bowel movements.

**bedside commode.** A chair with a dropaway seat, under which is a bedpan.

**bedsores.** Sores that occur when a person must stay in bed for a long time. They are caused by the continual pressure of the body rubbing against the bed clothes.

**blackhead.** An acne condition in which the oil clogging the pore becomes black.

**bland diet.** Special diet prescribed for people with digestive problems. Foods are cooked by baking or boiling and highly seasoned, high-fat, and gas-forming foods are eliminated.

**blind.** Being visually impaired to the extent that one cannot depend on sight for movement or learning.

**blood pressure.** Force of the blood as it travels through the blood vessels to all parts of the body.

**body composition.** The amount of body fat in relation to lean muscle.

**body language.** Nonverbal communication. For example smiling, slamming a door, or frowning communicate one's message to others without using words.

**bonding.** Formation of close emotional ties between parents and their infant.

**braille** (BRAYL). System of writing that leaves raised points on the writing surface so a blind person can feel the written letters and thus read what is written.

**breech birth.** Term referring to when a baby's feet or bottom come through the birth canal first.

**bulimia** (boo-LEEM-ee-uh). Eating disorder in which a person periodically eats large amounts of food, then vomits or uses laxatives and diuretics to get rid of the food.

**burping.** Patting or rubbing a baby's back to expel swallowed air that may cause discomfort.

**caffeine.** A mild stimulant found in coffee, tea, and many colas.

**calorie.** Unit of measurement of the amount of energy in food and the amount of energy one's body uses.

**cannabis** (KAN-uh-bis). A drug that changes moods and perceptions, causing confusion. Marijuana is an example.

**carbohydrate** (kar-bo-HI-drate). A nutrient used to provide energy.

**carriers.** Persons who can infect you with a disease even though they don't appear sick.

**casket.** Box-type container used for burial.

**cataract.** A clouding of the eye's lens.

**cerebral palsy.** Crippling disorder causing complete or partial paralysis of the muscles, especially those in arms and legs. The affected areas will be completely immobile or movements are weak and poorly controlled.

**cervix.** Narrow opening to the uterus.

**cesarean** (sih-ZARE-ee-un) **section.** Delivering a baby by surgical removal through an incision in the woman's abdomen and uterus.

**chancre** (SHANG-kur). Small painless red sore that appears in the first stage of syphilis.

**chemotherapy** (KEE-mo-THARE-uh-pee). Use of chemical agents in the treatment or control of disease. This is one method of treating cancer.

**circumcision** (sur-cum-SIH-zhun). Removal of the foreskin on the penis for hygienic or religious reasons.

**cleft palate.** Condition in which the roof of the mouth, or palate, did not close properly during fetal development.

**colic.** A condition in which a baby age two weeks to three months cries continuously for several hours, pulling the legs up to the abdomen, and at times passes gas. This often lasts from one feeding to the next.

**coma.** A very deep state of unconsciousness that lasts a long time.

**communicable disease.** Disease that can be easily spread from one person to another.

**communication.** Sending and receiving information, accomplished by both talking and listening to others.

**depressants.** Drugs that slow down body systems, initially giving a feeling of relaxation. Tranquilizers are an example.

**depression.** Feelings of sadness, hopelessness, helplessness, and/or ineffectiveness, often accompanied by anxiety or withdrawal.

**dermatologist** (DUR-muh-TOL-uh-jist). A doctor who specializes in skin problems.

**diabetes** (die-uh-BEE-tis). Chronic disease in which the pancreas does not make enough insulin.

**diagnosis.** Identification of the specific cause of a health problem by analyzing signs, symptoms, and results of special tests.

**diagnostic tests.** Tests taken to help detect or identify health problems or diseases.

**diaper rash.** Irritation of a baby's skin caused by dampness and bacteria in wet or soiled diapers.

**diarrhea.** Loose, runny, and frequent bowel movements.

**extended family.** Family in which not only parents and their children live under one roof, but also grandparents, aunts, or uncles.

**fad diets.** Diets that are popular for only a short time.

**fallopian** (fa-LOPE-ee-un) **tubes.** Tubes connecting the ovaries to the uterus.

**family practitioner.** Primary care physician who cares for people of all ages.

**famine.** An extreme scarcity of food that usually leads to starvation and death.

**farsightedness.** Having a problem seeing things that are close-up.

**fat.** As a nutrient, this is an oily substance in animal products and some plant foods that provides essential fatty acids, helps the body use fat-soluble vitamins, and provides energy.

**fetal alcohol syndrome.** Problems that affect babies born to women who drink excessive amounts of alcohol during pregnancy. Problems may include low birth weight, learning disabilities, distorted facial features, heart defects, and mental retardation.

**fontenelles** (fon-tuh-NELLz). Soft spots on an infant's head where the skull bones haven't yet grown together. The soft area is covered with a very tough membrane. As the skull grows the soft spots grow smaller; they usually close within the first one to two years of life.

**food jag.** Eating one food over and over, and perhaps excluding other foods.

**food poisoning.** Illness caused by eating food contaminated with harmful bacteria.

**fracture.** Broken bone.

**frostbite.** The freezing or partial freezing of the skin and underlying body tissues.

**funeral.** Ceremony in memory of a person who has just died.

**generic drug.** A drug that has the same chemical makeup and effects on the body as a brand name drug, but can be made by a number of different manufacturers. Generic drugs are usually cheaper.

**genes** (JEENZ). Tiny clusters of chemical units contained on chromosomes. Genes carry the directions for determining one's physical characteristics and traits. Genes control such hereditary characteristics as hair color, height, and blood type.

**genitals.** The body's sex organs.

**gerontologist** (jur-uhn-TOL-oh-jist). A person who specializes in the aging process.

**glaucoma** (glaw-KO-muh). Disease of the eye marked by increased, destructive pressure of fluids within the eye.

**gonorrhea** (gawn-uh-REE-uh). Very common type of sexually transmitted disease, initially characterized by a yellowish discharge and painful urination.

**grief.** The many emotions felt by the family and friends of someone who dies.

**gynecologist** (gine-uh-KOL-oh-jist). A medical doctor who specializes in the care of the female reproductive system.

**hallucinate.** To see things that are not really there.

**hallucinogens.** Drugs that give a temporary distortion of mental images. LSD is one example.

**hangover.** The after effects of drinking too much alcohol. Symptoms include headache, upset stomach, and dry mouth.

**health maintenance organization (HMO).** A prepaid group health care plan.

**heat cramps.** Muscle spasms that occur in the abdomen, arms, and legs as a result of overexposure to heat.

**heat index.** Measurement that indicates combined effects of heat and humidity.

**heatstroke.** Severe physical response to heat in which the victim has an extremely high body temperature and loses the ability to perspire.

**Heimlich maneuver** (HIME-likh muh-NOO-vur). First aid technique for clearing airway passage of a choking person.

**hemorrhaging** (HEM-ur-ij-ing). Very heavy or uncontrollable bleeding.

**hemorrhoids** (HEM-uh-roidz). Varicose veins in the rectal area.

**hepatitis** (hep-uh-TIE-tis). A viral infection of the liver.

**high blood pressure.** Also called hypertension. Chronic disease in which the force of the blood moving through the body's blood vessels is greater than it should be. This can cause damage to the heart and arteries, stroke, and kidney damage.

**HMO.** See health maintenance organization.

**holistic health care.** Treating the whole person—physically and mentally.

**hormones.** Body chemicals that cause certain changes to take place.

**hospice** (HAWS-pis). A program designed to help the terminally ill die with as much comfort and dignity as possible.

**hygiene** (HI-jeen). Personal grooming and health care. Includes care of skin, hair, teeth, eyes, and nails.

**hyperactivity.** Physical condition identified in children who are much more excitable, active, and distractable than their peers.

**hypertension.** High blood pressure.

**hypochondria** (hi-po-KON-dree-uh). Being abnormally concerned about one's own health.

**hypothermia** (hi-po-THUR-mee-uh). Gradual cooling of the body's inner core resulting from overexposure to cold. The body temperature drops several degrees below normal and the body systems and functions slow down. Death results if heat loss is not restored.

**identification.** Defense mechanism of acting like a role model.

**immunity.** The body's ability to fight off infection.

**immunization** (im-myoo-nih-ZAY-shun). Procedure in which immunity to a disease is produced in a person by giving that person a vaccine.

**incision** (in-SIH-zhun). A cut from a sharp object, such as a knife, surgical tool, or broken glass.

**incubation period.** The amount of time that passes between the time a pathogen enters one's body and the time the first symptoms of a disease appear.

**incubator.** Specially enclosed, see-through crib in which the oxygen supply, temperature, and humidity can be controlled. Incubators often have special armholes in the side so the doctor or nurse can reach in and care for the baby.

**infant.** A baby from birth to age one year.

**infection.** Result of bacteria or other pathogens entering the body.

**infectious disease.** Any type of disease that one can catch.

**insomnia.** Prolonged inability to get adequate amounts of sleep.

**insulin** (IN-suh-lin). Body hormone produced by the pancreas and needed to help blood sugar pass from the bloodstream into the body cells where it can be used for energy.

**insurance.** A system in which individuals or groups pay certain sums for a guarantee that their costs or the cost of their loss will be paid, at least in part, when the need arises.

**internist.** Primary care physician who cares for adults.

**intoxication.** Being drunk; the combined effects on the body of drinking too much alcohol.

**jaundice** (JAWN-dis). Yellowish discoloration of the skin and the whites of the eyes.

**labor.** Way a woman's body prepares for and reacts during delivery of a baby.

**laceration** (las-ur-AY-shun). A jagged cut, such as one received from getting tangled in barbed wire.

**larynx** (LARE-ingks). Voice box.

**latchkey children.** Children who come home from school and have no caregiver until their parent(s) come home from work.

**learning disabilities.** Disorders that can cause a child to have difficulty with reading, speaking, listening, thinking, and/or writing.

**legumes** (LEG-yooms). Edible seeds that grow in pods, such as kidney beans and peas.

**leukoplakia**(loo-kuh-PLAY-kee-uh). White, raised sores in the mouth. This condition can be caused by frequent use of smokeless tobacco.

**licensed practical nurse (L.P.N.).** Nurse who has completed a two-year nursing course and has passed a written exam.

**life support equipment.** Highly technical equipment that can sustain or revive someone in a near-death condition.

**liver.** The largest body organ, the liver is located mostly on the right side of the upper abdomen. It regulates the composition of the blood and is necessary for the proper digestion of food and absorption of nutrients.

**malnutrition.** Poor health resulting from not getting enough of the nutrients the body needs.

**massage.** Using the hands to rub and manipulate muscles in order to relieve pain, stimulate blood circulation, or offer relaxation.

**Medicaid.** A government sponsored assistance program that pays most medical bills of low-income people.

**Medic Alert tag.** Bracelet or necklace that tells about any health problems a person has, such as diabetes, epilepsy, or an allergy.

**Medicare.** A health insurance program for people 65 years and older and for certain disabled persons.

**menstruation.** A monthly discharge of bloody fluid released from the uterus and carried through the vagina to the vaginal opening.

**metabolic rate.** The rate at which one's body burns calories.

**metabolism** (muh-TAB-uh-liz-uhm). The sum of all the body processes, including breathing, circulating blood, and building and repairing cells and tissues.

**minerals.** Chemicals used to regulate body processes and which become part of the body's bones, tissues, and fluids.

**miscarriage.** Natural termination of a pregnancy before the fetus is able to live outside the uterus.

**mobility impaired.** Condition characterized by difficulty in moving part of one's body normally.

**mononucleosis** (mahn-oh-NOO-klee-oh-sis). A viral infection characterized by a severe sore throat, swollen lymph glands, and a feeling of tiredness.

**morning sickness.** Feeling of nausea, sometimes accompanied with vomiting, that occurs early in pregnancy.

**mourning** (MORN-ing). Process of separating oneself from a deceased love one.

**multiple sclerosis.** Disease of the nervous system that causes paralysis or weakness of the muscles.

**muscular dystrophy** (MUS-kyoo-lur DIS-truh-fee). Gradual degeneration of the muscles, causing difficulty in moving and in maintaining posture.

**narcotics.** Addictive drugs that dull the senses and relieve pain. Heroin is an example.

**nearsightedness.** Having a problem seeing things that are far away.

**neonate.** An infant in its first four weeks of life.

**neuroses** (noo-RO-sees). Mild mental disorders in which people over-react to mental and emotional stress. These people suffer from excessive fear and/or anxiety, but seldom lose touch with reality.

**nicotine** (NIK-uh-teen). A poisonous addictive substance contained in tobacco.

**nurture.** To take care of someone in a loving and emotionally supportive way.

**nutrient density.** Characteristic of foods rich in nutrients, but low in calories.

**nutrients** (NOO-tree-unts). Chemicals contained in food that the body must have to function, grow, repair itself, and make energy.

**nutrition** (noo-TRIH-shun). The food one eats and how the body uses the nutrients in that food.

**obesity.** Condition of being 20 percent or more over desirable weight.

**obstetrician** (ob-steh-TRIH-shun). A doctor who specializes in caring for pregnant women and delivering babies.

**occupational therapist.** Person trained to work with people to restore their abilities to live independently and earn an income.

**ophthalmologist** (off-thahl-MOL-uh-jist). A medical doctor who specializes in eye care.

**optometrist.** A person specially trained to test the eyes and fit corrective lens.

**orthodontist.** Dentist who specializes in straightening teeth.

**OSHA.** Federal agency responsible for setting and enforcing workplace standards.

**osteoporosis** (aws-tee-oh-pur-OH-sis). Wasting away or deterioration of the bone, making bones weak and brittle.

**ovaries.** Female sex glands where the eggs for reproduction are stored and where estrogen is produced.

**over-the-counter medicines.** Medicines that can be bought without a doctor's prescription.

**ozone** (OH-zone). A gas that helps shield the earth from the sun's harmful ultraviolet rays.

**Pap smear.** A sample of cells scraped from the base of the uterus and tested for cervical and uterine cancer.

**paralysis** (puh-RAL-ih-sis). Loss of feeling in and inability to move the affected part of the body.

**paranoia** (pare-uh-NOY-uh). Condition in which a person is excessively suspicious and distrustful of others and may have delusions of being persecuted.

**paraplegic** (pare-uh-PLEE-jik). Person unable to use his or her legs.

**passive smoking.** Occurs when nonsmokers breathe in the smoke from other people's cigarettes, pipes, or cigars.

**pathogens** (PATH-uh-jenz). Tiny disease-causing organisms.

**pediatrician** (peed-ee-uh-TRIH-shun). A doctor who specializes in infant and child care.

**peer pressure.** Pressure or influence exerted by persons in one's own age group to act or think in a certain way.

**penis.** External male sex organ.

**periodontal** (pur-ee-oh-DAWN-tl) **disease.** A disease in which the gums become inflamed and infected and teeth gradually loosen in their sockets.

**personality traits.** Characteristics that make a person different from every other person.

**pharmacist** (FAR-muh-sist). A person who is trained and licensed to prepare and dispense medications and drugs prescribed by doctors.

**phobia** (FOE-bee-uh). Severe, irrational fear of something that poses little or no threat.

**physical therapist.** Person trained to use treatment and exercises to help restore a person's muscle use.

**physical therapy.** Special exercises to restore normal movement to body parts that have been affected by injury or illness.

**pimple.** A small inflamed lump in the skin.

**pinworms.** White, threadlike worms that live in the digestive tracts of infected people.

**placenta** (pluh-SEN-tuh). Blood-rich organ on the wall of the uterus that provides nourishment to the developing fetus.

**plaque** (PLAK). Soft, transparent, sticky layer of film that forms on teeth when they are not properly cleaned, leading to tooth decay.

**PMS.** Condition preceding monthly menstruation characterized by severe abdominal cramps, headache, fatigue, and tension.

**poisons.** Substances that cause illness, injury, or death when they are taken into the body by swallowing or by being breathed in (inhaled).

**pollutants.** Substances that contaminate the environment.

**pollution.** Harmful changes in the environment that occur when unclean or dangerous substances are present.

**postpartum blues.** Also often called postnatal depression. Moodiness and depression that often sets in after giving birth, due to hormonal changes, tiredness, and change in lifestyle.

**posture.** The way one holds and carries one's body while standing, sitting, or walking.

**prematurity.** When a baby is born too soon—before the body systems are developed fully and the baby weighs less than five and a half pounds.

**premenstrual syndrome.** See PMS.

**prenatal.** Before birth.

**prescription.** Medicine that must be ordered by a doctor, who indicates exactly the strength and dosage that must be taken.

**pressure point technique.** Method of controlling very heavy bleeding by compressing the artery that leads to the wound against the underlying bone in order to stop the flow of blood to the affected body part.

**private practice.** This is when health care professionals have their own offices where they see their patients—they are in business for themselves, not with a group.

**progesterone.** A sex hormone that causes development of secondary sexual characteristics in males.

**prognosis** (prawg-NO-sis). The predicted outcome of a disease.

**projection.** Defense mechanism of putting the blame on someone else.

**protein.** A nutrient made up of amino acids and used by the body to build and repair cells.

**psychiatrist** (sie-KIE-uh-trist). Physician who specializes in mental health.

**psychoactive drugs.** Mind-altering drugs.

**psychological addiction.** Development of a mental and emotional dependence on a drug or alcohol that is often harder to overcome than a physical dependence.

**psychologist** (sie-KOL-oh-jist). A person trained to test for and treat emotional disorders.

**psychoses** (sie-KOE-sees). Severe mental disorders in which people cannot cope with life and withdraw from the real world. Schizophrenia is one type of psychoses.

**psychosomatic illnesses.** Physical illnesses that are caused by emotional upsets. Mind-body illnesses.

**psychotherapy** (sie-koe-THER-uh-pee). Involves an emotionally troubled person talking through his or her problems with a professionally trained therapist.

**puberty** (PYOO-bur-tee). The time in a young person's life when the reproductive organs become functionally active.

**pubic** (PYOO-bik) **hair.** Hair that grows around and just above the genital area.

**pulse rate.** Rate of the heartbeat felt in a throbbing blood vessel just under the skin.

**puncture wound.** A piercing cut down into the skin, such as one gets from stepping on a nail.

**pus.** Thick yellowish white fluid formed in wounds or pimples as a result of infection.

**quackery.** The practice of offering unproven methods of medical treatment.

**quarantine** (KWAWR-un-teen). Isolating or restricting a person, family, or localized group with a contagious disease to keep the disease from spreading.

**quickening.** Time around the middle of pregnancy when the expectant mother begins to feel fetal movement.

**rabies.** Deadly infectious disease that affects the brain and nervous system. It is usually transmitted through the bite of a wild animal.

**radiation.** The process in which energy is sent out in rays from atoms and molecules because of changes inside them.

**rationalization.** Making excuses to explain away one's behavior.

**RDA.** Recommended Dietary Allowances. A guide that specifies the amounts of nutrients and calories needed by people according to their age, weight, and sex.

**reference.** Person who will vouch for your character and abilities to a prospective employer.

**registered nurse (R.N.).** Nurse who has successfully completed a four-year college nursing program and who has passed a state board examination.

**repression.** Forgetting something ever happened in order to avoid pain.

**rescue squad.** Highly-trained medical technicians that give emergency care at the scene of an accident or other emergency situation.

**resistance.** The body's ability to fight off infections when exposed to pathogens.

**respiratory rate.** Measurement of how fast a person is breathing. Each time a person's chest rises and falls is one respiration, or full breath. The number of respirations in one minute equals the respiratory rate.

**respiratory system.** Parts of the body used for the breathing process—nose, sinuses, throat, bronchial tubes, and lungs.

**reversal.** Defense mechanism of acting or thinking directly opposite of the way one feels.

**Reye's Syndrome.** A very serious viral disease of infants and children. Symptoms include violent vomiting, hallucinations, severe headaches, and wild behavior.

**risk factors.** Lifetime habits and personal characteristics that increase one's chances of developing certain diseases.

**sanitation.** Keeping germs down to as small a number as possible.

**saturated fats.** Type of fats that tend to create higher levels of cholesterol. Foods high in saturated fats include egg yolks, beef, pork, lard, butter, and whole milk.

**schizophrenia** (skit-suh-FREH-nee-uh). A psychotic disorder characterized by disturbed and disorganized thinking, moods, and behavior.

**scoliosis** (sko-lee-OH-sis). Curvature of the spine.

**scrotum.** The external pouch of skin that holds the testicles.

**sedentary lifestyle.** Living habits that include very little physical activity.

**self-concept.** The image people have of who they are now and who they will be in the future. People with a positive self-concept feel good about themselves.

**semen** (SEE-mun). Whitish fluid of the male reproductive tract that carries the sperm.

**senior citizen.** Person who is 65 years old or older.

**separation anxiety.** Fear of infants and young children that their parent(s) or major caregiver is going to leave them and not return.

**sewage.** Waste products consisting of human wastes, food wastes, used laundry and bath water, and other substances.

**shock.** A serious medical condition resulting from the disruption of blood flow in the body.

**side effects.** The undesired effects a medicine might have on one's body in addition to the desired effects. A medicine to help a throat infection might have the side effect of causing a rash.

**SIDS.** See sudden infant death syndrome.

**signing.** Method of communicating with deaf persons by using special finger and hand movements. Also called sign language.

**smog.** A yellowish-brown combination of smoke, chemical fumes and fog.

**smoke inhalation.** Occurs when smoke fills a person's lungs and the victim cannot get enough oxygen to breathe.

**social security.** Government pension system into which a person pays a certain amount of each paycheck during working years and from which that person receives a monthly check upon retirement, after a certain age. Social security also makes payments to qualified persons who are permanently disabled or who are survivors of someone who paid enough into the system before death.

**sodium.** A mineral needed in very small amounts for maintaining water balance in the body and normal muscle action. Excess sodium intake has been linked to high blood pressure. Sodium is most commonly found in table salt and salty foods.

**soft diet.** Special diet for people with some types of digestive upsets or those who have trouble chewing. Includes semi-solid foods such as pudding, soups, and pasta.

**specialist.** A health care professional who practices in one specific field of health care.

**speech pathologist.** Person trained to work with people who have speech, language, or voice disorders.

**sphincter** (SFINK-tur) **muscles.** Muscles that control the opening of the bladder and bowels for elimination of body wastes.

**spina bifada** (SPINE-uh BIF-uh-duh). A birth defect in which the spine has not developed properly. The nerves in the spinal cord are exposed and may be defective, limiting use of the lower half of the body.

**splint.** Rigid material attached to the site of a possible fracture to keep the victim from moving that body part. This is a first aid measure used until the victim can get proper medical care.

**sponge bath.** For this, a basin of warm water is brought to the bedside of an ill or injured person. A washcloth is dipped in and out of this water for washing and rinsing the patient while he or she remains in bed.

**sprain.** An overstretched or torn part of a muscle or joint.

**sterility** (steh-RIL-ih-tee). Inability of a man or woman to reproduce.

**stimulants.** Drugs and other substances that speed up the nervous system, initially giving a false feeling of extra energy. Cocaine is one example.

**stress.** The strain put on the body by the way a person reacts to a situation.

**stress reaction.** The series of physical and emotional changes a body undergoes in response to a stress.

**stroke.** Occurs when blood flow to the brain is interrupted, resulting in brain damage. Whatever activity that area of the brain controls—such as speech, memory, arm or leg movement—is affected.

**stye** (STIE). Condition in which the roots of the eyelashes become infected and are red and swollen.

**sublimation** (sub-lih-MAY-shun). Defense mechanism of acting out one's feelings in a different, but safe, manner.

**substance abuse.** Using alcohol, drugs, or tobacco in ways that don't promote physical, emotional, or social health.

**sudden infant death syndrome (SIDS).** Also called crib death, this refers to when infants die during their sleep for no apparent reason.

**suicide.** Deliberate taking of one's own life.

**sun protection factor.** A rating that indicates the degree of protection a sunscreen lotion provides.

**sunscreen.** Lotion that can be applied to exposed areas of the body to protect the skin from harmful rays of the sun.

**support group.** A group of people with similar concerns or problems who join together to help one another.

**surgery.** Cutting into the body to remove or repair an unhealthy or injured body part.

**syphilis** (SIF-uh-lis). A serious sexually transmitted disease that has three stages that can appear, disappear, and then recur throughout one's lifetime.

**systolic** (sis-TOL-ik) **pressure.** Top number of a blood pressure reading. It indicates the peak pressure at the moment the heart contracts as it pumps out blood.

**tartar.** Hardened plaque that can get between teeth and gums and cause periodontal disease.

**technology.** All the scientific and manufacturing methods developed and used to provide for human needs and comforts.

**terminal illness.** Disease that has no cure and eventually causes death.

**testicles.** Male sex glands where progesterone is produced and where the sperm is made.

**tetanus.** Often called lockjaw, this is a serious, often fatal disease that occurs when certain bacteria that live in the soil get into a deep wound.

**tourniquet** (TOOR-nih-kit). A band of cloth or a belt placed just above a wound and twisted tightly to cut off blood flow.

**toxemia** (tok-SEE-mee-uh). Condition late in pregnancy in which the woman develops high blood pressure and swelling, especially in hands, feet, and ankles. Symptoms can worsen and it can develop into a very serious condition.

**toxic.** Poisonous.

**trimester.** Time span of three months. Pregnancy lasts about nine months, often divided into three trimesters.

**ultrasound.** Method of checking the health of a developing fetus by transmitting sound waves through the pregnant woman's abdomen. The echoes of the sound waves are transformed into a photographic image of the fetus.

**umbilical cord.** Long flexible tube connecting the fetus to the placenta; the lifeline of the fetus.

**urinal.** A container a bedridden man can use to urinate into.

**urinalysis** (yoor-uh-NAL-ih-sis). A test in which urine samples are checked to reveal how well the kidneys work, any signs of infection and other health problems.

**U.S. RDA.** Indicates the average amount of nutrients that will generally meet the needs of all people in a given age group.

**uterus** (YOO-tur-us). Female organ that holds the developing fetus during pregnancy.

**vaccine** (vak-SEEN). Small amounts of dead or weakened bacteria or viruses that are given to a person by mouth or injection so the person's body can build a resistance to the disease.

**varicose veins.** Bulging, knobby blood vessels.

**viruses.** Microorganisms that cause certain diseases, such as flu, chickenpox, and colds.

**visually impaired.** Refers to people who have difficulty seeing and whose sight cannot be corrected with glasses.

**vital signs.** A person's body temperature, pulse rate, breathing rate, and blood pressure.

**vitamins.** Complex substances in food that help speed up or regulate necessary chemical reactions in the body.

**warts.** Small skin growths caused by a virus.

**weaning.** Training a baby to drink milk from a cup instead of taking it from breast or bottle.

**wellness.** Process of becoming and staying physically, mentally, emotionally, and socially healthy.

**whitehead.** A form of acne that is a small whitish lump in the skin due to oil trapped in a pore.

**widow.** A woman whose husband has died.

**widower.** A man whose wife has died.

**wind chill factor.** Measurement that indicates the combined cooling effect of air temperature and wind speed.

**withdrawal.** Physical reactions of a person who is addicted to alcohol or a drug when he or she is deprived of that substance, even for a short period of time. Reactions can include nausea, shakiness, convulsions, and hallucinations.

**wound** (WOOND). Any break in the skin that might bleed.

**X-rays.** Rays with a short wavelength that enables them to pass through soft body tissues and allow dense body tissues such as bones and teeth to show up on film.

# Index

# Illustration Credits

**Chapter 9** **Page 202** Photo/Dave Schaefer; **203** Todd Carroll, Friendship House; **205** N. A. Peterson; **206** J. C. Roberts; **211** Vicky Kee; **212, 213** David Lancaster; **214** J. C. Roberts; **215** Barbara Caldwell; **217** David Lancaster; **218** David Whiting; **220** David Lancaster; **221** Courtesy of the American Red Cross.

**Chapter 10** **Page 225** U.S. Department of Agriculture; **226** David Lancaster; **228** N. A. Peterson; **230** *top* Copyright by the American Dental Association. Reprinted by permission.; **230** *bottom* Cinda; **231, 235** David Lancaster; **236** J. Berndt/Stock Boston; **238** David Lancaster; **239** © Ellis Herwig/The Picture Cube; **241** David Lancaster; **242** Gregg Goldman/Press Journal; **250** © Larry Lawfer/The Picture Cube.

**Chapter 11** **Page 253, 254** Photo/Dave Schaefer; **255** David Lancaster; **257** Richard Sullivan; **259** Visiting Nurses Association of Rhode Island; **261, 262, 265** *top,* **266** *top* David Lancaster; **266** *bottom* Sun Mark; **267** Photo/ Dave Schaefer; **269** David Lancaster; **271** Visiting Nurses Association of Rhode Island; **273** David Slater/Image Gate; **274** David Lancaster; **275** Daniel F. Clifford; **277** David Lancaster; **278** Visiting Nurses Association of Rhode Island.

**Chapter 12** **Page 280** Peter Southwick/ Stock Boston; **281** © Marilyn L. Schrut/Taurus Photos, Inc.; **283** Ability Magazine; **284** David Lancaster; **287** Whirlpool Corporation; **290** © Carol Palmer/The Picture Cube; **291** Photo/Dave Schaefer; **292** Wes Coulter; **293** UPI/Bettman Newsphotos; **295** Photo/Dave Schaefer; **296** UPI/Bettman Newsphotos; **297** Billy Allen/New York Special Olympics, Inc.; **298** © Rick Friedman/The Picture Cube.

**Chapter 13** **Page 300** Kerry Zabarski; **301** IBM; **303, 304** J. C. Roberts; **306** © Betty Barry/The Picture Cube; **307** Courtesy SCORE—Service Corps of Retired Executives. Photo by Orie Damewood.; **309** © Karen R. Preuss/Taurus Photos, Inc.; **310** Department of Health and Human Services/Social Security Administration; **311** © Marilyn M. Pfaltz/Taurus Photos, Inc.; **312** © Betty Barry/The Picture Cube; **314** David Lancaster; **315** © B. Griffith/ The Picture Cube; **316** David Lancaster; **319** © Milton Feinberg/The Picture Cube; **320** *left* Karl Schumacher/The White House; **320** *right* Academy of Motion Picture Arts and Sciences; **322** © Jeff Albertson/The Picture Cube.

**Chapter 14** **Page 324** Photo/Dave Schaefer; **325** Barbara Caldwell; **327** Frank Siteman/ Stock Boston; **329** J. C. Roberts; **332** The Dream Factory; **335** Donna M. Faull; **336** © Frank Siteman/The Picture Cube; **338, 340, 341** David Lancaster; **342** Michael Weisbrot/Stock Boston.

**Chapter 15** **Page 344** Courtesy of the American Red Cross; **346** P. C. Morse; **347** Ellis Herwig/Stock Boston; **348** David Lancaster; **350** Harry Wilks/Stock Boston; **351** *top* Peter Menzel/Stock Boston; **351** *bottom* Ellis Herwig/ Stock Boston; **353** Frank Siteman/Stock Boston; **354** Photo/Dave Schaefer; **355** David Lancaster; **356** Caterpillar, Inc.; **358** *top* Boston Edison, Pilgrim Station; **358** *bottom* Steven J. Strong; **363** Peace Corps/Niger/Frampton.

**Chapter 16** **Page 365, 366** David Lancaster; **369** Fred Bodkin/Stock Boston; **372** Eric Dusenbery; **378** Charles Hofer; **381** Yolanda Gatlin; **382** © William A. Kelley/Uniphoto; **383** WCVB-TV Boston; **384** David Lancaster; **385** George Bellerose/Stock Boston.